normal

AT ANY COST

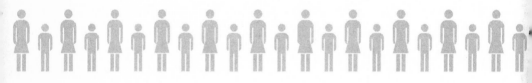

JEREMY P. TARCHER/PENGUIN
a member of Penguin Group (USA) Inc.
New York

normal

AT ANY COST

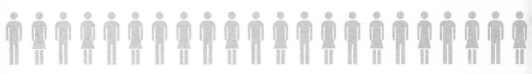

Tall Girls, Short Boys, and the Medical Industry's
Quest to Manipulate Height

SUSAN COHEN AND

CHRISTINE COSGROVE

JEREMY P. TARCHER/PENGUIN
Published by the Penguin Group
Penguin Group (USA) Inc., 375 Hudson Street, New York, New York 10014, USA • Penguin Group
(Canada), 90 Eglinton Avenue East, Suite 700, Toronto, Ontario M4P 2Y3, Canada (a division of
Pearson Canada Inc.) • Penguin Books Ltd, 80 Strand, London WC2R 0RL, England • Penguin Ireland,
25 St Stephen's Green, Dublin 2, Ireland (a division of Penguin Books Ltd) • Penguin Group (Australia),
250 Camberwell Road, Camberwell, Victoria 3124, Australia (a division of Pearson Australia Group
Pty Ltd) • Penguin Books India Pvt Ltd, 11 Community Centre, Panchsheel Park, New Delhi–110 017,
India • Penguin Group (NZ), 67 Apollo Drive, Rosedale, North Shore 0632, New Zealand (a division
of Pearson New Zealand Ltd) • Penguin Books (South Africa) (Pty) Ltd, 24 Sturdee Avenue, Rosebank,
Johannesburg 2196, South Africa

Penguin Books Ltd, Registered Offices: 80 Strand, London WC2R 0RL, England

Most Tarcher/Penguin books are available at special quantity discounts for bulk purchase for sales promotions,
premiums, fund-raising, and educational needs. Special books or book excerpts also can be created to
fit specific needs. For details, write Penguin Group (USA) Inc. Special Markets, 375 Hudson Street,
New York, NY 10014.

Library of Congress Cataloging-in-Publication Data

Cohen, Susan, date.
Normal at any cost : tall girls, short boys, and the medical industry's quest to manipulate height /
Susan Cohen and Christine Cosgrove.
p.   cm.
Includes bibliographical references and index.
ISBN 978-1-58542-683-6
1. Stature, short—Hormone therapy.   2. Stature, tall—Hormone therapy.   I. Cosgrove, Christine, date.
II. Title.
RJ482.G76C67   2009   2008040786
618.92'4—dc22

Printed in the United States of America
1   3   5   7   9   10   8   6   4   2

BOOK DESIGN BY NICOLE LAROCHE

Neither the publisher nor the authors are engaged in rendering professional advice or services to the individual
reader. The ideas, procedures, and suggestions in this book are not intended as a substitute for consulting with a
physician. All matters regarding health require medical supervision. Neither the authors nor the publisher shall be
liable or responsible for any loss or damage allegedly arising from any information or suggestion in this book.

While the authors have made every effort to provide accurate telephone numbers and Internet addresses at the time
of publication, neither the publisher nor the authors assume any responsibility for errors, or for changes that occur
after publication. Further, the publisher does not have any control over and does not assume any responsibility for
author or third-party websites or their content.

CONTENTS

INTRODUCTION

IN THE SUMMER OF 2003, a man approached an advisory panel of the Food and Drug Administration on his knees. Deno Andrews was a supplicant. More to the point, he chose to address the committee from the height he might have stood if doctors hadn't given him growth hormone throughout his childhood. Andrews's body didn't make enough of the hormone on its own; without years of injections he probably would not have reached five feet, or a lectern. In his thirties, 5'7" tall, he was asking the FDA to allow any extremely short child in the United States to receive the same injections that he got for his rare disorder. Potentially almost a million children who may have nothing wrong with their bodies except height.

Fixing short children is the right thing to do, Andrews said: "It is as right as getting corrective lenses for eyesight that is abnormal. It is as right as an insurance company paying to repair a dent in a car. It is as right as getting a tutor or extra help at school for a child who isn't performing well."

Some, however, perceive a difference between hiring an after-school instructor or correcting flawed eyesight and improving a healthy child's height as if banging out an unsightly dent. Where is that line, exactly, between normal and abnormal, disease and disadvantage, treatment and enhancement? Who gets to draw it? If someone is able and willing to pay to improve on heredity, do such boundaries even matter?

Normal at Any Cost describes more than fifty years of medical attempts to modify height in children. The broader purpose is to illustrate how the future might play out as medicine offers more and more opportunities to change inherited traits. Because over the last five decades, as physicians discovered ways to treat pathological conditions that make some people extremely tall or short, they also intervened in the lives of young patients who were normal and healthy, just far from average. Along the way, doctors made miracles and caused tragedies. They found themselves facing ethical dilemmas that reach far beyond the issue of how much height matters. They engaged in a running debate about what is normal; whether their prescriptions alleviate suffering or reinforce social prejudice; and how far they should go to accommodate the wishes of children, or the aspirations of parents. In a way, this small group of doctors has been on the front line of the future, along with the families of the tallest and shortest kids.

We tell this story decade by decade. It begins with girls whose mothers worried they would grow too tall to be happy, and who dutifully took massive doses of estrogen to stunt their heights. It describes how the pituitary gland, a pea-size organ that sits at the base of the brain and produces growth hormone, fascinated scientists who competed to harvest cadavers for the stuff that might make short kids grow. The book narrates the early days of treating children for dwarfism, until a strange disease seen in the elderly and among cannibals in a Papua New Guinea jungle struck down a young man in California. It follows scientists who raced to synthesize human growth hormone using the new technology of genetic engineering and in the process launched an entire industry, then details how that industry sometimes stepped over the lines of legality as it turned short stature into a market. The later decades include detective stories of a sort, as adults given treatments as children found one another, and as researchers tried to track down what became of these children. The final chapters show how, as ways to manipulate height expand, the government agencies that protect patients, the nonprofit organizations that speak for them, and the physicians who treat them have all been influenced by the pharmaceutical companies that sell to them. In the end, short stature is a multibillion-dollar business that is still growing like a weed.

Nothing in here should discourage a parent from taking a poorly growing son or daughter to be examined by a doctor. Growth is the primary indicator of health in a child. Also, this book should be read not as an indictment of technology or future treatments, but rather as an illustration of how quickly medicine can move from curing disease, to treating disability, to leveling disadvantage, to satisfying desires for perfection. Above all, *Normal at Any Cost* is not meant to negate the pain that children feel because of stigma for any reason, or to diminish the difficult decisions some parents must make.

This is a cautionary tale, however. Eugenics forever bears a terrible Nazi taint, associated with the extermination of "undesirable" populations. But eugenics—the word was introduced in the late nineteenth century—simply means intervening to improve heredity. The story of treating children to make them grow taller or remain shorter than nature may have intended suggests that the future of eugenics is not likely to involve totalitarian governments, mad scientists, or schemes to create worker drones and superbeings. Instead, it will take place through the individual decisions parents make on the basis of the options that doctors present, and the temptations that the genetic age of medicine might offer.

Consumers will drive eugenics, trying to make the best choices for their children's futures: debating over the dining room table or in the bedroom late at night about the right thing to do for a son, the best thing to do for a daughter. The choices will get harder. If past and present serve as guides, the difference between treatment and experiment will not always be clear, and the consequences won't always be what doctors, parents, and children expect. Finding information unbiased by conflict of interest won't be easy. Knowing a little history might come in handy.

We, the authors, are parents as well as journalists, and became interested in this story for different reasons. Christine Cosgrove is a medical writer who received pills as an adolescent in hopes of keeping her below six feet. Susan Cohen wrote about the early days of genetically engineered growth hormone and developed a career-long interest in bioethical subjects. In answer to the question someone invariably asks, Christine Cosgrove is 5'11" and Susan Cohen is 5'6".

PART 1

drug turns
young amazons
into beauties

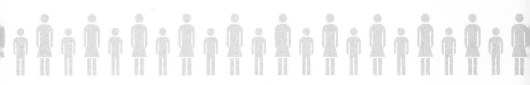

CHAPTER 1

"tallness can be a real handicap for a girl"

A FATEFUL TRIP TO BOSTON

A week before Thanksgiving in 1968, thirteen-year-old Laura Moore* and her twelve-year-old sister, Cathy, climbed into the family's Mercury sedan and left their small town in the southeastern corner of New Hampshire for a doctor's appointment in Boston. Normally, a trip to the big city was a festive outing for the Moore family and included the eight-year-old twins, Andrea and Scott. But that day the twins had been left behind with a babysitter, and the mood was tense even before Stuart, the girls' father, guided the car out of their hometown of Kingston and onto Interstate 93.

While her mother, Shirley, chatted reassuringly, Laura sat sullen in the backseat, gazing out the window. It was a cold November day. The fall colors that had lured throngs of tourists to New Hampshire a month earlier had disappeared, and a dusting of snow clung to the white pines and hemlock that forested either side of the interstate. Despite her mother's attempts to make conversation, Laura remained more or less mute. Cathy alternated between excitement

* The family name has been changed.

at the prospect of a day in the big city and anxiety; Laura's moodiness about the upcoming doctor visit was contagious.

The specialist they would see, Gertrud Reyersbach, maintained an office in an old brick building just off Copley Square. Although Reyersbach had never met the girls, she would decide that day if they needed hormone treatments—an idea that Laura barely understood but one which upset her in some way that she could not explain.

Laura and Cathy were not ill; they were tall compared with other girls their age. An eighth-grader, Laura measured 5'8" that fall, and Cathy, who was in sixth grade, was only an inch and a half shorter. On the basis of X-rays of their hands and wrists, their New Hampshire pediatrician had warned their mother a few weeks earlier that her daughters might grow to be unusually tall. Taller, in fact, than 97 percent of other girls—a height that doctors would consider treating.

The news hit Shirley hard. Measuring just over 6'1", Shirley might pass for a younger, quieter version of the late chef Julia Child, whose public television show, broadcast from Boston, had become a hit during those years. Perhaps because of her height, Shirley had developed a habit of lowering and angling her head, with its dark wavy hair, when listening to a conversation, giving the impression of intense interest and concentration. But a warm and gracious personality hadn't mattered during Shirley's teenage years, which haunted her as she watched her own daughters grow taller and taller.

PAINFUL MEMORIES

It could be said that the Moore family's journey to Boston that chilly, fall day in 1968 really began decades earlier when Shirley, born in 1930, was growing up in Dedham, Massachusetts. Shirley was big at birth and remained tall throughout girlhood. Although Shirley's mother—Laura's grandmother—was 5'7" and her father measured about 6 feet—not extraordinary heights for the time—family lore had it that Shirley's grandfather on her father's side had been exceptionally tall, and her mother's sister, Margaret, was 5'10". Shirley, it seemed, had inherited the "tall" genes from both sides of her family. By the time she was nine or ten, her mother had resorted to carrying a copy of Shirley's birth certificate in her purse to prove to disbelieving transit officials that her daughter was under twelve and could ride the bus for free. A few years later, as Shirley reached her full height, her older brother took to walking to school on the other side of the street. He was too embarrassed to be seen with his tall, lanky sister.

The culture of the times reinforced every bit of self-consciousness Shirley felt, and every anxiety her mother held about her future. In 1936, the writer Hugh Morris wrote, in *The Art of Kissing*, that the "man must be . . . taller than the woman . . . for he must give the impression of being his woman's superior (mentally and physically)." In 1942, when Shirley was twelve, the November issue of *Parents* magazine ran an article that would frighten the parents of any tall daughter. "Tallness can be a real handicap for a girl," the author warned. Protruding teeth in a tall girl "can get to feel like elephant tusks!" while "a pair of stubbed and run-over size sevens [shoes] look like the SS *Normandie* in her present unfortunate state." The writer advised parents to find a good dancing teacher for their tall daughters. "Extra inches mean she must have superior technique, but acquiring this skill in a public dancing class may be torture. She may find release in athletics if only she doesn't turn into an Amazon trying to beat the boys at their own games and in this way make up for the fact that she lacks the ability to be normally feminine."

Newspaper advice columnists also regularly offered suggestions. One in the *Los Angeles Times* advised a girl who felt she was too tall for her boyfriend to coif her hair "soft and low, wear low heels, wide belts, flared skirts and shallow hats with horizontal lines." John Robert Powers, founder of a well-known modeling and talent agency, had even more tricks up his sleeve. In his *Los Angeles Times* column, "Secrets of Charm," he advised:

If you are over five feet eight inches on the height measure, never let both arms fall straight down at your sides. That position only elongates and emphasizes your stature. Instead, always bend one or both of your arms from the elbow so that your hand comes to rest at the side-center of your waist. Or stick the fingertips of one hand in your pocket. Or place one hand at waist level behind your hip. With just such small gestures you can create a natural horizontal line that will cut your height as effectively as a flat-crowned hat, medium-heeled shoes and horizontally broken skirts."

Even girdles, he believed, could play a crucial role in downplaying a girl's height, although he did not make clear exactly how. "A tall woman's problem is eliminated by modern corsetry," he wrote. The right girdle could help any tall girl—"skinny, slender or stout"—build up a "mow-'em-down appearance."

Everywhere she looked, Shirley saw signs that her height was an embarrassment, a disadvantage, and something to be camouflaged. In the funny pages, a henpecked husband nervously looked up at his towering battle-ax of a wife. At the movies, directors made certain leading ladies always appeared shorter than their romantic leads. Although Ingrid Bergman, 5'9½", loomed over Humphrey Bogart and Claude Rains, her *Casablanca* costars, audiences in 1942 would never know it: both men stood on catwalks when they were filmed next to her.

Recognizing a growth market, so to speak, a few retailers began catering to women who were too tall for clothes off the rack. In 1948, Gimbels announced the opening of the Tall Girl Shop on the third floor of its New York City department store, guiding tall shoppers to the correct area with pictures of long-necked giraffes decorating the walls. Besides providing longer sleeves and lengths, the styling of these clothes aimed to hide a woman's height, not accentuate it. During the late 1940s and early 1950s, a 5'10" fashion designer, Peg Newton, made a name for herself with a line of glamorous evening gowns for tall women that "lopped off a few illusionary inches...by using larger pocket flaps, buttons and details than those on clothes made for average women," according to a *New York Times* review of her clothing.

A few young women did try to break ranks with the dominant culture and establish what might qualify as the first "tall pride" movement. Kay Sumner, a Disney animator who measured 6'2", tired of the practical difficulties of her height and formed a group called the Tip Toppers to agitate for everything from longer shoes and beds to higher door frames. By 1947, the group included 150 members in Los Angeles and had spawned fifteen chapters around the country. That year the *Los Angeles Times* reported that the women in the club did not try to camouflage their height, but flagrantly wore "high-heeled shoes, tall hats and gowns made from fabrics with vertical lines accented."

But even the Tip Toppers had a tough time with the 1950s and society's relentless embrace of conformity—especially once medicine could help alleviate their height problem. Women who had entered the labor force during World War II were encouraged to return home, marry, and raise children. Women who were well educated were expected to use the benefits of their education to run a household, not a business. A couple of years of teaching, nursing, or perhaps secretarial work before marrying were considered appropriate, but ultimately the only important goals for women were marriage, childbearing, and child rearing. It was not only the womanly thing to do, but patriotic, according to FBI director J. Edgar Hoover, who urged women to marry early and have children to fight communism. Failing to land a husband was considered a disaster; a woman who wasn't married (or at least engaged) by the time she was thirty was relegated to old-maid status. Despite the Tip Toppers, society's message remained unchanged: a tall woman could be admired, but a small woman was desired.

So, unsurprisingly, *Los Angeles Times* columnist Dr. Walter Alvarez wrote in the early 1950s that he'd received many letters from parents worried about their daughters' height and asking for advice. "I am sorry to say I know of no drugs which could safely be used to stop the girl from growing tall," he wrote regretfully. Instead, Alvarez, who was identified as an emeritus consultant in medicine from the Mayo Clinic, advised withholding food: "If I had a granddaughter who was

7

growing rapidly and threatening to qualify for the Los Angeles six-footer-girls club, I would suggest that she be fed enough for health but not much more than enough for that, and I would suggest that she not be stuffed with vitamins because some of them are stimulators of growth."

The same year, Shirley's social handicap was heading toward a new definition: disease. An entry in *Endocrine Treatment in General Practice*, a medical reference book edited in 1953 by New York physicians Max Goldzieher and Joseph Goldzieher, stated that tall girls who consult a physician because of their height "may have found it difficult to attract male companions." They warned: "These girls frequently develop severe somatopsychic inferiorities." In other words, they would feel bad about their height and themselves. At the time there was nothing to be done for these unfortunate girls except to irradiate the pituitary gland, which the authors mercifully advised against.

SAVED FROM SPINSTERHOOD

By the time Shirley had finished growing, at 6'1", she was taller than 91 percent of the male population: a potential social tragedy in a culture that insisted marriage was the only real role for a woman, and that a husband must be taller than his wife. Theoretically, that left Shirley with, at most, a pool of 9 percent of young men her age as possible mates. If she'd stopped growing at 5'9", about half the male population would have been taller.

Shirley's mother did her best to mitigate her daughter's height problem. She bought Shirley bathing suits with a skirt to "cut her height," and during the hot summer months she'd suggest she change out of shorts and into pants whenever she left the house, to hide her long legs. School dances were a particular misery; Shirley defined wallflower. By some cruel perversity, even the few very tall boys in her class seemed to prefer short girls, and in those days a boy would never escort a taller girl onto the dance floor. She was never asked to dance, so she stopped going.

Despite poor odds and her mother's fears, when Shirley was twenty-one, her brother introduced her to a fishing buddy from nearby Needham, and the two took to each other. Stuart Moore was a trombone player whose height barely topped Shirley's. But a somewhat unconventional childhood—his mother was a vaudevillian and his father was a violinist—may have allowed him to fall for a woman who was a little unconventional herself, at least in terms of stature. The two went together until Stuart enlisted in the Army in 1948 and was shipped to Okinawa. For the next four years he served his country playing in the Army band, while he and Shirley continued their relationship via the postal service.

By the time he'd finished his service and returned to the States, the two were eager to wed and begin a family. Stuart found a teaching job and the couple married in June 1952. On July 3, 1955, Stuart was giving a trombone lesson at a music camp in Maine when a telegram arrived announcing that his firstborn, Laura, had made it safely into the world. A few days later, Shirley bundled up the baby and traveled to Maine to introduce Stuart to his daughter. Blond, hazel-eyed Laura slept in a wooden drawer in their room in the camping lodge, serenaded from below by band music all day long and into the night.

The family grew quickly; fifteen months later, Cathy was born. By now, the Moores were living in Lebanon, New Hampshire, where Stuart was the director of the local high school music program. In 1960, Shirley gave birth to twins, Scott and Andrea. Like most parents, Shirley measured her children regularly, charting their growth. But unlike most parents, she had a special reason to worry: she had three daughters, and it was hard not to remember her own miserable teenage years.

By the mid-1960s America had become infatuated with the tall women who graced the covers of fashion magazines. At 5'10", Jean Shrimpton was perhaps the first to attain supermodel status. The leggy, big-eyed British model peered from the cover of *Newsweek* in 1965 and was the subject of stories in *Esquire, Ladies' Home Journal, McCall's,* and *Good Housekeeping* the same year. A few years later, an even taller German model with a mysterious background took center stage in the media: Veruschka was said to be 6'1", 6'4", or somewhere in between. The trend toward tallness had made it to Atlantic City as well; each year's Miss America seemed taller than her predecessor.

But in the real world, where women worked as waitresses, school-teachers, and secretaries, being tall bestowed few benefits. Finding shoes and clothes that fit was time-consuming and costly. Worse, the clothes that did fit were usually dowdy, hardly the dazzling couture worn by models on the covers of fashion magazines. As for jobs, one of the more popular and glamorous careers open to women at the time—airline stewardess—had stringent height restrictions: Women over 5'6" need not apply.

If the increasing height of models and beauty queens had little effect on Hollywood in the sixties, when leading men remained taller on film than their female costars, it had even less impact on the way Shirley felt about her own height. At thirty-eight, she still cringed when she overheard the remarks of children in line at the supermarket, at the beach, or on the sidewalk: "Mom, look at that tall lady!" Total strangers, usually men, felt free to comment to her directly: "Boy, you're tall!" Deep down she felt nothing had changed since her own youth: if a girl was too tall, her chances of finding a suitable mate would be severely compromised, and, like her mother before her, she worried about her daughters.

AND ONE PILL MAKES YOU SMALL

Laura, who seemed to take after Shirley's Scottish-Swedish side of the family with her straight blond hair and soft, round face, was almost always the tallest in her class all through elementary school. When her Girl Scout troop, decked out in the familiar green uniforms, sashes, badges, and berets, marched down Lebanon's main thoroughfare in a holiday parade, it was easy to spot ten-year-old Laura: she towered by a head over all the other Scouts.

Then, when Laura was eleven, Shirley received from her mother's sister Margaret an article clipped from the Sunday edition of *The Boston Globe*. The front-page story, headlined "New Treatment Helps Tall Girls," had caught the eye of Shirley's 5'10" aunt. "Too late for us!" Margaret scribbled in the clipping's margin, but she wondered if Shirley should consider the treatment for Laura.

"Girls who normally would grow to an awkward 6 feet or more are being held to 5 feet 9 through therapy at Massachusetts General Hospital," began the article written by the *Globe*'s medical editor. The story explained how synthetic estrogen given in large doses could accelerate puberty, thereby causing growth to slow dramatically and cease sooner than it would normally. The article quoted Dr. John Crawford, then an associate professor of pediatrics at Harvard Medical School and the chief of the endocrine-metabolic unit at Massachusetts General Hospital. The reasons for therapy varied, Crawford explained in the newspaper article: "The tall girl generally is admired by our society, but the girl who grows too tall—six feet or more—finds difficulty buying smart clothes, obtaining certain jobs (airline hostesses) or selecting suitable dance partners." True enough, thought Shirley, but the treatment seemed so unnatural that she set the article aside and didn't give it another thought.

She had almost forgot about the newspaper clipping heralding the "new" therapy, until a year and a half later she took Laura to the clinic in Exeter for her regular checkup. There, the pediatrician brought up the subject of Laura's height and suggested there were ways to prevent her from growing too tall. Shirley remembered the article then and, reassured by the pediatrician's enthusiasm for the treatment, agreed to have both daughters evaluated by a pediatric endocrinologist, a specialist in diseases involving hormones. The first step, however, would be to X-ray the girls' left hands and wrists. X-rays, the pediatrician explained, would show how much space remained between the epiphysis—the end of a long bone—and the shaft of the bone. In children the long bones are separated from the epiphyses, commonly known as growth plates, by a layer of cartilage that gradually turns to bone as the child grows. Growth is nearly finished when the epiphyses and the shafts finally fuse, generally when a child reaches the end of puberty.

Pediatric endocrinologists predict height by comparing the X-rays of their patients with those considered average, or standard, for healthy children of various ages. In this way doctors determine a child's bone age, which often does not correspond exactly to the child's chronological age, and estimate how much growth is left. If X-rays of thirteen-year-old Laura's left wrist more closely matched those of the average eleven-year-old girl in the atlas, it would mean that Laura still had a considerable amount of growth left. If they more closely resembled those of a fourteen-year-old girl, it would indicate growth was nearly complete.

The girls' wrists were duly X-rayed at the hospital in nearby Exeter and sent on to Gertrud Reyersbach, the specialist in Boston recommended by the pediatrician. In early November, Shirley received a short letter from the doctor.

"According to the best of our knowledge, Laura's final height should be 5'11", give or take half an inch either way. Looking at the X-ray of her hand and wrist, I would guess that it would be nearer 6 feet than 5'11"," wrote Reyersbach. "If we want to do something, we should start pretty soon."

Shirley and Stuart talked it over. Stuart left most of these kinds of decisions to his wife—she ran the household and he ran the high school's music department. Aside from music lessons for his children—they all played wind or brass instruments—he interfered rarely, particularly with medical questions. Although he'd been raised as a Christian Scientist, whose practitioners generally do not believe in doctors, Stuart rejected the religion as an adult. As far as he was concerned, doctors were professionals who had many years of training. Just as Stuart wouldn't expect doctors to know how to conduct an orchestra or a marching band, he didn't feel he should second-guess their diagnoses or treatments. In an era when television doctors were uncomplicated heroes, and faith in medical progress, especially American medicine, remained unquestioned, Stuart's attitudes were in keeping with the times. American researchers had halted polio, and the U.S. Food and Drug Administration had been widely hailed for protecting the American public from the thalidomide tragedy that struck European babies in the early 1960s. The doctors believed this treatment would be good for their girls, and Stuart and Shirley believed the doctors knew best.

If Laura's parents and the pediatrician were concerned about her height, one person, at least, was not. Laura. For the most part, she never noticed that she was considerably taller than her friends. When she did, she didn't mind. In fact, she rather liked it. She had no desire to become a ballerina—a profession that endocrinologists writing in medical journals warned would be closed to young women over 5'6". Nor did she care to become an airline stewardess. Laura was interested in her dolls, particularly her Barbie. She spent hundreds of hours playing with the dolls and sewing elaborate outfits for them. Slightly dyslexic, she struggled with math, but did well in arts and crafts and other creative subjects. Throughout elementary school, she'd been a contented girl who enjoyed all the activities of childhood.

When conversation about her height turned serious, and the pediatrician sent the girls to be X-rayed, Laura began to feel uneasy. She told her parents she didn't want to see the "special" doctor in Boston, but Shirley reassured her that it was for her own good. How could Laura know, thought Shirley, what it would be like in a few years when her height would make her social life a misery? Children who needed braces didn't want them, either, Shirley told herself, but good parents took them to an orthodontist anyway. That's what parents did. They made decisions for their children that their children were too young to make. Treatment wouldn't be cheap, Shirley knew, especially for a family of six getting by on a teacher's salary. But if it gave her girls a chance to have a more normal life, it would be worth it.

EXAM AND DIAGNOSIS

Stuart parked the car, and the family found its way to the Dartmouth Street office building and ascended in a clanking, metal-caged elevator. The girls and their parents were ushered into the doctor's office. Dark wood and a wide, deep desk dominated the room. Gertrud Reyersbach was small-boned and elegant; she seemed even tinier in the company of the tall Moore family. Although she'd lived in the United States for more than twenty-five years, she still spoke with a thick German accent.

To Laura and Cathy, the doctor with her short gray hair and nononsense navy blue suit seemed old. Cathy remembers her as "nice"; Laura's memories, perhaps tempered by the events of that day, are less charitable. "Old," "wrinkled," and "skinny" are the words she uses to describe Reyersbach, who would have been fifty that year.

After a brief meeting, Laura was led into an examining room to undress. The doctor told Shirley she needn't accompany Laura; the exam would only take a few minutes. In this physical exam, Reyersbach was looking for signs of puberty—breast development, pubic or underarm hair—indications that Laura's body had begun the process of maturation that can take anywhere from one year to four years to complete, timing largely determined by heredity. Breast development is the first sign of puberty's onset, and occurs on average a year or so before the peak growth spurt, which is fueled by a girl's increased production of estrogen. Menstruation typically begins about two years later, indicating puberty is nearing an end and that it won't be long before the epiphyses fuse and a girl stops growing. A leading proponent of the use of hormones to stunt the growth of tall girls would later describe estrogen therapy as "turning tortoises into hares." In other words, speeding girls into puberty and through it quickly would allow their bodies less time to grow tall.

In the examining room, Laura felt a little like a tortoise trapped on its back. Stripped to her underpants, anxious and embarrassed, she said nothing as Reyersbach examined her stomach, her arms, her hips, and her legs. The doctor pronounced Laura's breasts to be "tiny creatures" and patted her repeatedly on the head, shoulders, and back reassuringly. Then she told Laura she could get dressed.

Back in her office, she told the girls and their parents that Cathy did not need treatment, at least not right away, but that Laura, based on the results of the X-rays and physical exam, would benefit from the therapy. Cathy heaved a sigh of relief, while Laura choked back tears. Reyersbach advised starting Laura immediately on hormones and scribbled a prescription for diethylstilbestrol, a synthetic estrogen. As Laura's body adjusted to the medication, she explained, the dosage would be increased gradually. She predicted Laura would begin menstruating within a few weeks or months and told Shirley to make certain Laura was prepared. Laura would need to take the medication daily for at least two years. There were no side effects, she reassured the family, except for one: Laura's nipples would probably turn darker, from pink to brown. But that would be a small price to pay compared with growing to a height of six feet.

Back in the car, Laura began to cry. She told her parents she didn't want to take the pills. Shirley reassured her that the medicine wouldn't hurt her but would only make her stop growing—which she would appreciate later. No, sobbed Laura, she didn't want to take them and she wouldn't take them. She was mad at her parents and mad at the doctor. To cheer her up, her parents suggested a trip to Howard Johnson's for Laura's favorites: fried clams and pistachio ice cream. It worked, at least temporarily. Laura calmed down and the family drove home. For the next two years, Laura would dread the visits to Reyersbach. Although the family rarely ate out, because of the cost, to make those visits easier for Laura, her parents always included a little extra incentive—a meal out.

The day after the Boston trip, Shirley took Reyersbach's prescription to a local pharmacist, who also happened to be a neighbor. As he read the script, he frowned and asked Shirley why the physician had prescribed diethylstilbestrol, also known as DES, for Laura. He knew DES was the first inexpensive synthetic female hormone to become available to doctors, and that they prescribed it to pregnant women to prevent miscarriage in doses ranging from 5 to 10 milligrams a day and sometimes higher. It was also used for treatment of advanced prostate and breast cancer. Still, in 1968, the pharmacist knew that the drug was not approved by the FDA for use in young, healthy girls.

Whatever else the pharmacist may have known about DES, he didn't tell Shirley, but he did question Laura's need for the drug. Shirley patiently explained the concept of the treatment, and the pharmacist, rather grudgingly, filled the bottle with pills. Over the next few months the dosages increased; by February, Laura was swallowing 10 milligrams daily—one hundred times the amount of estrogen in a high-dose oral contraceptive.

Just as Dr. Reyersbach had predicted, during these first few months of treatment Laura's periods started. Her nipples turned darker. But in the months and years to come there were other changes, too, for which the doctors had prepared neither Shirley nor Laura.

CHAPTER 2

playing god with hormones

DES, THE WONDER DRUG

The small-town pharmacist who reluctantly filled Laura's prescription had reason to be concerned. Although the drug had been on the market for about thirty years, even the British scientist who had developed the compound worried about its safety.

The history of the development of DES began in the late nineteenth century with doctors and researchers in Germany, Britain, and America eager to unlock the secrets of mysterious "internal secretions," later called "hormones": how they worked in the female body, how they regulated menstrual periods and pregnancy and then ultimately failed, leading to menopause. They knew that understanding these processes would yield powerful knowledge about human growth and reproduction. By the early 1900s, after dissecting the ovaries of rats, rabbits, whales, and monkeys, and distilling the urine of pregnant animals and women, researchers believed they'd found the "female principle." They named it "estrogen" for its importance in the estrous, or menstrual, cycle.

But collecting and distilling urine to eke out tiny amounts of estrogen was time-consuming and expensive, and the final product could only be injected. In 1938, Charles Edward Dodds, a British scientist and physician, developed a chemical formula in his London laboratory that was inexpensive to produce and could be delivered in pill form. He named his compound diethylstilbestrol, or DES. It bore little resemblance to the hormone females naturally produce; in fact, its molecular composition was far closer to another blockbuster chemical invented the same year—DDT, the powerful insecticide.

Nobody, including Dodds, knew why his drug worked like the estrogen a woman's body produced, but it did. What was more important at the time was that Dodds had beaten his closest competitor, a German, in synthesizing the drug. Dodds, like other British scientists, had feared that if the Germans succeeded first, they would patent the powerful new compound, keep its formula secret, and capture the market for the large German pharmaceutical companies. British regulations demanded that research funded by the government could not be patented. As a result, Dodds published the formula for diethylstilbestrol in the journal *Nature* on February 15, 1938—enabling anybody to copy the compound and produce it.

Dodds's successful chemical synthesis, three times more powerful than estrogens derived from plants or animals, would help set the stage years later for hormone replacement therapy. Yet Dodds had reason to be cautious about the drug's potential to cause harm. The original stilboestrol, as it was called in Britain, was a light powder that drifted about the laboratory during the manufacturing process. The British workmen who made it unintentionally inhaled the powder. Some developed breasts. "They had problems putting their braces [suspenders] on," reported one of Dodds's collaborators. Researchers quickly discovered that mice exposed to the drug developed cancer of the mammary glands. So did rats. When given to pregnant mice, the reproductive organs of their offspring were malformed.

But Dodds's early fears about the drug's potency got lost in the excitement of discovery and commercial possibilities. DES, as it came to be known, could be manufactured cheaply and sold at a healthy profit by any drug company. In the United States, companies like Eli Lilly, Abbott, Squibb, Winthrop, and Upjohn were eager to market it; they set out to win FDA approval by joining forces and compiling evidence for the drug's efficacy. They were doubly successful: not only did the FDA grant approval in 1941 for the drug's use in several conditions, despite warnings from cancer specialists and Dodds himself, but working together for the first time, the companies set the stage for the formation ten years later of Big Pharma, the pharmaceutical industry lobby that would become so powerful later in the century. And although the synthetic estrogen was now officially approved for vaginitis, menopausal symptoms, and suppression of lactation, as with all drugs, physicians had freedom to prescribe it as they saw fit, for so-called off-label uses.

Company doctors encouraged physicians to experiment with DES, and two Harvard Medical School clinicians, a married couple, began treating their diabetic pregnant patients with the drug in the belief it could prevent miscarriage and improve pregnancy outcomes. They did not test it on pregnant animals, nor did they compare the results with those of a control group of women not receiving the drug. Their prestige, along with the encouragement of the drug's manufacturers, helped launch this new therapy for expectant mothers. In 1947 the FDA approved its use in pregnancy. Prodding by the manufacturers also encouraged the FDA to approve diethylstilbestrol to fatten farm animals in order to make them more profitable at market. That same year, a pharmacology encyclopedia's entry under DES noted that although to date "no national catastrophe has been recognized...it is perhaps too early for any deleterious effect on the incidence of carcinoma of the female generative tract or breast to appear."

DES was put to use almost immediately as a "wonder drug" for women experiencing difficulties during pregnancy. In the mistaken belief that insufficient estrogen levels caused miscarriages and premature births, an estimated five million pregnant women were eventually treated with it. Dodds was knighted for his scientific achievement, but insisted in his later years that he never meant for the drug to be used except as a replacement for natural estrogen in situations where disease or some other conditions required removal of a woman's ovaries.

During the years that Dodds was laboring to synthesize estrogen, doctors in Germany had discovered the female hormone could also be a valuable tool in the treatment of giantism, a disease of the pituitary gland that makes children grow extraordinarily tall. Estrogen could halt giantism in a girl by forcing her into puberty and closing the growth plates. It did not take long for some physicians to realize that the same concept might work in healthy girls who did not suffer from a disease, but were simply tall because their parents were. In the early years of the twentieth century, German and Austrian scientists and physicians were considered the best in the world, and many of America's top physicians journeyed to Europe to study with them.

TREATING TALL GIRLS AT MASS GENERAL

The doctors at Massachusetts General Hospital, in particular, applied what they learned in Europe to treat tall girls, and became the leading experts in the practice. One of those doctors was Fuller Albright, who is sometimes referred to as the father of modern endocrinology. Albright is often credited with furthering the treatment in the United States in the 1940s, along with some of his younger colleagues, including Laura's doctor, Gertrud Reyersbach.

Reyersbach had been born into a prosperous Jewish family in 1907 in Oldenburg, and as a bright and independent young woman, she trained in pediatrics and endocrinology at medical school in Göttingen. But the rise of Nazism limited her opportunities to practice medicine. In 1937, she and her widowed mother fled to the United States, where a few years later she joined the staff at Massachusetts General Hospital. There her interests and expertise in endocrinology meshed well with those of the older doctor, Albright, who had studied in Germany in the 1920s, and with those of John Crawford, the doctor touting the treatment for tall girls in the newspaper article that Laura's great-aunt had sent to Shirley.

Crawford, the youngest of the three, had graduated from Harvard Medical School, joined the Army, and served in Berlin as a doctor. A Boston-born New Englander, he was an indifferent student as a child, but was fascinated with moths and butterflies, which he collected and classified. When it came to being a physician, a colleague wrote, he was both a "scholar and a scientist." He too found his niche in the budding subspecialty of pediatric endocrinology. After his Army service, he returned to Boston in 1947 and began his career in pediatric research at Massachusetts General, one of the most prestigious medical institutions in the United States and the teaching hospital affiliated with Harvard Medical School.

These doctors at Massachusetts General treated perhaps a half-dozen tall girls with estrogen, beginning as early as 1946 with a rapidly growing girl whose menstrual periods had commenced but whose growth plates showed no sign of closing. They were concerned from the start, however, that interrupting the delicate messaging system of the reproductive system by halting ovulation might alter it irreparably, might even affect fertility. But the menstrual cycles of the handful of girls who were treated in the late 1940s and early 1950s returned to normal shortly after the drug was withdrawn, which reassured Crawford and his colleagues that it caused no long-term harm. In addition, the girls' families reported their daughters were easier to live with and their grades improved—an added bonus.

From the start, this treatment that aimed to alter an inherited trait—height—was controversial in the United States. Doctors at the Johns Hopkins Hospital, a rival academic medical center in Baltimore, were less likely to treat tall girls than those at Massachusetts General. But alternative treatments were few and could be considered barbaric. Even so, desperate parents felt compelled to resort to these alternatives, and reputable doctors accommodated them.

For example, in 1965, when seventeen-year-old Carol Walters had finished growing, she was 6'6", a height that her family found unacceptable. Carol's younger sister and a younger cousin were given estrogen to stunt their growth, but the new hormone therapy came along too late for Carol. Instead, surgeons in northern California removed six inches of bone from both legs. She was hospitalized for six weeks while surgeons performed the two shortening procedures. A year-long recuperation at home followed, which included eight months in a wheelchair before learning how to walk again. Two years later, doctors determined she needed more surgery to shorten her quadriceps muscles. She spent the following summer in bilateral leg casts. Despite years of physical therapy, however, she was never again able to run, skate, squat, stand on tiptoe, or dance.

Compared with such an ordeal, swallowing a pill once a day seemed a miraculous advance. Word soon got out about the initial successful treatment at Massachusetts General. Additional families began asking for help with their tall daughters, and the Boston doctors treated them with little publicity or fanfare. But that was about to change.

THE AUSTRALIAN CONNECTION

In 1956 a pediatrician from Australia arrived at Massachusetts General to learn more about some of the endocrine treatments being developed for use in pediatrics. Norman Wettenhall, a tall, ginger-haired patrician from Melbourne, would eventually build his international reputation on the use of estrogen to stunt the growth of Australian girls. He would do more than any other doctor to popularize the treatment that Laura would reluctantly embark on more than a decade later.

Melbourne in the middle of the last century was a large, socially conservative city that had grown up along the sluggish, brown Yarra River. Miles of mostly well-kept suburbs grew up and out around the city's center. The most exclusive was—and still is—Toorak, where Wettenhall's ancestors settled on a large tract of land when they arrived in the late nineteenth century, not as convicts but as aristocrats. Society was important in Melbourne, and the large, close-knit Wettenhall family had always been prominent and important.

Growing up in this privileged environment, Norman Wettenhall developed self-confidence and exemplary people skills at an early age, prompting his father, a physician, to suggest a career in diplomacy. But he turned instead to pediatrics, with a special focus on growth and puberty. His interests were not confined to medicine, however, but ranged from art and history to natural science and ornithology. Like Crawford, who was drawn to moths and butterflies as a child, Wettenhall developed a passion for birds. Near the end of his life he sold what was considered the finest collection of Australian lithographs, prints, and books about birds and natural history in order to set up a foundation devoted to preserving the environment. Birds, he believed, were excellent indicators of environmental conditions, and the more that was known about them, the better people could understand the needs of the entire ecosystem.

Given his interest in the natural world, it seems incongruous that he would champion a treatment that relied on synthetic estrogens to override the genetic instructions that determined a girl's height. Yet Wettenhall was a man of contradictions. Despite his wealth, he pinched pennies in ways that sometimes surprised colleagues. He belonged to the snooty Melbourne Club, which limited its membership to those of one race (white), one sex (male), and one religion (Protestant). But colleagues claim he treated everyone equally. He was somewhat aloof, but was described as kind and gentlemanly by patients and fellow physicians.

In the mid-1950s, this well-to-do pediatrician traveled to America to learn more about conditions like hypothyroidism and congenital adrenal hyperplasia, disorders that cause extreme short stature. Pediatric endocrinology was a fledgling specialty in those days, without a formal curriculum or society. It lured pediatricians like Wettenhall who had an interest in science.

Pediatrics, which had developed after World War I, was considered a "softer" specialty, one that had difficulty distinguishing its role from that of the general practice physician or obstetrician who up to that time routinely treated children. Research on childhood growth and development in the early decades of the twentieth century, however, gave pediatrics a shot in the arm. Standards for height, weight, and behavioral development provided pediatricians with a special knowledge base and gave birth to the well-baby conference. Unlike other doctors, pediatricians regularly saw patients who were not ill; they monitored growth, and spent much of their time answering the questions and calming the anxieties of parents who increasingly turned to these experts for help in child rearing. (Some doctors complained that all this weighing and measuring actually sparked anxieties, evolving into a "fetish" that drove a mother to try to "standardize" her child.)

When endocrinology combined with pediatrics, pediatric endocrinologists inherited this focus on development in healthy children. But the new subspecialty of pediatric endocrinology managed some of the sickest children and rarest disorders, and therefore worked within academic medical centers. There it also inherited a very different tradition from endocrinology, which had its roots in scientific and technical innovation. Endocrinologists were miracle makers.

During the years between the world wars when Wettenhall was growing up, scientists had begun to discover the amazing powers of hormones and how they controlled metabolism, reproduction, growth, and disease. In 1922, researchers at the University of Toronto discovered insulin, the hormone produced in the pancreas that regulates the body's use of sugar. The results were extraordinary: diabetics just hours away from death received one injection of this new miracle drug and recovered almost instantaneously. A decade later, a stunned crowd of rheumatologists from around the world sat in a darkened room at the Waldorf-Astoria hotel in New York City and watched a film in which patients crippled by rheumatoid arthritis climbed out of bed and danced after receiving an injection of cortisone, a hormone made in the tiny adrenal glands sitting atop the kidneys and extracted by physicians at the Mayo Clinic.

In hormone research, scientists and doctors were making names for themselves while transforming medicine and the pharmaceutical business. If there was a downside to the miracles wrought by these discoveries, which were literally snatching patients back from the precipice of death, it may have been that some physicians became "too confident of their powers, and some laymen too certain that their doctors had a quick fix for every sickness," wrote one medical historian. It tended to "replace one kind of religion with another, one set of priests with another." Much as deciphering the genome captured the attention of the world at the end of the twentieth century because it offered such promise for the future, so did hormone research in the middle of the century.

Massachusetts General was one of only two places in the United States where doctors trained in the new field of pediatric endocrinology; the other was Johns Hopkins School of Medicine in Baltimore. Pediatric endocrinology clinics had been established in the 1940s at these two elite medical institutions, and both attracted children with rare endocrine disorders, providing researchers with a rich pool of what some called nature's experiments—children from whom doctors could learn much about how the body works. These institutions trained the first generation of pediatric endocrinologists, who, in turn, largely trained those generations that followed.

Wettenhall spent time at both institutions. At Johns Hopkins, he worked alongside Lawson Wilkins, who was considered the pioneer of pediatric endocrinology. In Boston, he trained with John Crawford. Wettenhall's visit happened to coincide with the 1956 publication of the first study on the use of estrogen to inhibit growth in tall girls. In the *Journal of Clinical Endocrinology and Metabolism*, the New York endocrinologist Max Goldzieher claimed success in halting the growth of fourteen girls between the ages of nine and sixteen who were "growing excessively." Goldzieher reported that on average, the girls gained only two more inches once treatment commenced, although he did note that younger girls grew considerably more than those who received estrogen at age twelve or older. A year later, Laura's doctor, Reyersbach, published a brief article in the *American*

Journal of Diseases of Childhood on the subject of treating tall girls with hormones.

Aware of Goldzieher's work, Wettenhall returned to Melbourne not only with the training to become Australia's first pediatric endocrinologist but also with a solution for that country's unhappy tall girls. For an ambitious young doctor, it was an area of research that seemed wide open. He noted in a later publication that there were some 41,000 Australian girls destined to grow taller than was socially acceptable; if only a small number of them desired treatment, that meant there would be plenty of subjects for a larger and more thorough study than had ever been undertaken. Max Goldzieher's study was the first, but it was too small to be very meaningful. Furthermore, because the New York doctor hadn't predicted how tall the youngsters would have grown if left alone, it was difficult to say how effective the treatment had been. In the next few years, several additional reports on treating tall girls found their way into medical journals, but again, these studies reported on only a small number— in one case only two patients. To compound the problem, the types of estrogen used varied, as well as the delivery method and dosage: some doctors implanted pellets of estrogens; some injected the hormone; others prescribed oral Premarin, estrogen made from the urine of pregnant mares. Various methods of predicting height were used. With so many variables, it was impossible to know whether the therapy actually worked or which therapy worked best.

Wettenhall decided to undertake a more precise and rigorous study, one that would establish how many inches estrogen treatments could shave from a girl's predicted mature height. He was perfect for the job: he was equipped with a scientist's curiosity and a fastidious obsession for detail and also a ready and eager clientele. His family and friends inhabited Melbourne's traditionally conservative upper middle class, most of whom believed that girls who were too tall would suffer the same misfortunes as their American counterparts. Not only would a girl's ballerina dreams be dashed, but also her marriage prospects would be limited to a small pool of suitors. Like Americans, most Australians in the 1950s and 1960s couldn't imagine a tall woman marrying "beneath" her, and parents in Wettenhall's social circle had the leisure to worry about it and the means to pay for whatever might alleviate these worries. It didn't take long before anxious mothers were ushering their daughters into the offices of this prominent physician for an assessment of their girls' potential height and treatment. Nurses at private girls' schools in Melbourne sent notes home to parents of tall girls, suggesting medical attention might be in order. Pediatricians aware of the work Wettenhall was undertaking referred their tall patients to him. Even dentists, on the basis of looking at girls' teeth, offered referrals to Wettenhall. It seemed everyone was on the lookout for tall girls in need of treatment. None of them could imagine a time when girls might want to grow up to be tall women, nor could they foresee the cultural changes that would occur over the coming decades.

HEIGHT PREDICTION: A MURKY CRYSTAL BALL

The biggest challenge facing Wettenhall in his quest to study the effectiveness of estrogen on limiting height was the ability to predict the mature height of an individual girl, with and without treatment. Parents, of course, have always wondered how tall their children would grow, and in 350 B.C., Aristotle had an answer: he observed that a child's body at age five had attained about half its adult height. In the centuries that followed, painters and sculptors developed a better understanding of growth and height than doctors or scientists as they attempted to render the human body at various ages on canvas or in stone.

It wasn't until 1759 that a child's growth was accurately charted. That year, a Frenchman with an interest in science became the father of a baby boy. Curious, Count Philibert Guéneau de Montbeillard measured his son at birth and every six months thereafter until the boy finished growing. By doing so, he provided the first record of an individual child's rate of growth over time, a pattern that clearly showed years when the boy grew slowly and years when he grew rapidly, including the period of the pubertal growth spurt.

By the early twentieth century, parents were measuring their children against doorjambs, while pediatricians weighed, measured, and plotted the results on standardized charts at well-baby visits. The charts, based on the growth of thousands of children, provided guidelines for how normal children grow. Typically, between birth and age one, a child gains between seven and ten inches. That slows to four to five inches between the first and second year, and about two to two and a half inches per year from age two until puberty.

Deviations in growth rate are not unusual during the first three years of life. Small babies born to tall parents tend to catch up during this period; likewise, large infants of small parents grow more slowly. But by age three a child generally settles into what is called a "channel"—the space created on a standard growth chart between lines that mark "centiles," or percentiles, in intervals of five: five, ten, fifteen, twenty, and so on. A child who falls in the fiftieth percentile is average: half the children her age will be shorter, the other half taller. If these early years were a swimming pool with lanes marked along the bottom, the swimmer, or child, would be expected to stay in her lane after about age three. Children may cross lanes, or growth channels, again during puberty, particularly if they enter it earlier or later than average, which will affect the timing of their growth spurt. But between the early years and puberty, children tend to grow at a relatively constant rate of two to two and a half inches per year, and doctors become concerned if a child leaves his "lane," or channel, for a lower or higher percentile. The only way to know if that happens, however, is through accurate, regular measurement, something that pediatricians' offices often do poorly.

Even assuming accurate measurements, charting a child's growth is one thing, but predicting how tall that child will grow is quite another. At the time Wettenhall began to experiment with slowing growth in girls, pediatricians advised parents to simply double the height their daughter had reached by the end of her second year. This do-it-yourself method of height prediction was often off by several inches, but more complicated methods employed by radiologists and pediatric endocrinologists for predicting the height of an individual child in the 1950s and 1960s were not much more reliable.

Yet, accurate height prediction was absolutely crucial to the practice of treating tall stature in girls. If a physician couldn't reliably predict how tall a girl would grow without treatment, how could he know if a girl should be treated? How could a doctor claim to shave two inches off a girl's predicted mature height of, say, six feet if in fact he didn't know for certain she would grow to six feet without medication? And if height prediction calculations could be exact only within an inch or two, how would a doctor know if estrogen therapy reduced her final height by an inch or two, or not at all?

Two scientific methods of prediction emerged during the middle of the twentieth century, one American, the other British. The first, known as the Bayley-Pinneau method, was devised by American developmental psychologist Nancy Bayley and relied on the same book of X-rays used by Laura's doctor to determine her bone age. Bayley's method made use of the previously developed guide *The Radiographic Atlas of Skeletal Development of the Hand and Wrist*, which consists of page after page of ghostly photographs of the X-rayed hands and wrists of healthy upper-middle-class children taken in Cleveland during the 1930s. In this atlas, the various bones in the hands and wrists of very young children appear as small white continents floating in dark seas. Year by year, however, the bony structures grow closer together. Like the reverse of continental drift, the islands of finger, palm, and wrist bones expand until they merge. The dark areas, which represent space to grow between the bones, almost disappear in the X-rays of the oldest children.

Once a child's bone age was determined, a pediatric endocrinologist referred to Bayley's mathematically derived tables to estimate what percentage of mature adult height the child had already achieved and how much more growth could be expected. Her method became widely used in the United States and around the world.

In 1962, James Tanner, a British physician and growth expert, developed a different system for determining bone age and predicting height. It, too, relied on X-rays of the hand and wrist, but required the radiologist to carefully examine individual bones and assign them points in order to come up with a final maturity score. This British method was more time-consuming than the American, but its supporters, primarily radiologists in Great Britain, declared it to be the more accurate of the two.

But neither method was flawless: critics found drawbacks and potential pitfalls to both. All types of errors were possible, from inaccurately measuring a girl's height to incorrectly positioning her arm during the X-ray, which could alter the appearance of the epiphyses. A precise reading of bone age based on X-rays, experts admitted, was somewhat subjective in the first place.

Others questioned how well the hand and wrist represented skeletal maturation. While they were easier to X-ray and would not expose a child to a great deal of radiation, linear growth rate potential might be better calculated from X-rays of the legs and back, where most growth occurs, they argued.

It also appeared that what was the "average" standard X-ray for one population of children was not necessarily the average for another. The British system, at least in this first of several versions, was based on data of children from working-class families in England, who tended to mature later than children in other parts of England and the world because of poorer nutrition and living conditions. Conversely, the X-rays displayed in the American atlas were those of children from the middle and upper classes, who, because of good nutrition and a high standard of living, matured earlier than children from other backgrounds. Not only do children mature at different rates because of their genes and family economic status, but populations differ. A child in Denver, one researcher discovered, matures more quickly than a child in Scotland.

Even the British and American scientists who devised the two competing methods admitted they were far from foolproof. "Although our predictions seem to be the best available to date, they nevertheless leave a lot to be desired.... We do not know what causes the remaining unpredictability," Tanner wrote in 1975.

Similarly, Bayley pointed out that her tables were drawn from a small group of children—only 103 girls and 89 boys—and included margins of error large enough to make it impossible to state accurately that an individual tall girl grew less than predicted because she was given estrogen. (One astute observer pointed out that because Bayley's tables were based on the data of 103 girls of all heights, her predictions for those above the ninety-seventh percentile were based probably on only three girls.)

Recognizing the importance of prediction to Goldzieher's findings, Bayley investigated the use of estrogen to stunt the growth of fourteen tall girls and concluded that Goldzieher's patients would probably have stopped growing when they did without treatment. Using the example of one of her patients who was initially predicted to reach 5'9½" and who topped out at 5'8", she concluded that the difference was within a margin of error for her own method of height prediction.

Because Wettenhall understood the necessity of the most consistent, accurate measurements possible of his patients, he turned to an anatomist at the University of Melbourne, Alex Roche, who had been involved in growth studies in Australia since the early 1950s. Roche developed a third method of predicting height that involved X-raying a child's knee, a more complicated procedure and one that never became as popular as the American and British methods. Wettenhall and Roche collaborated for years, beginning in the 1950s. In 1962, Wettenhall established the Endocrine Clinic at the Royal Children's Hospital in Melbourne. Some girls were treated at this public facility, others through his private practice.

READ ALL ABOUT IT!

In 1964 at a conference in Australia's capital, Canberra, Wettenhall presented the first of several papers based on his experiences treating twenty-five tall girls. A flurry of newspaper articles reported on his success. On September 18 (coincidentally, Wettenhall's forty-ninth birthday), the *Sydney Sun* ran a front-page story with a one-and-a-half-inch headline: "Girl, 13, with Figure 35-24-35."

"Last night," wrote the reporter, "I met and talked with two of Australia's growth-controlled girls. They are happy, pretty teenagers who have been prevented from growing embarrassingly tall by daily doses of the artificial female hormone stilboestrol. But now these schoolchildren have the bodies of women." A photograph of the full-figured thirteen-year-old patient, identified only as Miss X, ran beside the story on page one. The article described Wettenhall's pioneering new form of growth control. "His work made world medical news this week after its recent successes had been revealed in a report issued in Canberra by the National Health and Medical Research Council. Since 1959, this doctor, with the full knowledge and consent of the girls and their parents, has treated about 25 too-tall girls with stilboestrol."

A similar story ran the same day in a sister publication, the *Daily News*, with an even more sensational headline: "Drug Turns Young Amazons into Beauties." The story focused again on Miss X, and also a sixteen-year-old, Miss Z, who was a ballet dancer. Both girls described their speedy ride through puberty, and the rapid change from childlike bodies to those of mature women.

"Oh, I like my new shape, but the change was certainly quick. It was all over in less than twelve months," said Miss Z. The estimated mature height for Miss Z, the ballerina, who was 5'4¾" at thirteen, was 5'7¾". According to the article, 5'6" was the maximum allowable height for a ballerina. "'If you are taller than that, you stand over six feet high when you go up six inches on your points,'" she explained. "'When mother took me to the specialist he put me first on one tab-

let a day, then two and finally three. This treatment has gone on for
about three years now and I seem to have stopped growing at five feet
five-and-a-half inches.' "

Readers were fascinated with the story of Wettenhall's apparent success, although some clearly questioned the need to devote
resources to a problem they deemed minor compared with the vexing
social and economic problems of Australia in the mid-sixties. In a
political cartoon that appeared the same day as the stories, the car-
toonist showed a citizen pointing to a giantess so enormous that only
her feet and legs appear. Emblazoned on her skirt were the words
"rising prices, fares, food, taxes." The citizen appealed to a professor
standing outside a science building. "Have a go at this one—NOW."
A radio personality known for his short poems broadcast one that
turned out, years later, to be prescient:

This idea of limiting growth of tall girls
Is an idea that might well be skittled.
It may, of course, appeal to a few,
But no girl, really, likes to be be-littled.

While some were fascinated or amused by these articles, others
voiced their dissent. The then president of the Australian Tall Girls'
Club, a Mrs. Pat Nisbet, who measured 5'10", was quoted as saying
she thought the treatment was "interfering with Nature," and that she
wouldn't be in favor of it "unless a girl was going to be exceptionally
tall—and by that I mean six feet, six inches, or so."

DISTURBING SIDE EFFECTS

Although accounts in the news media about the new treatment rarely
mentioned side effects, almost all girls experienced some. Weight gain
afflicted many girls, as did heavy periods, depression, moodiness, and
nausea similar to morning sickness. Some developed ovarian cysts,
and at least one was diagnosed with thrombosis—a blood clot in the

leg. Another suffered from galactorrhea, spontaneous lactation. Wettenhall suggested that dieting could control the weight gain, and nausea could be mitigated if girls started on a low dose of stilbestrol that was increased gradually rather than begin with a high dose. While these side effects were rarely mentioned in the news accounts, two positive side effects—clearer skin and less greasy hair—were hailed as significant benefits.

Besides the side effects, there were the office visits, which some girls found disturbing. Wettenhall did not believe in gowns. Patients were instructed to strip completely. A few minutes later the doctor walked in the door and the exam began. There was a large mirror in the examining room. He told the girls to stand before the mirror so he could point out their breasts and pubic hair in order to reassure them that their sexual development was proceeding as it should.

George Werther, a pediatric endocrinologist who worked closely with Wettenhall beginning in the late 1970s and who considered the older, established doctor as his mentor, was uncomfortable with this aspect of the examination. From time to time, Werther would see Wettenhall's private patients when the older doctor was away. "I remember being shocked when I walked into the examining room and there was this tall girl standing there completely naked. Norman had trained them to do this and argued that it made the exam easier, more efficient perhaps. Now, of course, it would be seen as terribly insensitive. I thought perhaps it had to do with his training in the Navy." For some girls the regular visits, once every few months, also included a pelvic exam. Although pediatric endocrinologists normally do not perform pelvic exams, Werther believed Wettenhall thought these were necessary to examine changes in the vagina and vulva brought on by the additional estrogen that was being administered.

Despite Wettenhall's charming bedside manner in the office and the people skills he displayed throughout his life, he was apparently incapable of putting himself in the place of the girls he examined. Years later, many remembered those exams vividly. One woman visiting Melbourne with her husband not long after she married suffered a panic attack when she realized she was not far from Wettenhall's office, where she'd been examined years earlier. She grabbed her husband's hand and pulled him down the street in a frantic effort to leave the area.

Another Wettenhall patient described in detail the embarrassment of being measured in the basement of the anatomy department at the University of Melbourne. This was common procedure, and virtually all girls who consulted with Wettenhall about their height experienced the same ordeal. The woman's grandmother brought her to the basement, where they were shown into an anteroom adjacent to the examination room. She was instructed to undress completely, put on a robe, and leave her clothes with her grandmother. There was no changing room. After she was weighed and measured, she was told to remove her robe and begin a lengthy process that included more measuring and photography while she was nude.

Various parts of my body were measured separately with a tape measure and with calipers. Two or three people (I recall two women and a man) were occupied with this activity. I believe I recall them measuring my inner leg and my pelvis. I think I recall them commenting among themselves about my bone structure, the bone angles, et cetera. I think I recall having parts of my skin marked with a marker, and someone telling me that it would wash off with soap.

Then I was photographed, I think this took a long time, I think they took long shots of my whole body and close-ups of various body parts. I don't know if they moved around me or if I was directed to change my position. I think I was told to raise and lower my arms and spread and close my legs.

Then I was led (I remember following behind) to the other end of the room. I don't remember being told where I was going or what would happen. The people who had worked on me until now left and returned to the far end of the room. I suppose to avoid the X-rays. I stood at one end of this narrow area and at the other end was the X-ray equipment and some men—maybe two or three.

They were definitely men, there was more than one, but I don't think I could see them clearly.

I stood in a marked-off circle with crosses showing where to place my feet so that my legs were separated from the groin down. I had to hold my arms at my side but not touching my sides. The X-raying took a long time, when it was done they told me to turn so I was facing them side-on, then again so my back was towards them and I was looking at the opposite end of the room at the people who had measured me. I think they were sitting around a table. Then I turned again and they did the other side.

It was when they were X-raying my back that I did away with myself utterly. . . . I became what these people were telling me that I was—a non-person, they were adults, they were doctors and scientists.

The terrible, terrible. . . shame that I experienced was, I knew, totally unwarranted. They were scientists, they were completely disinterested in me and my body. . . .

I believe I remember that one (of the men on the other side of the room) looked over at me, and I kind of smiled, as if I could be doing this thing without feeling a thing, as if it was all natural and a matter of course. I was pretending that this was so, and it wasn't long before the pretending was all that mattered. . . .

There was a peephole in the X-ray area through which my grandmother could choose to look, but she had no way of seeing the measuring and photographing area. As far as I know, she was completely unaware of what happened in that section of the room.

After the X-raying, I was given back the robe and sent back to my grandmother to dress. I clearly remember how it felt to take possession of my clothes and put them on and how it was to have them on again. I still felt naked. I had to wait while she spoke to some of them, I think they said we'd be notified of the results in about two weeks. She drove me home and on the way she talked about a dinner party she was planning, she was a very social person, very proper and big on manners.

I went home and my father asked "How was it" and I said "Fine." My brother teased me and the adults joked about how lucky I was to have missed a whole day of school. I felt numb. When I went to bed I curled myself into the smallest ball—I have slept that way often since then.

CHAPTER 3

two girls, two continents

A NEW PATIENT

The Australian newspaper articles that failed to mention the physical exams and the negative side effects the girls endured brought a deluge of new patients. One was Janet Cregan-Wood, slender and dark-haired with pale, light-freckled skin. She was eleven years old and measured just over 5'8". Her mother, Peg, had read the articles and, like Laura's mother, Shirley, remembered the teasing she'd endured as a tall young woman. She made an appointment with Dr. Wettenhall.

Janet was a private patient, so instead of being treated at the hospital clinic, she saw Wettenhall in his private "rooms," as doctors' offices are called in Australia after the British fashion. His rooms were located in the poshest part of downtown Melbourne, not far from the Melbourne Club. In fact, the office looked a bit like Janet imagined the Melbourne Club: dark wood, formidable furniture, and stuffed birds. On this first visit, Janet recalls Dr. Wettenhall sitting behind a very large desk covered with family pictures. He seemed kind and gentle, he spoke softly and smiled easily. He took a detailed medical history, carefully entering notes on a large index card. Besides height, weight, and other medical findings, he often jotted down conversational clues. If, for instance, a patient had just gotten a new puppy, or was about to have a birthday party, he would note it on her card. At the next visit he'd invariably ask, "How's Rex doing?" or "How was your birthday party?" Such carefully planned thoughtfulness or interest endeared him to his patients and their parents.

At Janet's first consultation, Peg was instructed to take her to the University of Melbourne's anatomy department, where proper measurements would be taken under the supervision of Wettenhall's collaborator, Alex Roche. The measurements took place in a large, cold room where various adults in white gowns instructed Janet to sit, stand, or kneel. Using calipers, they measured her skin, fat, breasts, and nipples. Like the other girls, she was photographed while standing on a brightly lit platform, naked, with her legs and arms apart.

Janet's final height was predicted to be just over 5'11". She and her mother agreed to begin treatment, but it was short-lived. Under Wettenhall's care her weight quickly ballooned. Her periods became so heavy that she needed to wear rubber pants to school. Even so, sometimes she had to run home in the middle of the day to change her clothes. Older adolescent boys were propositioning her, not realizing that despite her mature figure she was still a child. Less than a year after she began swallowing the DES tablets she quit—the side effects were too overwhelming to continue. Unlike the happy girls described in the newspaper articles, Janet sank into depression. She developed an eating disorder. Her depression became so severe, she was hospitalized. A few years later, her mother burned all the photos of Janet during those years. The pictures reminded them both of a very difficult and unhappy time.

Nevertheless, in the 1960s Wettenhall was making an international name for himself as a leading authority in growth suppression. Other pediatricians in Australia were following his lead and prescribing DES—even in remote areas, far from the tony suburbs of Melbourne. Not only did aspiring ballerinas who lived in Sydney and Melbourne need to watch their height, so, apparently, did girls who lived in rural areas. "Perhaps the most common concern of tall girls is that they feel conspicuous, especially when they live in a small community," Wettenhall wrote in a 1965 paper. A few years later he suggested another reason for treatment: "A very tall person...may have difficulty in establishing heterosexual relationships."

A CAUTIOUS FEW

Wettenhall's research was also attracting notice in North America and Europe. Many doctors remained leery, citing possible unknown long-term side effects of high-dose estrogen therapy. An editorial in the *British Medical Journal* in April 1963 ended with these words: "This form of treatment, which causes an unnaturally early puberty as an inevitable side effect, cannot at present be recommended." A few years later, another doctor, quoted in *Pediatrics*, questioned the ethics of the treatment: "I wonder what right we have as physicians to 'move' a girl toward the mean of average height, since the girl's adjustment as a tall adult woman may be a very favorable one."

Lawson Wilkins, in his first textbook on pediatric endocrinology, warned physicians to "resist parents who were frequently alarmed and excessively worried because they have been told by well-meaning friends, teachers, or doctors that the child has a 'glandular disorder' even though the child fell within the normal parameters of adolescent development."

But mothers—and it was usually moms, not dads, who obsessed about the height of their daughters—could always find doctors who would treat their girls. In Boston, New York, San Francisco, Los Angeles, Chicago, and Houston, families were referred to pediatric endocrinologists, mostly affiliated with large and prestigious teaching institutions. One San Francisco–area pediatric endocrinologist remembers a parade of tall mothers who came to her office asking for treatment for their daughters. "They all belonged to something called the Tip Toppers, a club for tall people, and they all told me that their daughters' lives would be ruined if we didn't give them this treatment. Well, of course, these mothers were all quite tall and they had found husbands." Two decades after Kay Sumner's tall pride movement, the Tip Toppers, it seemed, had capitulated.

In other areas of the country where there were no pediatric endocrinologists, pediatricians, internists, or gynecologists assessed and treated tall girls.

At the root of the controversy between those doctors who thought estrogen therapy was worth the risk and those who balked was the definition of disease. Was tall stature in a girl a medical problem or just a social disadvantage? John Crawford at Massachusetts General eventually treated some three hundred tall girls over several decades beginning in the mid-1950s. He believed that by treating their emotional suffering—how they thought of themselves—he *was* treating disease. Parents traveled from all over the country to ask him for help with their tall daughters. Most were upper-middle-class families; some had been turned away by other pediatric endocrinologists.

"I was the radical," said Crawford, with a touch of pride. He never wrote prescriptions for girls who didn't want the treatment, but for those who did, he believed it was the right thing to do. Over time, he also came to believe that the girls he treated were different from those who did not want treatment, and were more apt to make something of their lives. "They wanted more control. They pursued their education and wanted careers," he recalled. He denied obesity was a problem among those he treated, but rather affected the girls who refused treatment. Early fears about fertility were dismissed. Although Crawford never did a follow-up of his patients, he believed that the girls he treated were more apt to marry later and put off childbearing to pursue careers. "The girls who wanted treatment were just different from the start."

Just across town at Boston Children's Hospital, the attitudes toward prescribing estrogen to tall girls remained more conservative. Dr. Roswell Gallagher, who was considered the leading authority on adolescent health, headed Children's Hospital's Adolescent Unit, the first such clinic to specialize in the treatment of this age group. Gallagher urged restraint in treating tall girls. In his textbook *Medical Care of the Adolescent*, first published in 1960, he argued that estrogen administration should be considered only in girls predicted to be taller than six feet. Gallagher wrote that prediction methods were not perfect, and that anxiety on the part of a tall mother "may be based less on what heights are unusual today than on those which might have made one conspicuous in her generation." He advised doctors, parents, and daughters to wait before making a decision. "It would seem that efforts to limit a young girl's height should never be made unless there has been a preliminary period of at least three months during which time several sessions have been devoted to attempting to get the girl to accept herself as she is, to relieving the mother's anxiety, to reassuring the girl, and to settling the physician's own mind as to what may be the best course to follow. To do less is likely to result in paving the way for one anxiety to replace the one you attempted to remove."

With what seems like extraordinary insight, Gallagher added: "At this time of life the patient herself may have little interest or concern with her body; yet it is her body, what she is going to be, which we contemplate changing, and we surely would be reluctant to attempt a change based primarily on a mother's wish for this child. That would seem to be extending her part in this person's design and shape to a point which usurps another's rights."

He also opposed performing pelvic exams on adolescent girls unless it was absolutely necessary, and then he suggested it be done under anesthesia so as not to traumatize the patient.

Yet the work under way in Australia gained followers and momentum. The pediatric endocrinology community was not a large one, and word of Wettenhall's research traveled via national and international conferences. As his studies were published, more clinicians began seeing tall girls; parents in the Netherlands, Germany, France, Switzerland, and the Scandinavian countries also began clamoring for treatment for their tall daughters.

LAURA TAKES HER MEDICINE

In New Hampshire, Laura was dutifully swallowing her pills, but unlike those girls John Crawford said he encountered in his Boston practice who wanted to get ahead and have careers, Laura drifted in the opposite direction. She grew moodier. Her relationship with her parents began to deteriorate. To Shirley, whose fears stemmed from her own mother's attitudes decades earlier, worries about Laura's height were legitimate concerns of a mother who wanted the best for her daughter. For Laura, those fears translated into painful criticism of her appearance.

To compound the problem, Laura began to gain weight—just like Janet Cregan-Wood in Australia, just like the livestock that farmers routinely fattened with DES. Now she was not only tall, she was large. One day at the beach, the summer after she began taking the pills, her father made a negative remark about her appearance in a bathing suit to her sister Cathy. In a moment of sibling rivalry, Cathy told Laura, and Laura was devastated. In her attempt to regain her old, thinner figure, she tried starving herself. This was the beginning of eating disorders that would plague her for years. "When my father told me to eat—that I looked emaciated—it was the best thing anybody could say to me. It made me feel great to be called emaciated."

During those difficult years, Laura could have thrown away the pills without telling her mother. But she didn't. "I was an obedient child," she explained. Deep down she trusted her parents, who thought this was important. And her parents trusted the doctor.

In December 1969, perhaps in response to unsettling concerns emerging about DES, Dr. Reyersbach switched Laura from the synthetic estrogen DES to Premarin, estrogen made from the urine of mares. She was also instructed to take Pranone, a synthetic form of the natural progestin hormone produced by females, four times a day for five days every twenty-eight days. Pranone would protect the lining of her uterus and create a monthly "period," although the treatment itself prevented her from ovulating. Soon afterward, Laura began to complain that her stomach hurt. Over the next six months she grew sicker; she was plagued with chest pains and nausea, and vomited frequently. Doctors were unable to diagnose the cause. Shirley and Stuart feared that the therapy to limit Laura's height had become so distressing to her that she'd developed an ulcer, but doctors found no evidence of one. Because of her youth, doctors overlooked another possibility—gallstones. Nearly a year after the stomachaches began, Laura was rushed to the hospital for emergency gallbladder surgery. In those days, removing a gallbladder required surgeons to make a lengthy incision. Laura's scar ran from her midsection around her side and to the middle of her back. Hospital staff told Shirley they'd found sixty-three gallstones—a hospital record—in her fifteen-year-old daughter.

Shirley remembered reading that women who took birth control pills were at risk for a higher incidence of gallbladder disease. She asked Reyersbach if the estrogen prescribed for Laura might have been responsible for the gallstones, which were unusual in someone so young. Reyersbach reassured Shirley that there was no possible connection. But Shirley wasn't sure.

Laura's lengthy incision eventually healed, though leaving a nasty scar, but her relationship with her parents did not. With one hundred times the normal amount of estrogen surging through her body, she abandoned her dolls and, as she puts it, "went nuts for the older brother of her best friend." The two became inseparable, and she began spending more and more time away from her family, preferring the home of her nineteen-year-old boyfriend, Dan, and his family. Dan's mother and sisters were tall, although not as tall as Shirley, and when Laura confided in them that she was taking hormones to stunt her growth, they were horrified. Their reaction helped Laura justify her anger about the treatment, and further alienated her from her parents. Laura wasn't worried that her height would impede her ability to find dancing partners or a job as a stewardess. Despite measuring 5'10½", she'd had no trouble finding a cute boyfriend, further proving to herself that her parents' attempts had not only been psychologically and physically painful but needless.

Laura had changed, and Shirley and Stuart could not understand it. The hormone therapy that was supposed to ease their tall daughter's social and psychological adjustment had backfired. She lost interest in school. When exhortations to shape up failed, Shirley and Stuart resorted to restrictions. Laura ignored them. Clad in bell-bottoms and an Indian-bedspread blouse, her blond hair long and straight, Laura spent more time on the back of Dan's motorcycle than she did at home or high school. Finally, in 1973, she moved out. "The day I turned eighteen—the very day—after three years of a bad relationship with my parents, I walked out the door. That was it. I didn't see them again for quite a while."

The times had changed, too. The social landscape familiar to Shirley and Shirley's mother had altered. The civil rights movement, the women's movement, the antiwar protests, the sexual revolution of the late sixties and early seventies, all had made the country—even a small town in New England—a different place than it had been a generation before. Rules of behavior that guided Shirley and her mother were more and more often deemed irrelevant by girls growing up in the 1970s. Newspaper stories about women burning their bras had replaced advice columns like those John Robert Powers had written two decades earlier stressing the importance of proper corsetry to help disguise a height problem.

In 1970, when Melbourne native and feminist Germaine Greer's revolutionary book *The Female Eunuch* was published, the first female jockey rode in the Kentucky Derby. In 1971, the inaugural issue of *Ms.* magazine landed on the newsstands. In 1973, *The Joy of Sex* hit the bestseller list, and the Supreme Court ruled on *Roe v. Wade*. During the early years of the decade, height and weight requirements for police and fire departments were adjusted to allow women and minorities to compete equally for those jobs. Men were allowed to become flight attendants, and height requirements, like the term "stewardess," faded like a jet stream. Perhaps the most influential change for tall girls occurred in 1972, when Title IX banned sex discrimination in schools. Its effect on sports programs for women was profound: in 1971, the number of women involved in collegiate sports was 29,977; a little more than three decades later, that number would increase to 2,953,355.

DES: A MEDICAL DISASTER

In 1971, the year Gertrud Reyersbach felt Laura had reached her final height—just under 5'11"—and eased her off the hormones, two physicians at Massachusetts General published a devastating article in *The New England Journal of Medicine*. They had recently diagnosed a cancer of the vagina, clear-cell adenocarcinoma, in seven girls between the ages of fourteen and twenty-four. This type of cancer appeared rarely, and only in older, postmenopausal women. Girls who didn't die of the disease required hysterectomies as well as multiple surgeries to replace cancerous vaginal tissue with skin grafted from healthy parts of their bodies. As these cases presented themselves, the doctors were perplexed. Why were they suddenly seeing this disease in young women?

It was the mother of one who suggested that perhaps the DES she'd been prescribed when pregnant had caused the malignancy in her daughter. The doctors were horrified. The drug had been given to millions of pregnant women to prevent miscarriage as early as 1938, and physicians were still routinely prescribing it. The doctors quickly confirmed the link between clear-cell adenocarcinoma and DES, and published their findings. Nobody addressed how large doses of DES might affect pubertal girls given the drug to stunt their growth. Decades later, a doctor instrumental in discovering the DES-cancer link could not recall whether he or anyone else in his department at Massachusetts General discussed possible dangers with colleagues in the pediatric endocrinology department who were treating tall girls. It was assumed that the drug damaged only developing fetuses. Furthermore, because DES was sold under more than two hundred different names, few parents knew it was the same drug their tall daughters were swallowing.

The DES catastrophe developed despite numerous warnings, including those of its inventor, Dodds, that should have prevented it. As early as 1953, a study at the University of Chicago compared 840 pregnant women given DES with 806 pregnant women given a placebo and found that DES had "no beneficial effect whatsoever" on preventing miscarriage. In fact, the women who took DES had more miscarriages and lower-weight babies. Still, the FDA did not declare the drug ineffective for pregnancy until 1962. And although the FDA issued a safety warning in 1971 after the cancer connection was revealed, *The Wall Street Journal* reported that 11,000 prescriptions were written in the United States for DES in 1974.

DES was used as a lactation suppressant in new mothers, as a morning-after pill to prevent conception, for hormone replacement in menopausal women, for breast and prostate cancer treatment, and as a treatment to stunt the growth of tall girls. In some cases, the daughters of mothers who were exposed to DES in utero were exposed a second time to this powerful drug because they were growing too tall.

Yet even as the DES tragedy unfolded, pediatric endocrinologists prescribed other forms of estrogen to stunt tall girls, not because they were concerned about using the drug in young women, but because DES had acquired a bad reputation. They switched to Premarin or ethinyl estradiol, another synthetic estrogen that is a component of many birth control drugs. In Australia, Dr. Wettenhall continued to publish the results of his studies. In a 1975 article in the *Journal of Pediatrics*, he reported that he'd treated 168 girls and reduced their height *on average* by less than one and a half inches, although he noted that the average for girls who began treatment before they began menstruating was slightly greater—just over one and a half inches—than for girls who commenced treatment after menarche. Those girls, on average, saw a height reduction of just under an inch, ignoring the margin of error in height prediction that was greater than the result he claimed to have achieved. Still, he reported, "for girls worried about the problems of excessive tallness, the saving of even one centimeter—the equivalent of less than half an inch—can be appreciated."

Side effects such as nausea and weight gain could be easily controlled, he wrote, by reducing the initial amount of estrogen the girls received and working up to higher doses gradually. Dieting could counteract the weight gain. He noted that three girls had developed ovarian cysts requiring surgery, while another developed a blood clot in her calf. Other clinicians reported "annoying hypertrophy," or an enlargement of the labia minora, as well as a rise in cholesterol and triglyceride levels during treatment.

Although the treatment remained controversial in the United States, Wettenhall's study was by far the largest, and he was considered an expert on the subject. In 1976 he wrote the chapter on tall stature for the third edition of Roswell Gallagher's classic, and previously more cautious, textbook, *Medical Care of the Adolescent.* Despite the changing height restrictions on airlines and fire and police forces, and the storm over DES, Wettenhall's chapter in the 1976 version of *Medical Care of the Adolescent* suggested treating girls whose predicted height was 5'10", even shorter than that suggested reluctantly by Gallagher fifteen years earlier. By this time, estrogens were widely used throughout the world, although doctors in Europe preferred ethinyl estradiol, while most pediatric endocrinologists in the United States tended to use Premarin, which was used primarily as hormone replacement therapy for menopausal women.

While more and more girls received treatment, the proof that it worked as well as clinicians claimed was still lacking. No less an expert than Alex Roche, the anatomist who had worked closely with Wettenhall, published a book on the subject of height prediction in 1975. In the introduction he ended with the words of Aldous Huxley:

Why is it that no fortune-tellers are millionaires and that no insurance companies go bankrupt? Their business is the same—foreseeing the future. But whereas the members of one group succeed all the time, the members of the other group succeed, if at all, only occasionally. The reason is simple. Insurance companies deal with statistical averages. Fortune-tellers are concerned with particular cases. One can predict with a high degree of precision what is going to happen in regard to very large numbers of things or people. To predict what is going to happen to any particular thing or person is for most of us quite impossible and even for the specially gifted minority, exceedingly difficult.

While Wettenhall continued making the case for treating tall girls, controversy bubbled up again. Five years after the DES bombshell, studies reported that estrogen given to postmenopausal women had substantially increased their risk of uterine cancer. It didn't take long before a connection was made to the tall girls. If postmenopausal women taking estrogen were at greater risk of developing uterine cancer, why wouldn't the same be true for young girls who were given even higher doses of the drug?

In an article that appeared on February 11, 1976, in *The New York Times* about the possible risks, one pediatric endocrinologist suggested that tall girls were treated for only a couple of years while postmenopausal women took hormone replacement for a much longer period. Another reason that young girls were unlikely to be affected, suggested John Crawford of Massachusetts General, was that the pituitary gland in menopause continues to secrete ovarian-stimulating hormones but gets no response from ovaries that have "worn out." When women took estrogen after menopause, "cells that are normally never stimulated to divide again are asked to do something not in their behavioral program. The chronic overstimulation of cells to divide is at least a rationalization for endometrial cancer."

Others were becoming increasingly nervous about the practice, however. Dr. Claude Migeon, director of the pediatric endocrine clinic at Johns Hopkins University School of Medicine, observed that "the furor is making everybody edgy and concerned." Some pediatric endocrinologists were taking greater pains to explain that long-term side effects were not known. Kaiser Permanente Medical Center, for example, required parents to sign a form that read in part: "The doctor has explained to me the action of the medication and possible side effects. I understand that estrogen causes rapid sexual development. Currently we know of no long-term ill effects although long-term experience with this medication in children is lacking."

Two months later, a longer story about the treatment ran in *The New York Times Magazine*. It described the case of a girl, taller than average, whose mother first took her to a pediatric endocrinologist when she was seven years old. At that visit, pediatric endocrinologist Jennifer Bell estimated the girl's final mature height to be between 5'9" and 5'10". The girl's parents considered that an acceptable height. A year later, at a second visit, the girl had grown another four inches. Bell adjusted the girl's height prediction up another half-inch. At a third visit nine months later, the girl had grown an additional two inches but her sexual development had slowed. Bell worried that with puberty temporarily stopped, the girl could grow even taller—perhaps to six feet. That was unacceptable to both the girl and her mother, who said: "I don't want a basketball player for a daughter. I want a normal girl."

The girl and her parents decided to start estrogen therapy a month after her tenth birthday. After twenty-seven months the girl's final height was 5'6½". Curiously, although she and her parents believed that height to be "perfect," soon after she began to consider a career as a model. Then she feared that she would be too short.

Times readers responded not unlike some of the dissenting Australians who first read about Wettenhall's treatment in the 1960s. Letters to the editor, mostly written by tall women, expressed outrage. One writer, a tall woman who said she was teased about her height in school, likened the treatment to foot binding and pointed out that "school corridors are filled with laughter about a big bust or no bust, ear-to-ear braces, fat legs, thin legs, glasses, pimples," and so on. She said she emerged unscarred as a tall teen because she recognized that other attributes besides her height were important.

The *Times* article caused a reaction beyond its readers, however. In December 1977, the Lawson Wilkins Pediatric Endocrine Society and the National Institute of Child Health and Human Development cosponsored a conference in Santa Ynez, California, on the use of estrogen in children. More than twenty doctors, primarily pediatric endocrinologists, from around the world attended; some, including Crawford, submitted papers, and these were published in a special supplement to the journal *Pediatrics* the following year.

In an introduction to the supplement, Dr. Maria New, chairman of the conference planning committee, wrote that the conference "was conceived at a time when prescribing estrogens had become controversial among physicians and the public. The treatment of tall girls to limit growth was sufficiently newsworthy to appear as an article in *The New York Times Magazine*. The occurrence of adenocarcinoma in the daughters of women treated prenatally with diethylstilbestrol was the subject of congressional hearings. It seemed the right time to bring together experts on the risks and benefits of prescribing estrogens to analyze what was known on the subject and to make recommendations on the use of estrogens in treating the young."

The conference committee's recommendations reflected more concern about long-term side effects than had been expressed in journal articles up to that time. The conference concluded that height prediction remained subjective and uncertain. Moreover, there was no evidence of psychosocial benefit to the girls who took the medicine. "Little is known of the psychosocial benefit derived from treatment, and comparison has not been made with girls who have not been treated. Since this therapy is instituted for psychosocial reasons, it would seem urgent that studies be done to evaluate the psychosocial benefit of treatment [versus] no treatment," the article stated.

The conferees compared the use of estrogen to treat girls with a chromosomal condition called Turner syndrome, which causes inadequate production of estrogen, with its use to treat tall girls who are producing normal amounts of estrogen on their own. The group noted that estrogen treatment carried risks: girls born with Turner syndrome, who received estrogen because their ovaries make little or none, developed uterine cancer at an earlier age than the general population. In addition, the doctors noted recent studies which showed postmenopausal women given estrogen suffered higher incidences of uterine cancer, and use of DES in pregnant woman caused vaginal cancers in some of their daughters. Considering estrogen's carcinogenic effects, the group wrote:

> The human experiment has been conducted. Enough girls have been treated with estrogen over a long period of time from a young age

so that we should be able to evaluate the risk. The answers to our questions will probably not be made more readily available by turning to animal models. Rather, we should carefully follow up those children who are treated for tall stature with high-dose estrogens as well as those children receiving replacement therapy for agonadism (Turner syndrome). The follow-up should include endometrial biopsy, if possible, as well as evaluation of liver function and cytology [health of the cells] of the vagina.... It must be emphasized that it is necessary to conduct close follow-up of those children undergoing long-term, low-dose estrogen therapy as well as those who have in the past received high-dose, short-term therapy.

But very few doctors followed up these patients. Girls like Laura were treated for a few years and then left home, got jobs, or went to college. Few mothers were as diligent as Shirley, who stayed in touch with Gertrud Reyersbach for five or six years after Laura's treatment ended. Few, if any, physicians attempted to track down patients years later to ask about their health, let alone suggest they have endometrial biopsies or liver function evaluations. Doctors likely to see these girls in the future—gynecologists or internists—were in most cases unaware of the childhood hormone treatment.

LAURA MARRIES . . . AND MISCARRIES

In December 1979, at the age of twenty-four, Laura married Steven Cooper. Within a few months she was pregnant. But during the third month of her pregnancy she began to bleed heavily and miscarried. For Laura, the next decade began as the previous one ended: with a miscarriage. Laura recalls she "spotted through the whole pregnancy and was very nervous." After this second miscarriage she was referred to a specialist.

"I went through a battery of tests to try to determine what was wrong, and whenever I mentioned I had taken these hormones when I was a girl they all looked at me like I had rocks in my head. I really got some strange looks when I told doctors about the treatment." In fact, Laura's gynecologists had never heard of the height-reduction therapy; that was the purview of pediatric endocrinologists.

"Then I went to a doctor in Boston, and he did some major laparoscopy work and found endometriosis, fibroids, and a history of ruptured ovarian cysts. I had had bouts of just being doubled over in pain and didn't know what it was, and then it would go away. The doctor in Boston wanted to try fertility hormones, and I said no. I just said forget it—I'm not taking any more of this stuff. I didn't want the side effects."

Shortly afterward, Laura, then in her early thirties, became pregnant a third time. History repeated itself, and the pregnancy, which was physically painful, ended in miscarriage after three months. Depression, which had plagued her on and off for years, seemed to settle in for good. Her marriage suffered. "My husband just distanced himself from me and from the whole experience of the miscarriages. It was not a good marriage at that point. It was a bad time. Luckily I had my mother, and she was great in helping me through this."

PART 2

helping the
dwarfed children

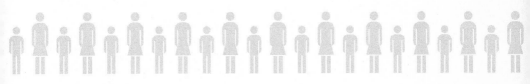

CHAPTER 4

"a gland lost is a gland wasted"

GIANTS, MIDGETS, AND THE MASTER GLAND

While some physicians worked to save tall girls from an awkward adolescence and an unmarried future, many more focused on children who did not grow enough. By the late 1950s, medicine had known for half a century that the pituitary gland held the key to growth, and yet, as triumph followed triumph in endocrinology, making a small patient taller remained frustratingly beyond reach.

People in ancient times knew about the pituitary gland at the base of the brain, though they had named it in the mistaken belief that its role was to discharge mucus, or *pituita*, rather than to regulate growth. They invented imaginative theories over the centuries to explain how human beings got taller. Some early medical books suggested it had something to do with a child's "moistness." This solved the mystery of why people stopped growing: when children reached adolescence and young adulthood their bodies "dried out" and solidified.

In the late nineteenth century, physicians began to realize the pituitary's importance. In 1887, a doctor in a Prussian clinic described an unfortunate musician with acromegaly, which is what giantism is called when it occurs in adulthood. Since the growth plates are closed, adults don't get taller, but their extremities, facial features, and sometimes their internal organs enlarge. The patient was forced to switch from the violin to the flute as his fingers swelled, only to give up the flute as his lips grew, and finally to relinquish music altogether as his eyesight failed. For the first time, a physician linked this disorder of excessive growth to a pituitary tumor. Not long afterward, other medical scientists found either tumor-ridden or atrophied pituitaries when they autopsied people they called midgets—adults who are normally proportioned but the size of small children. Conditions at both ends of the yardstick seemed to point to the gland's central role.

In the United States in the early 1900s, Harvey Cushing was already on his way to becoming the twentieth century's most famous neurosurgeon when he removed a pituitary tumor from a patient with acromegaly. The man made an amazing recovery. On the basis of his astute observations of his patients and their symptoms, Cushing concluded that the pea-size gland secreted what he called "the hormone of growth." Cushing correctly theorized in his landmark 1912 monograph that lack of this hormone during childhood made some people abnormally short. On the other hand, too much during childhood might make a person abnormally tall.

The public paid to gawk when freak shows displayed these so-called giants and midgets—an association that eventually made the label "midget" offensive to those people it described. As Cushing understood, midgets were actually hypopituitary dwarfs; they had a form of extreme short stature caused by what he called "hypopituitism," meaning their pituitaries did not produce enough of the hormone essential to growth. The condition didn't appear to be inherited, and it didn't cause the shortened limbs that characterized some other forms of dwarfism.

Cushing was optimistic about potential treatment for this hypopituitary dwarfism. Doctors of his era could already replace other missing secretions with glandular extracts, a practice they hailed as organotherapy. They could cure the thyroid deficiency that otherwise left children mentally stunted—or cretins, in the era's parlance. If stunted height resulted from a hormone deficiency, someday it surely could be cured by replacing the hormone.

Hard evidence for Cushing's optimism didn't come soon, however. It wasn't easy to find and purify this single hormone among the many different ones—no one knew exactly how many—that the pituitary secretes. It took until 1921, when one of Cushing's former students, the anatomist Herbert Evans, along with a colleague at the University of California, Berkeley, detected growth hormone in cattle. They made extracts from the front lobes of beef pituitaries and shot them into rats. The rodents grew into giants compared with their littermates—establishing that there is growth hormone secreted in the anterior of the gland's two lobes. These giant rats were proof that, with hormones, man could alter nature's plans.

Drug companies spotted potential profit. They stoked the public faith in animal hormone extracts, touting them for everything from exhaustion to senility to neuroses. Like multiple vitamins, some products offered a cocktail of ingredients: bits from thyroid, pituitary, and lymph glands, along with a dash of ovary or testis, spinal cord or brain. Pharmaceutical houses peddled these concoctions for general weakness and for "imperfect functioning," particularly sexual.

For physicians eager to mine organotherapy in order to build up a practice, the claims for pituitary extract made it seem like pure gold: the erectile dysfunction drug and amphetamine of its day, combined. Drug companies listed among the indications for which pituitary might work: "epilepsy, persistent somnolence, menstrual migraine, amenorrhea [lack of menstrual period], delay in the menarche, and impotence." A couple of London society doctors took to prescribing it to their rich patients for vague malaise.

As a brilliant neurosurgeon and true scientist, Harvey Cushing derided what he considered quackery in the newly emerging specialty of endocrinology, which had formed its first society at the end of World War I with the eager sponsorship of companies selling these organic extracts. Cushing charged that the companies lured what he termed "a credulous profession" with the temptation of "endocrine goldfields." He satirized this rush for riches as "glandward ho!" and scathingly predicted its course:

"Children are either too short or too tall, too fat or too lean. Their adolescence is too early or too late; they have too little or too much hair. They are intellectually backward or stupid, even defective or epileptic....The basal metabolism, laboriously calculated, is found to be a little low or a little high. All this needs attention and can be corrected by some whole-gland extract, usually with a pinch of thyroid thrown in." Cushing even zeroed in on the Alice in Wonderland possibilities presented by the combined potential of growth hormone and luteinizing hormone that triggers puberty: "The Lewis Carroll of today would have Alice nibble from a pituitary mushroom in her left hand and a lutein one in her right and, presto! She is any height desired." He had no idea how very prescient he was.

Doctors began to dabble in organotherapy for height. A British physician wrote in his 1927 endocrinology textbook that he'd prescribed glandular extract to a thirteen-year-old boy he thought might be hypopituitary, but then decided to wait, since the patient was short and fat but also showed signs of entering puberty. Within three months the boy "shot up, slimmed down and was captain of his school," even without benefit of medicine. This doctor had the honest insight that if he'd proceeded with treatment, he might have credited a natural growth spurt to pills: "a little uncritical organo-therapy." It was meant as a cautionary tale to other endocrinologists. And many did remain cautious, wondering if the pills might actually stunt growth.

In fact, pills neither stimulated growth nor prevented it. Herbert Evans, the Californian credited with discovering the growth hormone (GH) that Cushing theorized, also firmly established that, as a protein, it is broken down by the digestive tract just like meat and other proteins. That fact struck a blow to anyone considering pills for height. Growth hormone has to be injected.

Evans continued to refine GH from cows and, with University of California colleague Choh Li, in 1944 isolated and purified enough bovine growth hormone for experiments on humans. But while laboratory scientists could inject rats, bulldogs, and dachshunds—and grow giant rats, bulldogs, and dachshunds—clinical practitioners had no luck accelerating growth in children thought to be hypopituitary dwarfs. Since there are different causes and hundreds of types of dwarfism, doctors speculated that perhaps not all these patients actually were "hypopits," as endocrinologists casually called them. Or the extract wasn't pure. Or perhaps they just hadn't hit upon the correct dosage of hormone. Occasionally, a doctor thought the shots might be having an effect, and wrote up the treatment as promising—but not convincing. Why didn't it work?

A DWARFED CHILD GROWS!

In the laboratory, scientists isolated GH from a Noah's ark of species—pigs, sheep, oxen, whales—in their search for understanding the pituitary. They described it as the master gland, since it controls most of the body's endocrine functions, including reproduction and metabolism as well as maturation and growth. Each press report of their research achievements brought the scientists letters begging for help for dwarfed youngsters, as well as pleas from adults, mostly men, dissatisfied with their height.

One of these laboratory scientists was a chemist at Yale University who made the wire services when he isolated GH from oxen. His name was Alfred Wilhelmi, and he would go on to play a central role in the history of treating short children. But in the late 1940s, when he wrote to his fellow chemist and competitor Choh Li, he sounded mostly amused at the requests he was forced to field from short men:

"A short time ago there was a news story on this work," Wilhelmi wrote to Li in Berkeley. "It is now at the mercy of all the nation's re-write men, and some rather odd versions of it have come back to me in clippings.... One of the consequences has been that we have been getting about two letters a day from people who wish to grow taller. I have been sending numerous private little lessons in the physiology of human growth in order to discourage these hopefuls. It is a very odd experience." Wilhelmi explained to his unhappy adult correspondents that hormone could not add an inch to height once the growth plates close.

But even in children, who had room to grow, bovine hormone did nothing, and Wilhelmi was one of those who finally showed why. Unlike insulin or cortisone, which can be taken from pigs and used in people, growth hormone turned out to be species specific. This contradicted a long-held medical belief that all hormones are interchangeable between mammals. It came as a shock that what makes a piglet or a calf or a lamb grow does not help a boy or girl. Wilhelmi's experiments demonstrated that human growth hormone did not work in rats; bovine growth hormone, which did work in rats, did not work in fish. That explained why studies found no changes in the growth rate in pituitary dwarfs given animal growth hormone preparation, even over long periods.

But anxious families still brought their short kids, especially sons, to the pediatrician for help. In the early 1950s, doctors treated short boys with anabolic steroids, which include synthetic testosterone. In large enough doses, this shoved boys into puberty, virilized them, and sparked their pubertal growth spurts so they would get taller faster. But the pills could also speed them *through* puberty—and, in the same way that estrogens advanced everything at once in the tall girls including bone age, testosterone could prematurely close the epiphyses in short boys. Adolescent height might be gained at the expense of ultimate adult height. The same thing happened with short girls, to whom doctors gave small doses of estrogens to stimulate growth, trying to achieve the opposite effect they aimed for with massive doses in tall girls. They tried thyroid preparations in some patients, which only benefited those children whose thyroids were, in fact, malfunctioning. Big doses of thyroid made children grow but also rapidly advanced bone age. Sometimes, hoping to achieve a balance between accelerating growth velocity and sacrificing final adult height, they tried several treatments at once.

Their lack of success, and disappointment, became evident at the First International Symposium on Growth Hormone in 1954, when a scientist wrote: "Growth hormone, to date, has shown discouragingly little clinical promise.... The limits of our yardsticks must be heeded."

But it was not a matter of lowering expectations. It was a matter of finding closer relatives than cows or pigs or sheep. In the late 1950s, pharmaceutical companies using rhesus monkey kidneys while developing vaccines for polio collected and donated the animals' pituitaries for research. This turned out to be a rare opportunity for Maurice S. Raben, a physician and laboratory scientist on the staff of the New England Medical Center and Tufts University in Boston, where he'd developed unique methods for extracting and purifying pituitary hormones. Raben experimented with a preparation of the monkey GH; injected, it made another monkey grow, showing that the problem in trying to stimulate growth in primates had been the use of hormone from cows and pigs. Monkey GH would stimulate human growth as well.

Yet from the small simian glands, Raben eked out just precious amounts. It was exciting work, but farming monkeys for human use was obviously impractical. Across the country, Li—perhaps gazing out upon the vast Pacific—at one point imagined that he might be able to modify whale GH to more closely resemble the protein in people, noting that one whale pituitary produces more than fifty times as much growth hormone as a human gland. The solution, however, lay not in the ocean but in the morgue.

In 1958, Raben made a historic report. He'd extracted growth hormone out of pituitary glands removed from human cadavers, and used it on a child. Before Raben's experiment, the seventeen-year-old boy was only about 4'2" tall, showed no signs of puberty, and had gained less than an inch in the previous year and a half, far less than he should have. Because of these symptoms, Raben diagnosed him with pituitary dwarfism.

The July 1958 issue of the *Journal of Endocrinology and Metabolism* contained a paper from Lawson Wilkins, the country's preeminent pediatric endocrinologist, describing his failure to see any effects in young patients who took various bovine GH preparations for years. Just one month later, the same journal published Raben's short letter describing how he had injected human growth hormone, or hGH, into the teenage boy, at first twice and then three times a week. The boy grew at five times his previous rate, even slightly faster than a normal child, and gained 2.1 inches over ten months. Raben's achievement represented miracle making almost on the order of insulin and cortisone; he may not have saved a life, but he had made a human dwarf grow.

Having established that hGH therapy worked, Raben helped doctors eager to try it out on children who needed it. Those who knew Raben described him as a gentleman. He was "a smart and quiet man who seemed to know almost everything," in the words of a colleague, yet allowed other people to finish expressing their opinions before he spoke up to explain his own. Raben sent his precious primate GH to other investigators instead of making them wait for him to publish his method for preparing it, a generosity that the colleague noted was characteristic. In those days, unlike later, physicians did not seek to patent their discoveries.

In the years following his publication, Raben collected thousands of human pituitaries that were gathered during autopsies from around the country. He stored them in acetone—more commonly used as nail polish remover—until, a few days each spring, when he turned his laboratory into a processing factory. On those days the pungent odor of the harsh acid he used, not to mention the potentially explosive fumes of the ether, filled surrounding laboratories, and drove scientific neighbors out of the building. He sent the laboriously extracted hGH to endocrinologists for experimental use in kids with hypopituitary dwarfism.

Raben didn't need to speculate that doctors also might now be able to make other very short children grow as well, just as bovine growth hormone could transform normal rats into giants. Families were perfectly able to make that leap themselves, as were other doctors. A textbook in the 1950s noted that endocrinologists had experienced "a radical change in attitude" since the discoveries of cortisone and thyroid hormone and no longer limited themselves to using endocrine treatments only for demonstrable deficiencies but "freely in a great number of diseases." As with estrogens, diseases didn't always go in search of cures. Sometimes cures went in search of diseases.

Except there was not enough cure to go around, even for the few thousand children—no one really knew how many—who might have severe growth hormone deficiency in the United States. It took one human pituitary gland, extracted, pulverized, and processed, to produce enough hGH for one day's treatment for one young patient. According to Raben's pioneering experiment, a hypopituitary child would require shots at least three times a week, and for years, to achieve normal height. To spur the growth of a single boy or girl, doctors had to collect not dozens but hundreds, even thousands, of glands. They needed lots and lots of cadavers.

THE WORLD'S FIRST PITUITARY BANK

Across the country in California, Choh Li also was processing human growth hormone. His work required cadavers, too.

Unlike Raben, Li was not a medical doctor; he was a chemist who focused on molecules rather than patients. Li needed bountiful harvests of pituitaries so that he could decipher the chemical structure of hGH. Once he understood the basic building blocks, he hoped to make a synthetic version of it, just as chemists were able to synthesize estrogen, testosterone, thyroid, and other hormones. In San Francisco, Li teamed with a local clinical endocrinologist and helped organize a novel way to boost the supply of glands to his laboratory, as well as to children stunted by growth hormone deficiency.

"The world's first Pituitary Bank has been established at the University of California Medical Center, San Francisco," a press release grandly announced in 1960. Even in the inaugural press release, the clinical endocrinologist who directed the bank, Roberto Escamilla, felt compelled to explain that this "would not be an appropriate treatment for all short children." He didn't state it would not be an *effective* treatment for all short children. Nobody knew. There hadn't been enough hGH around long enough to experiment, although there was no shortage of doctors who were eager to try.

The world's first Pituitary Bank clearly wanted to publicize its need for donations without setting off a stampede of families to the University of California medical center demanding growth hormone for their short children. The press release suggested thyroid extract for those growing poorly because of inadequate thyroid function, and testosterone to stimulate growth in some boys. "And many families worry unnecessarily about children who simply are at the lower end of the normal height range," the release cautioned.

The bank would serve "normally formed midgets or near midgets" who lacked only one thing to bring them into normal height range: sufficient human growth hormone. UCSF could already brag about a few success stories. For example, an eleven-year-old girl stopped growing, then received hGH injections and shot up four and three-quarters inches her first year of treatment. Interestingly, with all its information on hGH, the press release failed to mention Maurice Raben's historic achievement, published as a letter to the *Journal of Endocrinology and Metabolism* two years earlier. Perhaps UCSF wanted the world to know that it also had been testing the treatment since 1957, and with even better results. Then again, major scientific achievements typically aren't announced in letters to the editor; some suspected Raben rushed to get to print first. This academic jockeying provided a subtle reminder that scientific glory was at stake, not just inches.

No one had higher ambitions than the brilliant chemist whose work was the reason for the Pituitary Bank's founding. Li had already distinguished himself by purifying ox growth hormone with Herbert Evans in 1944 and, even more significant, by isolating growth hormone in both monkey and human pituitary glands in 1956. Born in China, one of eleven children, Li struggled to prove himself and the value of his University of Nanking undergraduate degree when he first immigrated to the United States. The University of California, Berkeley, granted him probationary status to begin graduate work and he earned his Ph.D. there in 1938, then joined Evans's staff at a time when anti-Asian sentiment made both work and housing difficult to find.

Slim, tall (5'11"), driven, he started his professional career in a closet-size basement lab on the Berkeley campus where steam pipes threatened his research. Li's wife later described how her husband would leave bed in the middle of the night to go open the laboratory windows so that the pipes wouldn't overheat his experiments. He worked, she said, literally day and night, through lunch and sometimes dinner.

The University of California appointed Li to head its Hormone Research Laboratory in 1950, a lab that would eventually move across the bay to the medical school campus at UCSF, where it would occupy the whole floor of a building and attract scientists from all over the world. In the 1950s and 1960s, Li's career focused on the hormones of the anterior pituitary. Many speculated he was destined for a Nobel Prize. In his drive to decipher hormones, Li was interested in every pituitary. He even negotiated with the Philadelphia zoological gardens to send him sections of glands from an exotic list that included red kangaroo, black-faced chimpanzee, Bengal tiger, white-handed gibbon, monkey-eating eagle, and European badger.

But human patients with growth hormone deficiency desperately needed pituitary glands from human bodies unless someone could find a way to make hGH in the laboratory. If Li could decode the complicated structure of human growth hormone and produce a chemically identical version, hGH could be commercially produced instead of laboriously harvested. If abundant and widely available, synthetic hGH might turn out to be useful in treating everything from cancer to obesity and aging as well as height, Li suspected. In the meantime, he was willing to let doctors use a little of the cadaveric hGH he processed so they could study which groups of patients responded to the hormone therapy, and at what doses. Such information would be vital not only to treat short children, but also to obtain FDA approval for any commercial product that resulted from his hGH research.

There was tremendous public interest in making kids taller. In 1958, the physician heading UCSF's metabolic unit had been embarrassed to find his experimental treatment of a short girl with Turner syndrome transformed into a hyperbolic newspaper account. Under the headline "New 'Growth Drug' Means Hope for Girl Doomed to Lingering Death," a *San Francisco News* reporter described how the doctor used Li's growth hormone preparation to save a dying girl, quoting her father's effusive gratitude. The doctor swore he never stoked the reporter's over-the-top enthusiasm or told the girl's father her life was in danger from the chromosomal mutation that affected her height and fertility. The article also gushed that growth hormone would have the impact of "an atomic bomb" on medicine's ability to modify height, breathlessly concluding, "Hopes have risen anew for a world in which few children would be destined to be midgets, dwarfs, or even 'shorties.' "

The Pituitary Bank needed to milk this public interest. Li's work required a huge supply of fresh glands, but morticians had an unfortunate habit of embalming brains before autopsy, which made it difficult to extract any hormone to study. Plus, there weren't enough autopsies. Obtaining permission from relatives of those who died was not sufficient, since the glands by that time would not be fresh. The Pituitary Bank was designed to work like an eye bank, gathering pledges from people still living that their pituitaries were to be donated immediately upon death. That required a publicity campaign. A little drama was not out of order, if it didn't get out of hand.

Those working for the Pituitary Bank solicited pathologists throughout the ten western states, including those at public hospitals where the senile elderly died and bodies lay unclaimed. They thanked the participating pathologists with notes and parties, and proffered gifts of liquor at the holidays to the pathologists' assistants, called dieners. They courted the public with tearful stories about the children

whose lives could be transformed: a radio broadcast; a plug on network television's immensely popular *Arthur Godfrey Show*; an appeal
on local TV. They successfully prompted a Lions Club Auxiliary in
Eugene, Oregon, to appeal for donors to help the "dwarfed children"
who would otherwise live their lives as "midgets or near midgets." A
television audience was told that, ultimately, hGH might help extend
life. To other audiences, they acknowledged that the primary purpose
of the bank was to collect pituitaries for Li's research. A radio broadcast of the *University Explorer* devoted to the "Substance of Stature"
described Li's need for about ten grams of purified human growth
hormone from cadavers to determine the structure of hGH. To get
that much material, Li would need some 100,000 fresh glands. At
that point, the bank had been operating four years and had pledges for
only five hundred.

The bank was more successful with its collection drive—an
employee in fact drove hundreds of miles a year, visiting more than
forty hospitals, collecting glands from cooperative pathologists. Some
local coroners objected that it was illegal to take an organ from an
unclaimed body, leading one University of California official to joke
about body snatching. The Pituitary Bank began scrounging for glands
as far away as the Philippines and Hong Kong, Mexico and Panama,
and sought changes to clarify California law. Requests from people
who wanted growth hormone for themselves or their children or their
patients poured in from all over the world.

Demand could not be met. The bank adopted a motto: "A gland
lost is a gland wasted." A brochure for the public pleaded for contributions to help unfortunate dwarfed children, and declared that "at
present and probably for years to come, the dwarfed will outnumber
the donors." Yet even with cadaveric hGH unavailable for growth-
hormone-deficient children, a "central theme" of the Pituitary Bank,
according to its own records, was answering this question: Does
growth hormone do anything in patients who don't have growth hormone deficiency? They couldn't wait to try it.

A group of clinicians who received some purified hGH from Li experimented in 1959 on another girl with Turner syndrome. This patient produced plenty of her own hGH, but they gave her more, and her growth rate accelerated. They tried it in a boy with achondro-plasia, a genetic form of dwarfism characterized by shortened arms and legs. At fourteen, the boy stood a little over four feet tall and was entering puberty with a normal head size but disproportionate limbs. They didn't think it would help his condition, but they couldn't deny the boy's desperate and influential father, who had helped launch the Pituitary Bank. As expected, the injections proved unsuccessful.

Like the tall girls who endured humiliating examinations, the children and adolescents who were the subjects of these experiments repeatedly stood naked against a grid to be photographed, as was the practice of the time. Only their eyes were disguised by a blank strip to protect their privacy when their photos later were published in a medical journal.

One of these early subjects was a child who was just very short. Beginning in the early 1960s, UCSF doctors used Li's hGH to treat a boy diagnosed with a condition endocrinologists saw frequently—familial short stature. These were kids who inherited their height from their families. Kids who, like the tall girls, were normal but not average. Like the tall girls, these patients often had parents who harbored memo-ries of painful adolescences. Short mothers and fathers begged that their children be spared some of their own embarrassments and frustrations. So it was with great interest that the doctors took some of Li's precious purified hormone and gave one healthy but very short boy injections for ten years, sometimes as often as five times a week, during which he went from below the third to the fiftieth percentile in height for his age. He also went through his pubertal growth spurt, complicating interpre-tation of the result. But the researchers concluded with satisfaction that "his final height has been influenced by the administered treatment." Elsewhere too, from England to New England, physicians experimented with making short, normal kids taller. A boy here, a boy there.

"When you have a new drug or technology, you want to see what else you can do with it," explained Robert Blizzard, a pediatric endocrinologist who started his career in 1957, just in time to see what else you could do with human growth hormone.

THE NATIONAL PITUITARY AGENCY IS BORN

Bob Blizzard—who would later develop a shock of snowy white hair befitting his last name—grew up in a small town in southern Illinois where he had a sickly childhood and fond memories of the country doctor across the street who frequently came to see him. Blizzard "never wanted to do anything besides medicine," although at one point after serving in the Army during World War II and then graduating from Northwestern University Medical School, he thought he'd go to Montana, working as a pediatrician for half the year and fishing for the rest. But while starting his residency in Iowa in the early 1950s, an era when medicine was increasingly specializing and subspecializing, the doctor in charge urged him to find some special hobby within pediatrics that might interest him. Blizzard went to Baltimore to train at Johns Hopkins with Lawson Wilkins. At the time, there were about twenty pediatric endocrinologists in the entire United States, drawn to this pioneering branch of medicine.

From the start, Blizzard liked to experiment. While training with Wilkins, he saw children brought to Johns Hopkins because they were shorter than the third percentile or taller than the ninety-seventh when compared with others of the same age and sex. Doctors defined the bottom three percent as having short stature, and the top as having tall stature. Kids with short stature might simply be late bloomers, for which the medical diagnosis was constitutional delay. They might have primordial dwarfism—a catchall term used at the time to cover the many presumably genetic varieties of dwarfism, often involving physical abnormalities beyond height. Or they might have pituitary dwarfism, meaning they were growth hormone deficient. This was rarely inherited. Such children typically were normal size at birth but began to lag on the growth charts between ages one and four, and by adulthood grew only to four or a little over four and a half feet tall.

Examining short kids, doctors couldn't prove growth hormone deficiency: they had no way to measure GH in a person's body. But children who lacked it sometimes exhibited telltale features, unusual facial proportions or body fat distribution. They also usually looked much younger than their ages, though so did children who were constitutionally delayed. There was judgment and guesswork involved.

While in training in 1955, Blizzard examined a girl from Florida whom he thought was hypopituitary. In California, Li had just extracted growth hormone in his lab and sent some to Lawson Wilkins to try out on patients. Blizzard hospitalized the Florida girl for three months, with her mother staying overnight beside her, and tracked the effect of his injections on the child's metabolism, taking her blood and urine samples into the lab himself. Blizzard likes to say with a grin that this was "the first patient treated with growth hormone." Then comes the delayed punch line: "*bovine* growth hormone." She didn't grow. As it turned out, the girl was not deficient but resistant to the GH her body already made; she had a condition that would later be called Laron dwarfism. Even the human growth hormone that became available a few years after this experiment would not have made her taller, because her body couldn't use it. Blizzard believes this may have been the first documented case of growth hormone resistance but he didn't realize it at the time because, in a phrase that is a favorite of his, "one is a series of nothing." His patient stayed in touch, and let him know that although she stood below four and a half feet even as an adult, she eventually married a 6'2" Army sergeant and they had a normal child.

When Maurice Raben's historic letter appeared, Blizzard was one of those doctors eager to try human growth hormone in patients. While Li supplied it to a few internists and endocrinologists on the West Coast, there were two sources on the East Coast: Raben in Boston and Alfred Wilhelmi, who had moved from Yale to Emory University in Atlanta. Both scientists were willing to extract hGH if doctors could get them the pituitaries and if they could retain a third or so for their own research. Li, Raben, and Wilhelmi each had his own extraction method, developed while working with cattle, pigs, and rats.

To supply Wilhelmi with glands to process, Blizzard established a few small pituitary collection programs in hospitals in Ohio and Louisiana, enlisting parents of growth-hormone-deficient children to knock on the doors of pathologists and explain the situation: to treat just one child required 365 pituitaries a year. He managed to collect one to two thousand glands annually this way. "We were giving the pathologists two dollars [per gland] for the services rendered in collecting, storing and shipping the pituitaries," and to provide "a little encouragement," Blizzard recalled. Then he watched as other pediatric endocrinologists, "mostly newcomers, decided that they were going to do the same. And how were they going to get established? Well, they gave three dollars per pituitary." Individual parents also made arrangements to procure hGH for their children. A black market sprang up. Competition for pituitaries on the East Coast, in the words of another doctor, was "tooth and nail."

In a letter to the pathologist at an Ohio hospital, a mother testified to Blizzard's gratifying results. Her daughter Sandra had grown three and a half inches in the one year since treatment began "and hopes to reach five feet. She is now 4'3½" tall and is seventeen years old, in the last year of high school. We want to thank the doctors." But she also pleaded with the hospital to continue supplying pituitaries to physicians like Blizzard, "for they are in great need of them to carry on this wonderful work." A pathologist who answered her letter assured her they would collect glands for the group at Johns Hopkins, where Blizzard had joined the faculty after teaching for several years at Ohio State University. This, the pathologist wrote, was an "example of how doctors can work to benefit patients directly without government interference."

But the federal government was just what the doctor ordered. In 1962, representatives of the National Institutes of Health (NIH) came to Blizzard and said they would like to establish and fund a national collection program. Alfred Wilhelmi helped launch this effort. As part of the Endocrine Study Group at the National Institute of Arthritis and Metabolic Diseases, Wilhelmi was admired for the work he'd already done with GH from a variety of species. A former Rhodes Scholar married to another highly respected scientist (he wore sweaters she had handknit to the lab), he had already supplied the institute as well as Blizzard with some hGH. Like Li, Wilhelmi required pituitaries for his own research into various hormones, and hoped a national effort might convince morticians not to embalm bodies before autopsy. An early proposal for the national collection project noted that Wilhelmi's numerous contributions to the field need hardly be listed. But he was a chemist, not a medical doctor, and therefore not ideal to lead a program that would involve human patients. Blizzard had top credentials as a pediatric endocrinologist and experience organizing a collection project, plus the personal ability to pull people together. He is a man who makes lifelong relationships not just with patients but also with colleagues. Blizzard would have to convince individuals and groups that a collaborative effort could serve everybody.

There were a lot of interests to manage: Parents, children, doctors, researchers. Scientific glory, academic careers, medical practices, commercial potential. Advancing knowledge for the future versus treating children who needed it now. All competed over an organ the size of a pea.

The National Pituitary Agency officially began in 1963 at Johns Hopkins Hospital under NIH auspices. Blizzard, at the helm, hired a pathologist as executive director, and the College of American Pathologists also sponsored the program. Blizzard promised laboratory scientists and medical clinicians alike that he would protect their interests while making sure that hGH went into the hands of those who would put it to the best use. He was clear that the best use was what he called investigative therapy. The NIH, whose mission was research, was not legally allowed to operate a treatment program. Therefore, doctors who wanted to get their hands on hGH for patients would have to design experimental protocols and win approval from the agency's medical advisory board. This meant community pediatricians and endocrinologists had to refer their patients to the specialists, mostly academic pediatric endocrinologists, who had research credentials and a chance to successfully compete for hormone from the NPA. Doctors squawked. They saw the new agency as a roadblock to getting hGH. Some pediatric endocrinologists made up studies just to obtain growth hormone for patients, not bothering to write up the so-called experiment afterward. But unlike estrogen therapy for tall girls, hGH was not available to every pediatrician and the corner general practitioner.

Li and the UCSF Pituitary Bank grumbled about this new arrangement and, for a while, Blizzard grandfathered them in. Other small collection programs, including one at the Veterans Administration hospitals, merged with the NPAs. Testy letters flew back and forth between San Francisco and Baltimore. Li and Blizzard reached a gentleman's agreement that the Pituitary Bank on the West Coast and the National Pituitary Agency in the East would not solicit the same pathologists. But the new federal program was thirsty for hormone to distribute. Certain patients received top priority. Hypopits stood first in line. Among that group, girls were required to be shorter than boys to qualify. All of them would receive hGH free of charge. In order to stretch the limited supply to cover as many patients as possible, however, boys would be taken off treatment when they reached five feet, and girls would be cut off at a height below that. The rationale was that males are taller than females. But the cutoffs reflected and enforced cultural attitudes toward height and gender: short stature was worse for a male.

Even with these restrictions, hormone shortages interrupted treatment, sometimes for months. The NPA began collecting about 18,000 glands a year. Not enough for all of the hypopits, let alone for the requests pouring in to try hGH on everything from ulcers to schizophrenia. And Wilhelmi and Li were guaranteed to receive up to 25 percent of the collected glands for their work on structure, extraction, and synthesis. The agency realized it not only needed publicity but to organize the same highly motivated parents who had been willing to knock on the coroners' doors. In an era before direct drug advertising, enlisting patients as advocates and seeking publicity were not things doctors did comfortably. (Perhaps this was especially sensitive for a specialty born out of organotherapy and "glandward ho!" enthusiasms.) The first NPA newsletter admitted that most physicians would oppose such distasteful steps. The newsletter acknowledged their concerns: publicity could make them smell like quacks, deluge them with demands from parents, raise false hopes for the many who could not be helped.

But the statistics demanded action: In a country with some 1.6 million annual deaths, there were only about 100,000 autopsies in which the brain was removed. The newsletter complained that foreign residents and interns remained "without allegiance to this Anglo-Germanic tradition" of postmortems. While the NPA would work to educate medical staff, parents could be prompted to educate the public and their local hospitals about the need for glands, as well as to raise funds. The agency attempted to get the cause of hypopituitary children written into the scripts of popular television shows with such heroic fictional physicians as Ben Casey and Dr. Kildare, but without success. To overcome the medical community's suspicion of patient groups, Blizzard promised any lay organization would be well controlled.

The parents who joined Growth Inc., which Blizzard started with some families whose children he treated, did not join up to lobby the doctors or goad the government to move faster like some of the patient activist groups that came later; they simply wanted to help physicians to help their kids. This was, after all, the era of the handsome young Dr. Kildare and the gruff but warmhearted Ben Casey, who would risk anything, including his job, to defend a patient's interests. The group, which later became the Human Growth Foundation, met in the Long Island home of a couple whose son was a hypopituitary dwarf.

Among other members in those early days were Fred and Gwen Mahler, who had four children, two being treated by Blizzard. Fred was a pilot for TWA, Gwen a former stewardess forced into early retirement by airline rules, which at the time stipulated that hostesses could not be married. Blond, loquacious, bouncing with energy, she remained active in Clipped Wings, the organization of forcibly retired TWA stewardesses like herself. Gwen Mahler worked to convince Clipped Wings chapters around the country to raise money for short children, while Fred enlisted his fellow pilots to collect and fly pituitaries back to Baltimore, where the NPA would ship them on to the extractors. During his layovers in various cities, Fred would call on a local coroner, explain and plead his case to the dieners, then fly off with pituitary glands in jars of acetone in a box in his cockpit. Even temporarily preserved in acetone, the glands were better off refrigerated. A storm that threw Mahler off course would send him into a panic that the dry ice would melt and the pituitaries be ruined.

Other parents also energetically collected glands, including Lucille and Roland Sluder. They lived on Long Island, where Roland worked as a butcher at an A&P while Lucille stayed home caring for her father and her three children. The youngest, Linda, seemed like a normal, pretty little girl, but was so small at eighteen months that Lucille dressed her in doll clothes. People frequently called Linda a little doll. A stranger passing her out in the yard even stopped and said it to the toddler's face, assuming she was too young to understand. But Linda was older than her size led people to believe and she was independent. She literally stood up for herself and insisted, "I am *not* a doll." When Lucille realized her youngest child was not growing the same way her others had, she voiced her concerns to the pediatrician, who told her not to worry. But when Linda reached five, their pediatrician agreed that the Sluders should take her to be evaluated by pediatric endocrinologists and gave the family some names at Columbia-Presbyterian Hospital in Manhattan. They made that ride, by train or bus, repeatedly for four years, until the doctors finally hospitalized Linda, performed tests, and diagnosed her with growth hormone deficiency. She was nine. It was 1965, and scientists had developed a technique to measure growth hormone in the blood. The doctors were able to tell the Sluders that their daughter was not producing enough to make her grow to normal height.

After this diagnosis, the Sluders were told about a federal program that would provide them medicine. "It was wondrous, the answer to our prayers," Lucille Sluder thought. While the office visits would continue to cost money, the hormone came courtesy of the National Pituitary Agency, free of charge, which was important to the Sluders. Not that Lucille didn't ask questions, and not that they didn't pray for guidance before agreeing to inject something into their child; they were active Methodists who had met each other at a church youth group just after Roland's prolonged service in World War II. Doctors assured the couple that growth hormone was something the body was meant to have, and that it did not produce side effects. HGH did not sound experimental. Lucille felt reassured that it was natural and also that the federal government was distributing it. That meant it was safe. She learned how to administer the shots; three times a week Linda cooperatively sat still for the injection deep into her thigh. She never complained about either the shots or about being so small. She was a happy child and other children liked her, even catered to her because of her size.

As Linda accumulated inches, Lucille threw herself into helping other families obtain the same miracle. At the growth foundation meetings she heard heart-wrenching stories of severely stunted children who might also grow normally if only enough pituitaries could be collected. There was a need. There was a cure. But the cure was lying, too often unretrieved, in the morgues. She began to phone pathologists around Long Island, where both she and Roland had also grown up, and discovered most were pleased to help once they understood the problem and the program. She'd take her container with dry ice to the hospitals and gather the little bottles the NPA distributed with instructions. The Sluders kept a refrigerator in their basement just for pituitaries. Pilots like Fred Mahler would stop by to empty out the fridge.

While the pituitaries mostly went to Raben and Wilhelmi, there were other extractors, including Li (at the beginning) and later Brij Saxena at Cornell University, who slightly modified Raben's method.

They would pool the glands in large batches, grind them in a blender or pulverize them in a mincer, and dry them into powder which could be reconstituted to shoot into patients. They were like chefs who each had a slightly different way of cooking the same dish. They stuck to the methods they'd developed while working with animal pituitaries. Their preparations were crude, but they worked. The FDA agreed to regard pituitary hGH as an investigational new drug and to allow NIH to vouch for its safety and efficacy. The NPA would provide information on its processing and report any undue responses. The public, hearing dramatic pleas on behalf of dwarfed children, might have assumed this was a treatment program. But since the NPA described its goal as research, that relieved it of the kind of scrutiny, inspection, and regulation that the FDA performs for other biologic products like blood.

Wilhelmi and especially Raben, who was extolled as an indefatigable "national resource" who was "synonymous with hGH," also enjoyed international reputations. They answered requests from doctors on several continents, and exported the miracle abroad when asked, if sent pituitaries and allowed to keep a small portion of the hGH they extracted for their own research. (Li, on the other hand, had the reputation of hating to part with an ounce that he might use in his quest to decipher the molecular structure, although he did regularly send a little to a doctor in Paris who had pleaded for some to treat his grandson.) A patient in Brazil gratefully received Raben's product. A New Zealand pediatrician shipped glands to Atlanta, where Wilhelmi mixed them with an American batch, then processed and shipped some of the hGH to Auckland. When other countries, including England and Australia, established their own pituitary programs, they followed the recipes for extraction cooked up by either Wilhelmi or Raben. Even more than their preparations, they exported their methods.

CANNIBALS AND SLOW VIRUSES

These were heady times for pediatric endocrinologists. After decades of frustration, they could finally make hypopits grow. There was no reason to take notice of two coincidences in the year that was so auspicious for them, 1963.

The same year that the National Pituitary Agency officially got off the ground under the auspices of the National Institute of Arthritis and Metabolic Diseases, a different institute within the vast organization that is the NIH called for the world's first conference on slow viruses. When he later won a Nobel Prize, Daniel Carleton Gajdusek, the NIH pediatrician and virologist who meticulously described this unique group of illnesses, recounted how a district medical officer in New Guinea introduced him to the Fore people, thinking he would be interested in the odd neurological symptoms of a disease that afflicted many members of the tribe. Gajdusek lived among the South Fore, observing their customs. Later, he found that some of the tribal members' brains, at autopsy, showed a pattern of holes where neural cells had died.

Gajdusek eventually linked the disease, which the Fore called *kuru*, to their practice of cannibalism, a funeral ritual in which they ate the brains of their close relatives to honor them. Years passed and some of those who engaged in the practice began trembling, jerking, stumbling, and dying. The Fore blamed *kuru* on evil sorcerers, but Gajdusek suspected the brains they ate were somehow infectious, although he couldn't find evidence of a specific bacterial or viral agent. Along with others scientists, he eventually determined that *kuru* belonged to a group of neurological illnesses that could be transmitted but which could incubate for decades without symptoms. Hence the name: slow viruses.

By the time the conference took place on the Bethesda, Maryland, campus of the NIH, researchers suspected dozens of human and animal illnesses might be slow virus diseases characterized by the same pattern of destruction that led to their being grouped together as spongiform encephalopathies—infectious conditions that eat spongy holes in the brain. The list included scrapie, which afflicted only sheep, and Creutzfeldt-Jakob disease (CJD), which occurred sporadically in about one in a million people, striking in old age and inevitably killing its victim. Neurologists, who specialize in diseases of the brain and nervous system, rarely saw a case of CJD during the course of a career, although it had first been described in the 1920s. The condition's ungainly name derived from those of the two German doctors who independently reported it. Because it appeared only rarely and in the elderly, no one within the small community of pediatric endocrinologists was likely to have heard of Creutzfeldt-Jakob disease. Pediatric endocrinologists still had no particular reason to notice in 1968 when Gajdusek reported in the journal *Science* that he was able to take the brain material from a human CJD patient and infect a chimpanzee, or in 1969 when he showed CJD could be transmitted from one chimp to another. These dreadful diseases, it turned out, could arise spontaneously *and* also be transmissible. Gajdusek had spread the deadly CJD from one brain to another by injection.

The second coincidental event in 1963 was a paper published in a European medical journal coauthored by a Swedish biochemist named Paul Roos, describing his method for purifying pituitaries. He advocated running the hormone through a long glass column containing a gel filter that sorted out the proteins by size. Ultimately all that was left was a single protein, hGH. Roos used this method on frozen glands and ended up with a preparation much purer than Wilhelmi's and Raben's. But in the United States the NPA found frozen glands messy to deal with and expensive in terms of time and effort. Early shipments got lost and then arrived thawed or partially thawed, wasted, after all that strenuous effort to collect them.

Among the extractors, Li liked to work with frozen pituitaries, but he didn't send back much hGH to the program. Raben believed he could even eke some hormone out of embalmed pituitaries, but he mostly advocated for those preserved in acetone, which "simplified the collection of glands" since they could last for months refrigerated. After pulverizing them, Raben wrote, treating the pituitary powder "with acetone, ether, and hot glacial acetic acid provided strong bactericidal and viricidal action." He concluded that this "made the final product well suited for clinical use," although he also assumed it was "chemically impure," meaning it probably contained other substances along with hGH.

Since Raben wanted to spend less of his time processing pituitaries, Wilhelmi agreed to do more. He used an alkali (rather than acid) method on the acetone-dried glands, but also avoided gel filtration except for small laboratory studies. Roos's process was laborious, especially with large batches, and Wilhelmi asserted it would lead to low yields if applied to acetone-dried glands. The NPA wanted to squeeze out every drop of hGH it could, and remained focused on the urgent need to refine the collecting rather than the processing of pituitaries. The preparations that Wilhelmi, Raben, and others using their methods churned out of their labs worked. Growth hormone was natural. It made kids grow. It was not making them sick.

There was one sign, more bothersome than worrisome: some patients developed antibodies, which meant their immune systems were trying to fight off hGH as if it were an invading bacteria or virus, and a few of these children even stopped growing. It was surprising that people developed antibodies to a substance they were meant to produce. Physicians treating these children wondered if they might also have been made immune to whatever small amount of growth hormone their bodies secreted—that they had essentially been inoculated against their own GH—and would end up shorter than if no one had intervened. At least half a dozen clinics in the middle and late 1960s reported antibodies in patients who started to respond to hormone therapy and then stopped, especially children treated with hGH from Raben's lab. But some people given insulin or other hormones also developed antibodies. Perhaps certain kids were just more susceptible to antibody production. Still, doctors questioned whether the processing method was at least partly responsible; by contrast, it was rare for patients to develop antibodies after being treated with Roos's preparation, which had been adopted by commercial companies supplying Scandinavia.

In 1969, Alfred Wilhelmi, who processed glands for the NPA in his Emory University lab and was the linchpin of the federal growth hormone program, coauthored a paper describing a refinement in his method. He noted some of the antibody reports. He acknowledged that his preparation was only about 70 percent pure, and that the remainder probably included various proteins from the neural tissue that was often still attached to the glands before pulverization. He described a way to make a purer product, including the column filtration step that the Swede Roos had described six years earlier. But Wilhelmi and colleagues concluded that thoroughly refined hGH should be reserved only for the laboratory, for chemical and immunological studies where purity was essential. On the other hand, the impure hGH, which Wilhelmi termed "clinical grade," should remain the standard for use in patients, because it yielded more medicine from fewer glands. By "clinical grade" he meant the human growth hormone being injected for years at a time into the arms of such children as the Mahler siblings, Linda Sluder, a New Zealand girl named Debbie MacKenzie, and—a few years later, in a small town in South Dakota—a toddler named Tony Grossenburg.

CHAPTER 5

"no patient seems to have caught anything"

A BOY THEY WANT TO HELP

John Anthony Grossenburg came into the world full-term and healthy on June 26, 1970, in South Dakota. But he weighed only five pounds. From the start, his mother, Patsy, remembers, he didn't eat well "and he was just so little." The Grossenburgs are not tall. Patsy stands 5'3"; her husband, Mick, who is 5'8", recalls several aunts who never reached five feet. Still, their first child's slow inching on the growth chart concerned them. They questioned their family doctor, but he assured them everything was fine and advised them not to worry.

During his first year, Tony didn't crawl. "His head was big. If he tipped over he couldn't pick himself up," Patsy recounted. In his second year, he walked, but Patsy knew he didn't resemble other toddlers: "You could tell by looking at this little guy that he wasn't growing normally. People would stare, 'cause here was this little guy walking." His knobby knees appeared huge on his skinny legs, which didn't seem as if they would support him. He slipped a lot, but Patsy couldn't find shoes small enough to fit him. Patsy's mother sewed him clothes from patterns meant for dolls. The family lived in Winner, a town with a population of less than 4,000 that had earned its name by capturing a coveted place along the railroad line in the heart of South Dakota farming and cattle country. When Tony was twenty months old, the Grossenburgs drove him to see a doctor in a somewhat larger town. There, the pediatrician suggested another, longer, trip, to the world-famous Mayo Clinic.

Rochester, Minnesota, where the Mayo Clinic is located, is a ten-and-a-half-hour drive from Winner, and the family would get to know the highways well. In 1972, a young pediatric endocrinologist at Mayo examined John Anthony Grossenburg, who, at two years old, was 28½ inches tall, almost six inches less than average, and weighed only fifteen pounds, which was just about off the chart. They stimulated his growth hormone secretion by giving him insulin, then measured how much GH his body produced. A Mayo doctor wrote to the referring pediatrician that tests showed John Anthony was normal, meaning not growth hormone deficient, but below the third percentile in height, with a significantly retarded bone age, and noted that he'd been small for gestational age. Their impression was that he had intrauterine growth retardation: he had failed to grow normally in the womb for some unknown reason. Most such children catch up in the first few years, but some never do. The pediatric endocrinologist recommended a therapeutic trial with human growth hormone. He would apply to the National Pituitary Agency as part of an investigation into whether low-birth-weight children responded to hGH. What Patsy Grossenburg remembered hearing about her son was that "probably his pituitary gland isn't functioning normally" and if they gave him hGH, he would grow.

The family lived across the street from a medical clinic in Winner, and the nurse there gave Tony a shot in the buttocks with a long needle three times a week. Once in a while, when they took Tony up to a cabin they owned in the Black Hills, Mick gave his son the injections, but he found this difficult. The toddler seemed to respond, gaining two and a half inches in the first six months. Then the Mayo Clinic told them that because of the NPA's scarce supply of pituitaries, there was not enough hormone to continue uninterrupted. "They'd treat him, see if he grew, then reapply each time" for another half-year's supply of hormone, according to Patsy. But each time, Tony seemed to respond less. He grew only one and a half inches with the second six-month series of shots. The Grossenburgs wondered whether hGH was making a difference. Still, as Tony went on and off therapy four times over ten years, they never questioned that it was worth trying. "You think: Will he ever be able to sit in a regular chair at a table; will he ever be able to drive a car; will he ever be able to reach the buttons in an elevator? You want to help him."

As two younger boys came along, Patsy realized she babied Tony more than the others, lifted him into the car although she let his brothers climb in on their own. She felt protective. He was an intense, sensitive child who relished books. In elementary school, the girls wanted to hold him on their laps and he loved it, but it bothered the teacher, who thought he'd be better off being treated like everyone else his age. By middle school, things got tougher. In South Dakota every boy is expected to suit up for sports. A man who grew up in the state, former national television news anchor Tom Brokaw, once compared the hoopla of South Dakota high school team wins and losses to "what the native Sioux used to call the Winter Count, the big events represented by symbols painted onto a tanned buffalo hide." As for the town of Winner, its most famous resident to date probably remains Frank Leahy, the championship-winning football coach of Notre Dame in the 1940s and early fifties. In middle school, Tony Grossenburg remained tiny and uncoordinated. He had a bad complexion, and his mother's voice still sounds pained when she recalls his unattractiveness to girls during adolescence. He got along very well with adults, was outgoing and compassionate, and served as an altar boy at the Catholic church.

For almost ten years, the Mayo Clinic pediatric endocrinologist treating Tony Grossenburg remained enthusiastic and repeatedly applied to the NPA for growth hormone. "He wanted to be very aggressive," Patsy remembered. Her impression was that the treatments were "kind of like research" and "kind of like trial and error," but she pushed the doctor to do as much as possible for her son, and "he was, 'Go for it, let's try it, we might do wonderful things here.'" They'd drive to Minnesota, or sometimes have to hire a private plane and pilot, so Tony could be measured, X-rayed, and examined two or three times a year. "They would always check his bone age, spread-eagle and photograph him. They'd pull his penis up and measure it." The hormone was free, but the travel was "a hardship." Patsy Grossenburg kept meticulous files, including the cards recording the doctor's findings and recommendations from each visit—all thirty of them. As Tony's growth tapered off, the endocrinologist did not offer any explanation to her, other than the scarcity of hGH that interfered with treatment. "He just seemed to think if we got enough of it, it would have made him grow. And I remember calling him and pushing, asking what more we could do." When growth hormone was unavailable, the physician prescribed a brand of oxandrolone. The Grossenburgs understood that was a hormone, but not exactly what it did. It's a synthetic form of testosterone and spurs growth and sexual development, although it can also advance bone age. They trusted the Mayo Clinic. No other family they knew had a child whose growth was severely delayed, and the Mayo Clinic saw the rarest cases of everything, from all over the world. Overall, Tony enjoyed the attention, the sense that he was special, and even looked forward to the adventure of his trips to what he thought of as the "big city."

One trip remains especially memorable. The Grossenburgs arrived at the clinic and were greeted by a nurse who told them the young doctor they saw there had died unexpectedly. The older and eminent pediatric endocrinologist who met with them immediately took a more conservative approach. Particularly, Patsy recalled that he cautioned: "We've got to be careful. We don't want to do more harm than good."

Tony hit puberty early, but didn't experience the large growth spurt that usually accompanies it, especially in boys. When X-rays showed his epiphyses had closed, the physicians at Mayo Clinic stopped prescribing hGH. He was only about twelve. From what he understood of their explanation, his body made enough growth hormone but could not make use of it. He was a smart, outgoing, healthy young man who was going to remain only five feet tall. His parents were left to wonder whether the years of treatment had helped. They thought the shots probably made him grow more than he might have otherwise, but there was no way to know. Their other sons were below average height, but within the normal range. The Grossenburgs reassured Tony over and over that height didn't matter, that what counts is on the inside. Entering high school in Winner, he didn't believe them.

PITUITARY PROCESSING GRINDS ON

For children like Tony Grossenburg, the 1970s began with optimism. In January 1971, the University of California dramatically announced that Li and his associates had synthesized hGH for the first time. It had taken thirty-two years, dating back to the days when Li first had to prove himself as an immigrant and a scientist in a less-than-welcoming adopted land. The triumphant news, along with Li's photo, appeared in *The New York Times*. Congratulatory letters poured into San Francisco from all over the world—from Asian academics taking special satisfaction in his achievements, from friends and colleagues, from short men harboring erroneous fantasies they might still grow, from the Long Island chapter of the Human Growth Foundation thanking him for his contributions to humanity.

The university's press release recognized what scientists had known since the days of Cushing and Evans: that the term "growth hormone" is, in a way, a misnomer; that hGH is involved in many different vital functions and does much more than regulate growth. Therefore, the press office waxed as enthusiastic as some of the organotherapists of an earlier era: "Using the new synthetic hGH the answers may now be found as to why we grow to a certain height and then stop; what goes wrong with those who grow abnormally short or tall; why certain cells become runaway cancer cells; why some people maintain a normal weight and others are abnormally thin or fat; and many other heretofore unsolved questions." It raised the possibility that growth hormone could prevent obesity in people who eat too much, as it appeared to do when injected into rats who gorged. On this topic, the release coyly added: "Dr. Li is reluctant to speculate, but other scientists are optimistic in their opinions concerning possible human application."

It looked as if the shortage that had deprived growth-hormone-deficient children of many inches of height might soon end, as doctors had hoped for ever since UCSF's announcement, in 1967, that Choh Li had deciphered the structure of hGH. Just unlocking the structure represented an impressive accomplishment. As UCSF pointed out—human growth hormone was "the largest and most complex hormonal molecule that has yielded to chemical analysis," with close to two hundred amino acids, which are the building blocks of proteins. By comparison, the pituitary hormone that Li had synthesized in 1960 adrenocorticotropic hormone (ACTH), contained thirty-nine amino acids, and he'd had to reproduce only nineteen of them to make it biologically active. Li himself likened the difference in size between the two molecules, and the two problems, to the difference between exploring a cottage and exploring a mansion.

Now Li claimed not only to have figured out the blueprint but to have rebuilt the mansion from scratch. However, his initial report contained a mystery. The synthetic hormone created in Li's laboratory should have worked the same way as the purified hormone extracted from pituitaries, yet it appeared to be only 5 to 10 percent as active. Almost immediately after Li's announced success, a researcher at Harvard's Massachusetts General Hospital pounced on a pair of errors in sequencing the amino acids. He published his correction of Li's work within months. The UCSF lab had made a small mistake, missing two additional amino acids. But this represented a huge embarrassment to Li, who resented the implication that he'd been too quick to jump to conclusions and to claim credit. One science magazine described Li as "highly annoyed" with being corrected in print. He testily responded to his Harvard challenger—a lowly assistant professor of medicine—that he already knew about the error and had worked out a revision, charging that it was his critic who precipitously went public.

Academic squabbling aside, the fact remained that Li had not successfully replicated growth hormone for use in humans. He had made a groundbreaking contribution in isolating hGH and deciphering most of the human growth hormone molecule, but he would not be the one to synthesize it so it could be widely distributed. Though he would continue to explore other hormones and win prestigious awards, Li would die without capturing the Nobel Prize that many thought he deserved. Meanwhile, the world still needed to go about the frustrating and messy business of collecting pituitaries and rationing the use of growth hormone.

Each of the pituitary programs around the world established its own rules regarding who could receive hGH and for how long. Canada's supplies allowed treatment for six months of the year. In the United Kingdom, where children spent a year on and then a year off the shots, the official goal remained to boost kids with short stature to their full "genetic potential," including an experimental program to treat children who were not growth hormone deficient. But given the scarcity of the supply, the British program deemed it a reasonable compromise to get their patients to what program officials termed "socially acceptable height," and which they designated as the tenth to twenty-fifth percentile. The United States program began with eight months of treatment a year and a height cap of only five feet, then, as supplies increased through collection efforts to allow year-round treatment, raised the limit to 5'4" in girls and 5'6" in boys. Children with hypopituitary dwarfism got priority, but even in that group doctors measured their success solely in inches. Although growth hormone plays a role in so many body systems, the single goal of treatment was height.

While the world's growth experts anticipated the day when hGH might be abundant rather than rationed, a pediatric endocrinologist named Salvatore Raiti breathed a sigh of relief when Li's triumph turned out to be temporary. In 1970, the U.S. program recruited Raiti, an Australian working in England, as its new director. Blizzard and the NPA had found it difficult to convince someone to take the administrative job, which was an academic dead-end at a time when pediatric endocrinology was establishing itself as a subspecialty in medical schools, on faculties, and at university hospitals. Blizzard had generously but reluctantly stepped back to the helm of the NPA after the resignation of one administrator and the death of another, but he really wanted to focus on his full-time academic career as a clinical researcher and teacher. Meanwhile, Salvatore Raiti eagerly hoped to return to the United States, where he had done some training at Johns Hopkins with Lawson Wilkins. While waiting for his visa, Raiti heard about Li's synthesis and imagined his new job evaporating even before he started.

Instead, Raiti got to take over the NPA operation, with a joint appointment at the University of Maryland, and a goal to increase the supply of hormone. "The challenge was to get more pituitaries. Everyone was fighting for it," he recalled. Raiti inherited the program's three processors—Raben, Wilhelmi, and Saxena—though by this time Wilhelmi produced the most and held a special status. Raben was involved with other areas of research and no longer wanted to turn his Boston laboratory into a fume-ridden production plant. Raiti describes an "aura" that surrounded Wilhelmi, who was a basic scientist unlike the two other processors, who were both medical doctors, and who was treated by the NIH officials overseeing the pituitary program with a respect bordering on adoration. In the eyes of these public officials, as Raiti put it, Wilhelmi was *the* professor, *the* academic." On the other hand, they made it obvious they had no interest in Raiti, who ran the program, or in the day-to-day details. He met with the director of the National Institute of Digestive and Kidney Disorders just once a year and, according to Raiti, only at his own request. "He'd say once a year is fine."

The FDA didn't provide oversight, either. The FDA reviewed

commercial pituitary hGH products when several European manufacturers sought licenses to enter the U.S. market in the mid-1970s,
but not the National Pituitary Agency's hGH. As director of the federal program that sent growth hormone out to be injected into a few
thousand American children, Raiti said, "I think I went to the FDA
once. They were very kind to us." The program had no adverse incidents to report. Raiti would just write up two or three pages annually
to send to the FDA. "I'd get it back with a rubber stamp: 'Received.'
It's not that they turned a blind eye—but this was recognized as a
research effort, not commercial."

Along with these arrangements, Raiti also inherited the antibody
problem, which he downplays: "It was accepted...that up to ten percent of children would develop antibodies. It was not apparent at that
time it had anything to do with purification." In fact, some doctors
continued to publish evidence that the impurity of the program's hormone might be to blame, and to worry that the antibodies might stall
growth in some of their young patients. Studies in the early 1970s
revealed that some preparations "hardly ever cause the appearance
of antibodies, whereas others lead more often, or even regularly to
formation of antibodies." In every study, the Roos method—which
included gel filtration and which was used by the Swedish pharmaceutical firm KABI in its commercial pituitary hGH manufacture—
produced either the fewest antibodies or none at all.

In contrast, pediatric endocrinologists at the University of North
Carolina, Chapel Hill, detected antibodies in almost one-third of
thirty-seven hypopituitary children being treated there with NPA
hormone. When two patients displayed impaired growth, the doctors substituted KABI hGH. The result: "a dramatic resumption
of growth" in both children. Elsewhere, an investigator switched a
patient from a crude, cloudy Raben preparation to a clearer, more
refined Raben preparation, and reported the antibodies decreased or
disappeared.

In 1973, when Raiti oversaw a symposium on human growth hormone at the University of Maryland, UCSF pediatric endocrinologists

called for "more stringent quality control" after finding that 40 per-cent of children they treated developed antibodies to hGH. Among that group, 5 percent lost some ability to respond to the effect of the hormone shots. In fact, the most frequent cause of decreased growth rate in children receiving therapy at UCSF was the development of antibodies. These doctors, too, detected growth-inhibiting antibod-ies more frequently in patients receiving hGH prepared by Raben's or Wilhelmi's method than in those treated with Roos's method.

The possibility that injecting hGH could stunt rather than stimu-late growth in the long run particularly worried the British because of their experimental program to treat some children with short stature who were not growth hormone deficient. What if antibod-ies made these children unresponsive to their own hormone, and not just to hGH they got by injection? Treatment could cause more harm than good. The UK used processing based on Raben's and Wilhelmi's methods, and found both types of preparations impure, although the Raben type in particular seemed to interfere with growth in some patients. They concluded that this was "a strong argument against the free use of hGH in non-deficient, short patients." Therefore, they dis-continued prescribing it for children whose only diagnosis was short stature.

In 1973, the British, who were switching from the Raben method—with its harsh acid—to a refined version of Wilhelmi's, grew worried that this gentler processing might not eliminate viruses like hepatitis and meningitis. There is no documented evidence to date that pediatric endocrinologists worried about slow virus illnesses like Creutzfeldt-Jakob disease at this point, or had even heard of them.

Wilhelmi wrote to a colleague: "The question of virus in our hGH preparations has come up from time to time, especially since we use rather gentle methods in the isolation." He candidly went on: "We don't have advice or opinion from an array of experts. Our main evi-dence of the low hazard is that, in years of use of substantially more than a kilogram of clinical grade hGH, no patient seems to have caught anything."

While he emphasized that no child had gotten sick, he responded to the concern raised by a member of the steering committee of Britain's program by stating that in the United States "we are presently going to modify our procedure to include a step of filtration...and this, I think, will provide further assurance of removing virus from the system." But "presently" didn't mean right away. Gel filtration is a form of column chromatography, like Roos's slow and labor-intensive purification through tall glass columns, and Wilhelmi had resisted its use. In fact, he and coauthors had once referred to gel filtration as "tedious" in a paper that recommended his own method of producing clinical grade hGH for "simplicity" as well as for "high yield."

Not everyone remained satisfied by the argument that further processing would diminish the precious supply of growth hormone. In 1973, a South African chemist published a method for making hGH from acetone-stored glands that was 95 percent pure—using gel filtration—while almost tripling the yield. He found Wilhelmi's clinical grade not 70 percent pure, as had been claimed, but only 40 percent or 50 percent. An account of the achievement in the *Johannesburg Sunday Times* displayed the South African chemist grinning, with a jar of pituitaries in one hand and a flask of powdered hormone extract in the other. It described how he'd been motivated to make a purer product by his friendship with a pituitary dwarf.

In 1974, after a U.S. National Academy of Sciences National Research Council report recommended that the NPA processing be centralized, Wilhelmi took over the entire task from the other processors, including Raben, who died just a few years later. Wilhelmi did not change his methods, however. Whenever he was questioned about the antibody incidents, according to Raiti, Blizzard, and others, Wilhelmi responded that he could not purify the product any further without sacrificing the yield—that making it twice as pure meant serving half as many kids. Wilhelmi's word was still golden with NIH. Wilhelmi's standard answer was "he would lose a lot more hormone," Raiti recalled, "and he was the kingpin. He was God."

Pediatric endocrinologists in the United States didn't need studies to tell them the hGH they received from the national program remained impure. Instead of being nearly transparent as a purified hormone should have been, the product was the "color of Coca-Cola," remembered Wayne Moore, who was starting his medical career at the University of Kansas Medical Center. Moore felt so "offended" at the quality of the extract that he further processed the contents of each vial he used for his patients. When he was finished, it came out almost clear. He also undertook a study of the NPA product's effect in children and published his results in the *Journal of Clinical Endocrinology and Metabolism* in 1978. Moore's investigation determined that the hGH was even more contaminated than the South African chemist had discovered. It was only about 30 percent monomeric growth hormone, meaning the part uncontaminated by any other component, and this small fraction contained "most if not all of the growth promoting potential of clinical grade hGH." In other words, less than one-third of the drug being given to children did anything to boost height. Therefore, the higher yield was an illusion. "I don't think they knew. It floored me that nobody had paid attention to that. I purified the growth hormone myself and isolated the monomeric growth hormone. . . . The rest was biologically inactive," Moore said. The rest included other growth hormone molecules, damaged growth hormone, debris, or worse, unidentified protein. When Moore's paper appeared, Raiti appended a note at the end saying that even before this "excellent study," the agency had abandoned Wilhelmi's "former concept of clinical grade," and had employed a different method since December 1976.

Wilhelmi reached retirement at the end of 1976. As he prepared to leave the program, he finally agreed to use Roos-style gel filtration on one batch of frozen pituitaries in order to produce a purer hormone for those children who'd developed antibodies that interfered with their growth. By that time, the collection effort was netting six to eight times more pituitaries a year than it had at the beginning. Raiti had worked especially hard to eliminate embalmed glands, which yielded little or no hormone, and to collect frozen ones. Frozen glands proved productive for the companies KABI and Serono, which supplied hGH to some of the European pituitary programs. But frozen pituitaries required very careful processing to eliminate viruses, which can remain active even after freezing.

The scientist who succeeded Wilhelmi was Albert F. Parlow, a man obsessed both with the arcane details of extracting pituitary hormones and with doing a better job than his predecessor. Parlow won the contract for producing the NPA's growth hormone—he was the only bidder—and began in 1977. He is a crusty Princeton- and Harvard-trained physiological biochemist who collaborated with Wilhelmi at Emory University in the early 1960s. After a bitter falling out with Wilhelmi, Parlow moved to UCLA's Harbor Hospital and developed his own scientific niche: pituitary hormones in the laboratory rat. By the late 1970s, he'd spent more than a decade honing this expertise, extracting, isolating, and purifying hormones for research use from the tiny glands found in rodents. Parlow was eager to improve on Wilhelmi's methods, methods he found "very basic, fundamental, and forgive me, crude."

A grizzled eccentric in a white lab coat and a baseball cap, Parlow to this day is married to his laboratory—which he keeps locked and under camera surveillance. Parlow also remains harshly critical of Wilhelmi: "He was not skilled or versed in the technique of column chromatography. The technology that he used was the technology of the fifties. And as a person who was in his fifties, and the chairman of a department, and [who] wanted to do the human GH purification himself in a relatively small setup, it was beyond both his experience and his will to engage in this extra work involved in high purification of human pituitary GH." Basically, kids were growing. And they were not getting sick. The evident success enabled Wilhelmi to avoid changing, Parlow argued: "He rationalized that it wasn't necessary. He rationalized that it would be a loss of the precious material if it was subjected to high purification.... And because he had been such a driving force in establishing the system of collection of human pituitary glands, because he did have a large program of pituitary gland hormone purification with respect to domestic animals...he was not pushed."

There was tremendous satisfaction, even glory, involved in the work the NPA was doing on a shoestring budget, distributing the miracle drug for free, and Wilhelmi—who received multiple awards from the Endocrine Society in his lifetime—deserved much of the credit for launching the program. Some who knew and admired him believe Wilhelmi sacrificed his other work for the sake of helping these short children. Parlow, who readily admits hating him, charged that Wilhelmi got too caught up in making miracles: "He reaped an enormous amount of kudos from the fact that he produced this product which had such a dramatic effect on kids who could not otherwise grow."

Taking over in 1977, Parlow set up hundreds of glass columns in his Los Angeles lab. In each column he placed small amounts of pituitary at a time, and waited three to four days as the material dripped down and filtered through the gel sieves segregating proteins by their molecular size. He knew how to load and operate the columns, to keep the batches uniform, all from his work with rats. He and his assistants carefully washed and heated their glassware between batches to 400 to 500 degrees Fahrenheit for a good part of a day in a self-cleaning oven, scrubbing everything. The lab workers who processed glands wore caps and gowns and gloves and masks. They washed their columns between use, repacked the columns frequently, refreshed the resin periodically. Parlow's goal with human growth hormone was the same as it had been with animal pituitary hormones: "to produce the best product that was producible." Though he says he was "totally unaware" of Creutzfeldt-Jakob disease at the time, he believes this fastidious devotion also saved lives.

A HIGHLY INFECTIOUS DEMENTIA

The same year that Alfred Wilhelmi retired from processing pituitaries for the NIH, Carleton Gajdusek received a Nobel Prize for his work describing *kuru* among the Fore in New Guinea. Gajdusek's connection of cannibalism to transmissible dementia had established his NIH laboratory as the world's foremost research center on the new category of diseases being called slow viruses. In hindsight, it was as if two trains were speeding down separate tracks, unaware they were headed for the same junction. The pediatric endocrinologists rode one train; the experts in slow virus diseases rode another. It didn't do them any good at all that NIH operated the railroad.

Soon after Gajdusek and others in his lab demonstrated in 1968 that CJD could be transmitted from a human brain to a chimpanzee by injection, they found they could then transmit the disease from one infected chimp to another, even after the infectious material had been stored for several years. The material did not need to be injected into the brain. It could be delivered peripherally, which was how human patients received their shots of growth hormone, in the thigh or arm. Whatever the mysterious infectious agent causing CJD, it remained resistant to heat, formaldehyde, and ultraviolet radiation.

In 1973, this exotic area of research became personally relevant to one particular group of doctors, after a Boston neurosurgeon who developed a rare skin disease died; an autopsy revealed his brain eaten by the spongy holes characteristic of Creutzfeldt-Jakob disease. Gajdusek took some of the surgeon's brain matter and inoculated a chimpanzee and a squirrel monkey. Both developed CJD. Reporting this experiment to the Tenth World Congress of Neurology, in Barcelona, Gajdusek warned that the surgeon could have been infected by practicing medicine. At that point, however, there was no documented case of transmission of CJD from one human being to another.

The next year, Gajdusek and colleagues warned in print that, although the mode of transmission of CJD remained unknown, the evidence that brain tissue from people who had died of CJD remained highly infectious when shot into the arms of primates in his laboratory warranted precautions among doctors performing biopsies and autopsies of patients with presenile dementia. That included patients diagnosed with Alzheimer's, brain tumors, strokes, and other similar conditions—since doctors often missed CJD. The article, which appeared in the *Journal of Neurosurgery* in September 1974, noted that experiments had found high concentrations of CJD agents in the brain, but that all organs from CJD patients, no matter how they had been stored, should be considered infectious: "There is still no documented case of Creutzfeldt-Jakob disease in man caused by contact with contaminated tissues. We recommend the above precautions because of the still theoretical possibility that such an event can occur."

But the possibility had moved beyond theoretical. Infection of one human being by CJD-contaminated tissues from another human being had occurred—during eye surgery in New York City. In a four-paragraph letter to *The New England Journal of Medicine* that appeared in March 1974, Columbia University ophthalmologists reported the death of a female patient who developed CJD a year and a half after receiving a cornea transplant at age fifty-five. The cornea came from the body of a man who had died of pneumonia; later, at autopsy, he was found to harbor CJD. The letter noted this case might be the first evidence of person-to-person transmission of the terrible disease and ended with a warning that "there are wider implications to be considered in all transplantation programs." The next year, Gajdusek's laboratory published precautions in the *American Journal of Clinical Pathology* for autopsies of CJD patients.

Thus, by the mid-1970s, so much concern existed among neurologists, neurosurgeons, anesthetists, pathologists, and other medical and laboratory personnel about handling tissue potentially contaminated with CJD that some nursing homes and hospitals refused admission to patients with presenile dementia; some surgeons and anesthetists declined to perform procedures on patients they suspected of CJD; and pathologists refused to conduct some autopsies. Although the College of American Pathologists cosponsored the National Pituitary Agency, the program proceeded without apparent alarm in the United States, as did the programs in Australia, Britain, France, and everywhere else. Pediatric endocrinologists appeared unaware of any risk.

Accepting his Nobel Prize in December 1976, with a speech later published in the widely read magazine *Science*, Gajdusek made no mention of the worldwide harvest of pituitaries. He did raise other alarms: He estimated the occurrence of CJD at one per million per year in large population centers around the world. He acknowledged the corneal transplant case as possible evidence that "other tissue transplantation may also be a source of infection," and he mentioned two young Swiss epilepsy patients who had developed CJD after exposure to contaminated electrodes during a surgical procedure. In addition to the Boston neurosurgeon, two other medical doctors had died of CJD—a fact that, Gajdusek thought, "raised the question of possible occupational infection, particularly in those exposed to infected human brain tissue."

On the other hand, Gajdusek found no evidence that CJD could be transmitted by blood transfusion. Both the cornea transplant patient and the primates he'd injected with CJD had exhibited symptoms in only eighteen months. And in his list of substances that he believed inactivated unconventional viruses like CJD, he included acetone. These statements would have reassured doctors prescribing growth hormone, if any of them had reason to pay attention.

However, one scientist who did pay professional attention to slow viruses was already worried about pituitary hormone programs. A few months before Gajdusek gave his Nobel speech, a veterinary researcher in Scotland suddenly made the connection between pituitary extracts and potential CJD contamination.

The researcher was Alan Dickinson, a microbiologist and father of five children, and he lost sleep over the possibility that youngsters could be infected by their growth treatments. Around midnight on October 5, 1976, Dickinson lay awake contemplating how hGH was processed. He was an expert on scrapie, a fatal disease that had been recognized in sheep for hundreds of years. Theories over the centuries about how it struck its animal victims had associated scrapie with everything from lightning to loose ovine sexual habits—before it was recognized as one of the spongiform encephalopathies like *kuru* and

CJD in man. For some reason, Dickinson began thinking about the growth hormone shots given to kids that he'd heard about in 1961 when he worked briefly in California.

There were two issues: collecting and processing. Even if pathologists avoided harvesting pituitaries from those who died of CJD, what about those who died of other causes—who harbored the long-incubating disease but had not yet developed its symptoms? *Kuru*, for example, could remain undetected for decades. It seemed likely that at least some of the pituitaries being collected, especially since many came from senile elderly patients whose cadavers lay unclaimed, could carry undiagnosed CJD. Dickinson had infected mice with scrapie in his laboratory and found, in unpublished experiments, that their pituitaries became infectious, though less so than the brains.

The second question that kept Dickinson awake was this: If processors ground up one diseased gland in the pooled batches from which they derived growth hormone, would CJD survive? Dickinson knew the scrapie agent remained impervious to methods that killed other known viruses or bacteria. He'd tried to kill it with temperatures above boiling, intense gamma radiation, strong chemicals, and burial underground for years. It occurred to him that night in his bed on a farm outside Edinburgh that whatever infectious agent caused CJD might not be eliminated in hormone processing. It might even be concentrated by some methods. He sat up in bed with the realization. The next morning, he phoned the British Medical Research Council, which administered the growth hormone program in the United Kingdom.

The Medical Research Council, without any obvious sense of urgency, suggested Dickinson look into procedures at the two laboratories producing hGH for their program. Speaking to the processor at one lab, which used a refined version of Wilhelmi's purification method on acetone preserved glands, Dickinson cautioned that she and her staff needed to take care to avoid infecting themselves. Ironically, Dickinson expressed more concern about the method being used at the second laboratory: column filtration of fresh glands. He feared the columns might concentrate the infectious agent, and that there could be cross-contamination between batches if the strictest sterilization procedures were not followed.

About four months later, on February 22, 1977, Dickinson put his concerns down on paper, writing the council a careful letter. He suggested they test their processing on scrapie-infected mouse brains, that they assess the likelihood they were collecting glands that might contain CJD, and that they exclude glands from dementia patients. The program steering committee duly noted receiving this communication as well as the fact that, to date, no patient appeared to have gotten CJD from human growth hormone. The committee agreed, however, that the matter should be investigated further. They contacted two virologists in the UK for advice; both agreed the risk was real, though extremely small, and advised that the processing should be tested using laboratory animals as Dickinson had suggested. Both thought the pituitary program should proceed throughout the testing. The council decided the matter should be explored quietly, without alarming the public, or even alerting the pediatric endocrinologists who prescribed hGH to children.

A few days after Dickinson wrote the committee, the British medical journal *The Lancet* published a letter from Swiss neurologists reporting on the two epilepsy patients who had died of Creutzfeldt-Jakob disease after undergoing a procedure to measure electrical activity in their brains. The same electrodes had been used to probe the brain of a CJD patient, then sterilized with benzene, ethanol, and formaldehyde, and reused for testing the two epileptics. Their deaths represented the second and third documented cases of person-to-person transmission.

The British committee that Dickinson had challenged to investigate whether hGH might kill the children it helped make taller changed neither collection nor extraction practices. One of the virologists the committee had consulted noted that cadaveric hGH not only represented a low chance of transmitting CJD but might soon become unnecessary. A new technology, recombinant DNA or gene splicing, promised to make possible an unlimited supply of synthetic human growth hormone in the foreseeable future.

Dickinson later told an interviewer that he thought they were gambling. "The treatment was immensely satisfying, you see…because you're not dealing with a condition which is life-threatening, you're dealing with something which enormously modifies the quality of life. Immensely satisfying, and against that you set this nebulous inconceivable entity, Creutzfeldt-Jakob disease, and the name is even difficult to pronounce, and who are these people at this animal research institute raising a fuss? What a joke. Please." He agreed to perform the mouse experiments, although he could not begin right away. Once started, the tests could take years to produce results because of the long incubation time in the animals he would inject. There was no other way to test for the infectious agent.

Meanwhile, in 1978, someone associated with the Medical Research Council wrote to Gajdusek's laboratory at the NIH inquiring about the possibility that pituitary glands might be infected with CJD. Gajdusek was traveling. Colin Masters, an Australian researcher temporarily working in the lab, answered the inquiry and agreed that CJD might, indeed, be present in pituitaries and the tissue surrounding them, and that glands should not be collected from patients with dementia. The British sent Masters their purification protocols for the NIH to review. Asked decades later why he hadn't followed up on those protocols or, apparently, brought the question to the attention of anyone else at the NIH, Masters reportedly responded that he assumed the Americans already understood the potential risk: "Presumably the people who were running the pituitary programs should have been aware of the warnings that were being sounded in the medical press."

In Scotland, Dickinson went about his veterinary research still contemplating the growth hormone treatments he'd first learned about in California. He worried that the Americans and others running such programs had not been alerted to the issues he'd raised, according to an interview he gave Australian journalist Jennifer Cooke for her excellent book *Cannibals, Cows & the CJD Catastrophe*. The doctors who ran such programs around the world formed a small community. In 1980, Dickinson met the newly appointed chairman of Britain's National Health Services hGH committee and asked him whether this international community had been told yet about the CJD risk. Dickinson received a "blank look" in response, as he described it to Cooke, and so he went on:

" 'Just in case it hasn't happened,' Dickinson said, 'I think you ought to think about this issue and if necessary make sure that you have a quiet word, if this is the way to do it, with people using hGH.' " That year, 1980, Dickinson finally began his experiments into whether or not CJD survived the purification procedures adopted from the Americans and used by the British.

Meanwhile, children in England, Australia, New Zealand, France, the United States, and elsewhere dutifully took their medicine. Who wouldn't want to be taller if they could?

MAKING SHORT KIDS GROW

Among children like Tony Grossenburg, who fell below the third percentile in height and were labeled with short stature, tests found less than 1 percent were growth hormone deficient. Eighty percent were short with no known organic cause, a group that endocrinologists termed as having normal variant short stature or constitutional short stature. It was a basket diagnosis: kids small for no known reason, probably for a variety of different reasons, lumped into the same diagnostic bin. Their parents brought them to the doctors all the time. The tantalizing question remained: Would these short, normal kids also respond to growth hormone. If so, which ones?

At a Baltimore symposium in 1973, doctors presented what they had learned in the fifteen years since Raben's first successful treatment with cadaveric hGH, and what they still wished they knew. They'd found that growth hormone was part of a very complex chain of events involving other hormones—insulin, androgens, cortisol, and thyroid among them. They also had discovered that, potent as growth hormone is in determining height, there are other powerful factors in the body that either stimulate or inhibit the release of hGH. They hoped that two of these—growth hormone–releasing factor and what they would later called insulinlike growth factor—might someday be used to treat those children who did not respond to growth hormone shots or whose bodies did not respond to their own normal levels of GH. Endocrinologists didn't yet know how many factors there were, what they did, or how they could be used for treatment, nor did they fully understand the adolescent growth spurt. Because this system was proving much more complicated than they had anticipated, they had tempered some of their earlier great expectations that every child "with a statural deficit," as one doctor put it, might be made to grow with hGH alone.

But how to identify those they already knew could be made to grow with hGH? They still lacked a good test to sort out kids with growth hormone deficiency from those who were simply short or late bloomers, and they wondered whether there could be such a thing as partial deficiency. Measuring hGH levels in the blood did not suffice, because so many variables—from obesity to fasting to thyroid function to the stage of puberty to the stage of sleep to whether or not a child had just exercised—could affect the hormone's release. There were even rare children who grew poorly until removed from a deprived or abusive home. Once hospitalized, their growth hormone levels normalized spectacularly; their diagnosis was psychosocial dwarfism. On the other hand, even normal youngsters frequently had low or undetectable levels after fasting. And obese kids remained especially tricky to diagnose.

Pediatric endocrinologists would put their small patients through a variety of stimulation tests before measuring their GH levels. As a first step in the screening, children might be given glucose or estrogens. Their hormone levels might be measured while sleeping, or after strenuous exercise like bicycling or climbing stairs. If still suspicious, the physicians would progress to a more definitive and often more uncomfortable test. The most effective involved administering insulin, which induced hypoglycemia, or low blood sugar, and stimulated GH. This test was also dangerous; hypoglycemia can cause seizures, comas, and death. Other substances, like l-dopa and arginine, either failed to offer clear-cut results or provoked nausea or vomiting. Doctors chose their own combination of methods. Some liked to give the kids Bovril, a pungent British beef tea, which appeared to stimulate GH secretion. But most found they couldn't get even British youngsters who had seen and smelled Bovril before to drink it, let alone Americans. Other tests did not gain wide use because hospitals did not have the nursing staff to monitor children as they slept or exercised.

The main problem, however, remained that even the definitive tests weren't very definitive. Different tests produced different results in the same child. Therefore, the standard developed: a diagnosis of growth hormone deficiency should be made only if a patient failed at least two of the so-called definitive tests.

Even among the clearest cases of hypopituitarism, once treatment started, patients responded in varying ways for reasons doctors didn't fully understand. Most patients grew less in the second six months of therapy than in the first six months, and less in the third six months than in the second. Shorter, younger, and lighter-weight children seemed to react best. In some, bone age advanced faster than height. In others, it was the other way around.

Monitoring bone age, pediatric endocrinologists knew, was crucial. If diagnosis resembled an educated guessing game, treatment resembled a sophisticated balancing act. To catch up to peers, a hypopituitary child needed to grow not just more rapidly but more rapidly than normal kids, without unduly advancing the closure of the epiphyses, which could prematurely end growth. Some doctors at the Baltimore symposium wondered out loud how to judge when treatment was successful. One of the more conservative suggested that the only response that justified the possible risks and prolonged medical care even in growth-hormone-deficient patients would be at least a doubling of their growth rate.

When it came to short, normal kids, the equations became even more complicated. Would dosing them with hGH create antibodies that might interfere with the action of their own hormone, or cause other long-term, as-yet-unknown effects? John Crawford reported that he'd conducted an experiment at Massachusetts General on about forty short children with no evident hGH deficiency to see if doctors could boost their growth. He obtained unexciting results: "Only irregularly was acceleration of statural growth seen and to so small a degree as to be of little long-term practical importance to the child." Yet Crawford—the self-proclaimed radical who prescribed estrogen to hundreds of tall girls—remained optimistic about hGH treatment for a whole host of short kids, based on how it accelerated the growth rate in a few patients with constitutional short stature, Turner syndrome, and low birth weight, as well as the evidence nature itself provided that too much hGH made people gigantic. Crawford looked forward to the day of "unlimited supply" not just of hGH but other growth factors as well, so that "clinicians may be in a position to bring relief to many more short children than can be helped today." He was not alone. Another experimenter reported he had improved the growth rate in almost every type of patient given growth hormone, including those with familial short stature.

Only one speaker present at the symposium talked at all about the reasons why doctors treated short stature, whatever its cause: the psychosocial life of patients. He was John Money, a pediatric psychologist at Johns Hopkins University who worked with sexual and gender problems in endocrine and other patients. Money cautioned the physicians not to neglect the psychosocial side of their patients' lives, since he argued it would be absurd to spend hundreds of dollars on improving their bodies otherwise. The real difficulty that hypopituitary dwarfs faced was not height, it was the fact they looked child-like. Even when growth hormone therapy made them taller, they still suffered in adolescence, "for they do not reach the height that they would expect in their secret dreams." Yet Money said he had seen adult men who were five feet tall survive without too much stigma if they looked like sexually mature males. He urged families and doctors to treat youngsters according to their chronological ages, rather than according to how immature they looked. Not to keep them behind in school. Not to infantilize or juvenilize them. And to educate them about sex.

Then Money launched into a discussion about homosexuality and "erotic disabilities" that he believed were caused by a combination of prenatal hormones in the womb and the sense of identity children developed after birth. Money delivered the underlying message that extremely short men might be at special risk of becoming homosexual and that doctors could play a role in preventing this. "One of the most important things that we can do as professional people—and which we don't do very well yet—is to provide some kind of a social service that makes it easily possible for people with short stature to find one another, so that romance can bloom in its ordinary and normal way." To pediatric endocrinologists, it must have sounded more like a call for matchmaking than medicine, and out of their realm.

RACISM, SEXISM—HEIGHTISM

As long as pituitary human growth hormone remained scarce, doctors did not debate whether or not their goals were psychosocial, medical, or cosmetic. For the most part, they replaced a hormone in those who lacked it, just as they gave insulin to diabetics. Either that, or they advanced scientific knowledge by giving hGH experimentally. But even in the pituitary era and among those with hypopituitary dwarfism, endocrinologists measured medical success in inches. Increases in height are easier to calculate than gains in happiness, social acceptance, or life chances. Medicine assumed, as society did, that taller was better—at least if you were male. Though the prevalence of growth hormone deficiency was equal in both sexes, two-thirds of those brought to growth clinics by their parents were boys.

The few psychological studies of growth-hormone-deficient children, some conducted by John Money, seemed to confirm the belief

that extremely short stature put children at risk for profound problems: social isolation, infantilism, negative self-concepts, distorted
body image, difficulty in displaying aggression, feelings of incom-
petence, and deep disturbances in identity formation. Since growth
hormone deficiency is so rare, however, these studies based their conclusions on handfuls of patients, some of them with multiple hormone
deficiencies, and others whose hypopituitarism resulted from treatment for life-threatening medical conditions like cancer. The research
lumped different types of patients together and asked them questions
with psychiatric tests that had been developed to detect significant
mental illness. When the Human Growth Foundation held a symposium in Galveston, Texas, in 1979, to summarize what was known
about the social adjustment of kids with short stature, the answer
was: Not much. Basically, those who assumed such children suffered
psychologically looked for pervasive problems and found them; the
studies reflected the assumptions and biases of the researchers. Short
children whose parents did not worry about them, after all, didn't get
brought to growth clinics in the first place.

Yet even among studies that found hypopituitary dwarfism a psychological liability, the shortest stature didn't automatically condemn
a child to either a miserable adjustment or a personality disorder. One
such investigation of two dozen hypopits detected a host of "profound
psychological problems" yet also concluded that "hypopituitary children do not always have significant development problems. Several
children studied have done relatively well in mastering the emotional
tasks of development. These children came from families [that] made
conscious efforts to foster the children's sense of competence." Parenting could make a difference.

The idea that being short led to personality disorders derived
from the Freudian theory that body image is central to adjustment
and personality development. When adults did not make this adjustment successfully, they developed an inferiority complex, according
to the work that the Austrian psychoanalyst Alfred Adler did in the
1920s, which was widely popularized in the United States during the

1950s. A tall girl developed an inferiority complex because she felt unfeminine. A diminutive man had difficulty thinking of himself as powerful. His size made him defensive. Trying to compensate for his lack of stature, he could become a tyrant with a Napoleon complex— another of Adler's oft-cited concepts. As a character in Pat Conroy's 1976 novel *The Great Santini* put it, more crudely:

> Give me a guy less than five feet eight, Johnson, and I'll give you a real bastard nine times out of ten. It has been my experience that short men get a chip on their shoulder as big as an aircraft carrier. They're just pissed off at life and God and everybody else just because they're midgets.

Even if shortness did not inevitably lead to psychological disability, everyone knew it represented a social disadvantage, though the scientific evidence for this, too, remained slim and largely anecdotal. The seventies being a decade of isms and identity-based liberation movements, it was only natural for a sociologist in 1971 to coin a term for discrimination based on stature: "heightism." Even the English language seemed to embed this bias, with expressions like "short end of the stick," "shortchange," "shortsighted."

The classic U.S. study associating height with social status was published in 1968, when a psychologist divided his undergraduates into five groups and then presented the same man as a visitor to each group separately. Each time, he introduced the visitor with a different academic rank—ranging from student to lecturer and up the academic ladder to full professor. Afterward, the psychologist asked his undergrads to estimate the man's height. The higher the undergraduates believed the visitor's academic status to be, the taller they assumed he was.

Ms. magazine ran an article by Leonard H. Gross that summed up the plight of the short male, titled "Short, Dark, and Almost Handsome." Gross didn't disclose his adult height in the article (though the magazine published a picture of him at his bar mitzvah with a girl who stood a head taller), but he did describe the no-win situation for a male of below-average stature. He grew up knowing he could never breach the 5'7" or 5'8" barrier to become a firefighter or a cop, jobs that served as symbols of becoming a real man. Short boys could act accommodating and be labeled as "sissies," or act tough and be accused of trying to compensate for their lack of height. Short men had trouble being taken seriously; if they insisted on making their presence felt, people labeled them little Napoleons.

Worst of all, even though the feminist movement knocked down height restrictions that had been used to bar women as well as short men from some occupations, and even though women's liberation aggressively challenged traditional notions of machismo, nothing dented the preference among females for a taller mate. They'd give up on the dark and handsome long before they'd compromise on the tall. In his article, Gross called on women to make a feminist cause out of the plight of men who did not measure up, and to consider dating a shorter man. "The convention of every man having his little woman perpetuates male superiority in that the woman of the couple is symbolically more childlike," he argued. But this particular barricade did not come tumbling down.

Studies confirmed that women found taller men more attractive. This preference seemed so universal across time and national boundaries that one social psychologist called it "the cardinal principle of date selection." Some speculated it was a natural law, since males are taller than females in the human species.

Those looking for proof that nature invented heightism could point to the fact that while male and female monkeys, which live in trees, are equal size, male ground-dwelling great apes like the gorilla are taller and twice as heavy as females. Perhaps when human ancestors climbed down from the leafy branches, the females obeyed Darwin's theory of sexual selection and looked around for the males who could offer the most physical protection out in the open. Like peahens who choose to mate only with those peacocks exhibiting the longest, most glorious tails, a prehistoric grandmother would have chosen a taller male in order to pass tall genes on to her offspring. This also helped assure that her sons would be desirable, so they would pass her genes along to future generations. According to other theories, when early humans roamed as hunter-gatherers a man may have preferred a shorter woman because she required less food, or because she sexually matured sooner, as short females tend to do.

But thousands of years later, why did the male-taller rule still hold? Looking to evolutionary psychology, Finnish professor Marjaana Lindeman argued that height might once have signaled a man's "physical power, maturity, and dominance" and communicated his ability to provide for a family. Lindeman described the lingering preference for tall men as an irrational evolutionary leftover, just as useless as the fact that the hair on our arms still bristles when we're afraid, though it has been at least tens of thousands of years since our bristles scared off an attacker. But other experts speculated that heightism remained about domination. For example, a 1954 study by psychiatrist Hugo Beigel quoted a 6'1" male subject who said that his ideal mate would be a 5'3" female because he wanted her "to be dependent on me at all times."

Whatever its origin, the notion that a man should be taller than a woman he wants to date remained widely accepted by both sexes even as other once fixed ideas about male-female relationships were challenged. More men began doing dishes. Some even stayed home to tend babies while wives became primary breadwinners. Yet assumptions about height and the sexes resisted change. In 1966, two sociologists conducting a study of dating attractiveness assigned University of Minnesota freshmen dates by computer completely at random. Or almost. If the computer assigned a man to a woman taller than he was, researchers removed her IBM card and placed it back into the deck. It was inconceivable to them that a taller woman would go out with a shorter man.

These stubborn stereotypes suddenly received more than academic attention in 1977 when Randy Newman—a songwriter who enjoys making people laugh at bigotry with his outrageous lyrics, and who happens to be tall—released "Short People." He seemed to be rubbing salt in the psychic wounds. Short people "got no reason to live," went one lyric. "Short people got nobody to love," another teased. "They got little noses / And tiny little teeth / They wear platform shoes / On their nasty little feet..." Newman insisted that he was poking fun at the bigoted narrator in the song. The catchy tune played everywhere, becoming the No. 2 single in the country in December 1977. Some short people failed to see the humor.

In fact, they decided not to take it anymore and protested, charging that Newman picked on them because they represented the last discriminated-against group that someone could safely satirize. They complained they'd been picked on all their lives: called "shrimp," "shorty," and "midget" even by friends, who expected them to be good sports and laugh. They had been dumped into trash cans and pummeled at school, rejected for dates, and passed over for jobs. Their angry reactions caused some radio stations to ban the song; a 5'5" state legislator in Maryland introduced a bill to restrict it from being played in his state; *The Washington Post* published a photo of short people throwing eggs at the album; three songs parodying tall people boomeranged onto the airwaves. In the face of all this strong emotion, the popular press asked just how much discrimination people below average height actually faced, especially in the job market.

A flurry of articles concluded that height did affect both hiring and salaries. The articles relied heavily on two pieces of informal academic research:

A 1968 survey of one hundred graduates of the University of Pittsburgh Graduate School of Business discovered that their starting salaries rose with each additional inch of height, from $701 a month for the graduate most below six feet tall, to $788 a month for someone who hit 6'2".

As for getting hired in the first place, a marketing professor at Eastern Michigan University showed visiting corporate recruiters two candidates with equal qualifications for a sales job—one 6'1" and the other 5'5". He reported that 72 percent chose the taller candidate. On the other hand, when explaining his conclusions, the marketing professor revealed more possible factors at work than height alone, including gender and ethnic stereotypes, not to mention sales techniques.

"Some people think that the blond Teutonic giant that comes hulking into your office is more intimidating and therefore a better salesman," he was quoted telling U.S. News & World Report.

Conducting a survey of heightism in the job market for an article titled "Short People—Are They Being Discriminated Against?" U.S. News & World Report answered its own question. Yes. People of less-than-average height—men shorter than 5'9" (175.2 cm) and women below about 5'3½" (161.3 cm)—had faced bias "at one time or another in their working lives." The examples included a 5'4" male doctor who described struggling to be taken seriously in medical school and a man who had been turned down as a department store manager in Abilene because he was 5'6". Failing in his attempt at merchandising, the Texan turned to politics, eventually becoming a five-term mayor of Houston. But in politics, too, the taller candidate seemed to hold the advantage—winning 80 percent of presidential elections between 1904 and 1980.

These tales of disadvantage came from men who, unlike growth-hormone-deficient children, were normal height. They just weren't average. They didn't only want to be taller; they wanted to be tall. In fact, most American men wanted to be above six feet, preferably 6'2". Not every boy could hope to reach that perfect height, however. Not unless...

In the late 1970s, the FDA approved commercial pituitary growth hormone for use in this country, produced and marketed by two European companies, KABI and Serono. More parents might obtain prescriptions for their children. Still, the day had not yet arrived when hGH would be available to anyone who wanted it. Not quite.

Then the decade that began with Choh Li's overoptimistic announcement that synthetic hGH was almost at hand ended in 1979 with a press release from a small south San Francisco company, Genentech. Scientists there announced they had spliced the gene for human growth hormone into bacteria, and they had made the bacteria churn out human growth hormone. This time, the promise of a future unlimited supply of human growth hormone was true. The 1980s would see a new era in the history of treating children for height.

CHAPTER 6

"soon. very soon..."

AN INDUSTRY LAUNCHED

If 1958, when Maurice Raben announced he'd made a child grow, is the most important year in the story of treating height, the runner-up might be 1980. On October 14, Wall Street exploded with enthusiasm for Genentech's initial public offering. By the end of that first trading day, stock in the world's first true genetic engineering company had more than doubled its opening price, making history for an IPO by raising more than $38.5 million in hours. It also launched a new industry: biotechnology. As investors bet millions on gene splicing, Genentech began to stake its future on human growth hormone, the stuff that went to only a couple of thousand U.S. patients a year.

At the National Pituitary Agency, director Salvatore Raiti saw his program threatened, and argued the country didn't need more growth hormone. The NPA was supplying about sixteen hundred U.S. patients with free pituitary hGH. Raiti told reporters there was no waiting list, that all children who met the NPA's guidelines already received treatment. As supplies had increased, so had the five-foot height caps: boys got hormone until they reached 5'7", and girls 5'3". A little below average, but well within normal.

Only another four hundred or so patients bought cadaveric hormone from either Serono or KABI, the European companies licensed to enter the U.S. market for hypopituitary dwarfism. In spite of colorful ads and brochures, commercial manufacturers had found it difficult to turn up customers. Their products cost about $5,000 to $10,000 a year for a therapy that might last ten years or more, and they also faced opposition from pediatric endocrinologists. Bob Blizzard—who thought he had put an end to the competition for pituitary glands back in the black market days of the early 1960s—had prodded the Lawson Wilkins Pediatric Endocrine Society to condemn KABI's harvesting from bodies in American morgues. Defenders of the federal program argued that its growth hormone represented a bargain at $1.2 million annually, a cost of only about $500 per patient. Still, observers speculated that, in a country philosophically disposed to market-driven health care, eventually industry would pressure the government to step aside and let the commerce really begin.

HOW GENENTECH MADE GROWTH ITS BUSINESS

Genentech entered the growth hormone business almost by accident. When the scientist Herbert Boyer and the entrepreneur Robert Swanson cofounded Genentech in 1976, they thought they might apply recombinant DNA techniques to biological, agricultural, or even industrial uses, but they didn't know which ones. Boyer, a molecular biologist at UCSF, had codiscovered the process that allowed scientists to cut and paste parts of the genetic code of one organism into the code of another. Boyer also happened to have a son below average on the growth chart who had been hospitalized overnight and tested for growth hormone deficiency. The boy's levels measured normal, but through that experience Boyer learned that doctors gave pituitary hGH to some children—and rationed a limited supply. He said later that he'd filed away the idea recombinant DNA technology might some day expand the hormone's availability.

Robert Swanson, a businessman with venture capital experience, dreamed that Genentech would develop its own product, not just perform specialized research for larger corporations. He was a shorter-than-average man with bolder-than-average plans, willing to stride into the arena with the giant multinationals, the old established drug companies known as Big Pharma. Genentech was still a tiny start-up in a converted warehouse when Swanson tried to figure out what flagship product it could make, manufacture, and market on its own. This was both a business and a scientific question.

Hitting the road to find investors, Swanson liked to demonstrate Boyer's recombinant DNA technique with pop beads, using a child's plastic necklace. He'd break the circle of beads, pop in a new bead as if it were a gene borrowed from a different organism, snap the circle closed, and stuff the whole thing into a box representing the bacterium *E. coli*. It was a matter of picking the right pop bead, a gene that scientists could manipulate into bacteria that would respond to the new genetic instructions by churning out a protein.

Genentech successfully developed recombinant insulin in 1978 for Eli Lilly Company, to replace the need for relying on animals. Insulin worked as a pop bead, but not as a Genentech product; serving the world's vast number of diabetics who required daily doses represented much too large a production and marketing challenge, and Eli Lilly already dominated the worldwide market.

Swanson was raiding academic labs for some of the best and the brightest postdoctoral students at a time when government research funding dwindled. He lured them to work in the industrial city of South San Francisco, conveniently located between UCSF and Stanford, where he promised they could race for scientific glory and develop new products at the same time, while earning more money than in academia. Possibly much more, depending on how many races they won.

Wearing jeans and playing pranks on each other like college kids, the young scientists worked into the nights and through weekends, as *Star Trek* episodes blasted through the public address system, and quarter pitching contests congested the hallways. As the soaring stock value turned some of these share-owning young scientists into paper millionaires, Swanson joked that their games escalated from staking quarters to dollars. As for Swanson's worth, *Esquire* magazine described him as "not a very big man unless he's standing on his wallet."

One of the postdocs plucked from UCSF, a German scientist named Peter Seeburg, brought along test tubes of material from the university laboratory where he'd worked with two professors to develop recombinant human growth hormone. His professors had already filed a patent for biosynthetic hGH, and UCSF protested that the university hadn't given its former student permission to remove the test tubes. Seeburg countered that it was routine for postdocs to take the material they were working on, but Genentech quietly paid the University of California to settle the dispute. The two professors each got a share of the payment. Academic biologists typically pursued science for its intellectual and career rewards. Some of those who'd criticized Herbert Boyer for jumping over the wall into industry were surprised by how much money could be made in this genetic revolution.

Genentech established a team to explore whether or not hGH might be the right pop bead, while other teams investigated other possibilities. Surprisingly, hGH, which had dangled so tantalizingly out of reach for Choh Li to synthesize chemically, turned out to be not that difficult to synthesize biologically. The growth hormone gene proved even easier than the insulin gene to manipulate into bacteria successfully. Genentech's announcement that it had made recombinant hGH just beat out UCSF's.

To help finance its growth hormone project, Genentech struck a deal similar to the agreement with Lilly for insulin, but with KABI, the Swedish company that supplied most of the world's commercial pituitary hGH. KABI would retain worldwide market rights while Genentech undertook the research. State-owned, but for-profit, KABI almost hadn't gone into the growth hormone field because the market was so tiny and the pituitary collection process so difficult. But the Swedish government stepped in on behalf of the fifty or so

Swedish patients who needed treatment, and the company had found cadaveric hGH surprisingly profitable. Genetic engineering offered KABI the possibility that its scientists would no longer have to scour morgues the world over for 200,000 pituitaries a year, and the company believed it could sell as much as could be produced.

Genentech soon suspected it had found not only the right pop bead but also its flagship product. In 1980, it renegotiated its agreement, reclaiming rights to produce and market recombinant hGH in the United States. KABI could sell it everywhere else. Besides being doable scientifically, human growth hormone offered advantages as a trial run for a company that dreamed of producing pharmaceuticals. Though small, the market was already established. A sales effort would need to reach a community of only a few hundred pediatric endocrinologists, a physician audience, as marketers liked to put it, based mostly at major medical centers. So Genentech would not be competing with giants like Merck and Lilly, which had lengthy relationships with the country's hundreds of thousands of doctors. Perhaps most important, a lot was known about the natural form of human growth hormone, which meant shorter clinical trials and might ease regulatory passage. Swanson confidently predicted FDA approval in 1982 for biosynthetic hGH, which the company called Protropin.

The FDA requires a safety test before large-scale human clinical trials, so Genentech looked down the highway to Raymond Hintz, a pediatric endocrinologist at nearby Stanford University. Ray Hintz was an experienced researcher, bearded and avuncular—a man who obviously liked both a good joke and a good meal. He enjoyed pediatric endocrinology, with its mixture of treating "skinny kids, fat kids, short kids, tall kids," and was building his career in academic medicine. He'd never been asked to conduct such preliminary trials before, the kind that drug companies usually conduct themselves, and he realized that Genentech was a brand-new type of company, just "beyond garage stage."

In early 1981, Hintz lined up a handful of Genentech employees for shots. True, they were adults, but as he put it, "adults are just big pediatric patients." These guinea pigs included some of the company's top scientists and managers, but not Robert Swanson, who said he didn't like needles. Since this was a controlled study, Hintz randomly chose half of them to get pituitary hGH and half to get recombinant hGH. By day four, half the group suffered from fevers, chills, and headaches, and generally felt crummy. Everyone knew the pituitary hGH was impure. They grumbled: How could the NPA give this stuff to kids? But it was Genentech's Protropin, not pituitary hGH, that was making them sick. The bacteria had produced endotoxins that processing did not eliminate. It would take Genentech at least another six months to fine-tune its purification process before the company could move on to the next stage of human trials—to test whether or not biosynthetic hGH worked.

Though Protropin was purer than cadaver-derived hormone, it was not exactly like nature's. Protropin had 192 amino acids, rather than the 191 in pituitary hGH, an unanticipated result of the method Genentech scientists had used to trick bacteria into making human hormone. No one knew whether the extra amino acid, methionone, made any difference, especially whether it would cause immunological reactions in patients. This would take longer than Robert Swanson thought.

In 1983, Genentech figured out how to make hGH without the extra amino acid, so-called met-less hGH, but the company didn't want to delay the regulatory process further by starting the clinical trial process over. They would push ahead to get FDA approval for Protropin. Meanwhile, Swanson posed for photos in front of the manufacturing vats.

Having none of the production experience of the pharmaceutical giants, Genentech worked out its manufacturing problems on a small scale. Contamination sometimes forced them to fumigate the room by heating paraformaldehyde in a frying pan on a hot plate and then to evacuate the facility. Later, they worked in a cold room that was approximately two hundred square feet, where their basic equipment consisted of a mechanic's tool kit and some off-the-shelf air compressors. They eventually increased their yield of recombinant hGH one hundredfold. Swanson was quoted as telling his experts, "I want this safe enough to inject my baby daughter." Nobody had ever made a 99 percent pure protein on the scale they were attempting, and they knew the stakes. As a company researcher later wrote, they were well aware in those pioneering days that "even a very small mistake could lead to disillusionment among the investors and others who were following the fledgling biotech industry."

Finally, Genentech started trials in children to test whether or not its biosynthetic hGH worked. It boosted growth, but the children developed more antibodies to Protropin than they did to pituitary hGH. In September 1984, an FDA advisory committee asked Genentech for an additional year's worth of information on more kids. They wanted to make sure biosynthetic growth hormone proved as safe and effective as nature's own.

ANYONE WHO WANTS IT?

"Soon. Very soon..." promised a dramatic Genentech ad that ran over three pages in leading pediatric journals in 1984. "The new era in human growth hormone."

Pediatric endocrinologists knew biosynthetic hGH was on the horizon; they didn't need the ad to tell them that a new era loomed in which there would be enough to treat anyone in the world who wanted and could afford it. They expected Protropin to be both profitable and heavily promoted. They expected it to be misused and abused, too, based on the increasing underground market in commercial pituitary hGH, which adult bodybuilders took to add muscle mass and others hoped would forestall or reverse aging.

Though Genentech sought FDA approval of Protropin for the treatment of hypopituitary dwarfism, physicians frequently and legally prescribe drugs for unapproved or off-label uses, as they had with DES and the tall girls. Pediatric endocrinologists in the 1980s diagnosed only about 10 percent of the very shortest children, those two or more standard deviations below average, with growth hormone deficiency—the name they increasingly preferred to call the condition because parents recoiled when their children were labeled with "dwarfism." (The word "dwarf," one growth expert complained, had "a curiously sinister and magical sound in the ears of parents and patients." He advocated diagnosing all those in the bottom percentiles as having "short stature" instead.) Pediatric endocrinologists desperately needed to decide whether they would prescribe hGH for what they began to refer to as idiopathic short stature, meaning short stature of unknown cause.

As Genentech geared up to manufacture Protropin pending FDA approval, the National Pituitary Agency's stock of hormone from cadavers had become sufficient to essentially do away with height caps and to treat growth-hormone-deficient kids without interruption. Adding its 2,450 recipients and those enrolled in the Canadian national program, plus the families who bought the hormone commercially, there were about 3,000 North American patients. The minuscule market suited Genentech strategically as a starting point. A drug company could spare itself or postpone the additional large clinical trials required by the FDA if doctors believed that the pharmaceutical could safely and effectively be used for other conditions and prescribed it off-label. Clinical trials are expensive. And all drugs have some adverse effects. "The trick of marketing is to grow the market as large as possible without recruiting patients who will suffer toxic side effects that may endanger the product for everyone," explained Cynthia Robbins-Roth, a Genentech scientist who later became an industry analyst, writing in her book for investors. "A great clinical development strategy is one that allows a company to move quickly into a small market, then expand into related patient populations with follow-up studies."

Genentech officials candidly discussed their hopes for growing the market beyond growth hormone deficiency. The future, company vice president Gary Steele told a reporter in the fall of 1984, would be "little Johnny who is in the lowest percentile and is unhappy." Little Johnny could be short because his parents and grandparents were short, or he could even be temporarily short because he was maturing slowly and would sprout up in high school or in college, after years of jealously looking up to his friends.

Having already sunk some $15 to $24 million into biosynthetic hGH even before FDA approval, and anticipating its investment would stretch to the $30 to $50 million a drug typically cost to bring to market, Genentech never planned to stop with a few thousand customers. "We're really committed to this in terms of more than hypopituitary dwarfism," said Steele, who was vice president of product development. "The strategy is to start there with a carefully defined market. . . . Clearly our strategy is to move beyond that to constitutionally delayed short stature." These included the shortest 3 percent of children, "short because of a variety of medical, genetic, or environmental factors." That meant more than a million American children. And why, ultimately, halt at the third percentile? As a Genentech marketing man, John Reher, volunteered for the same article: "If my child was in the fourth percentile, I'd wonder why he shouldn't be worked up."

To begin with, Genentech questioned the definition of growth hormone deficiency, exploiting the difficulty of measuring GH levels and the lack of knowledge about what levels are normal. The body releases the hormone sporadically, peaking at night, which is why doctors sometimes hospitalized children for expensive overnight testing. They combined this with stimulation tests, just as in the 1970s, but still remained unsure of how well these reflected the body's real-life response. Various laboratories used different methods to interpret these responses, adding even more uncertainty.

Some pediatric endocrinologists suggested that patients actually fell along a continuum and might be only partially deficient, yet benefit from treatment. The traditionally accepted cutoff for growth hormone deficiency, 7 to 8 nanograms (ng) of hormone per milliliter of blood, was arbitrary as an adequate response to the tests, they argued; it had been dictated by the scarcity of pituitary hGH, and should be raised to 10 ng. The medical community went along. With this redefinition alone, the number of kids diagnosed as growth hormone deficient might be closer to 10,000 or even 15,000 than 3,000. And Genentech hoped to see the diagnosis expand further. As Steele explained, the country would see "the supply of growth hormone defining what the deficiency is. It's an evolving definition."

Genentech's next step was to find other conditions for which the product might be useful. Beyond treating deficiency, the company conducted trials of hGH in girls with Turner syndrome and in adults with muscle-wasting after surgery, and contemplated its use in treating burns and healing wounds. A multicenter study investigated hGH treatment in three hundred short normal children who did not test deficient, yet measured below the third percentile for their age and had a low growth rate. These represented the ultimate prize, kids who were short for whatever reason. The company's marketing man John Reher waxed enthusiastic: "We hope we'll find normal-variant short stature. Or growth-hormone responsive short stature." In other words, short, healthy kids whose diagnosis was that they grew faster on Protropin. "The dilemma then becomes not so much for us as for the physician."

DOCTORS FEEL THE PRESSURE

The dilemma for physicians was that hGH might make normal, healthy kids taller. And healthy kids with normal hormone levels represented the vast majority of those brought to the pediatrician with concerns about growth.

The primary reason for suspecting hGH would make even a normal child grow was giantism, the condition that results when a pituitary tumor pumps out too much growth hormone in childhood. Because of this, even in the days of extreme scarcity, experimenters had investigated other uses for pituitary hGH besides growth hormone deficiency. Raymond Hintz's personal favorite was the title of a

1971 paper by British growth expert James Tanner: "Effect of Human Growth Hormone Treatment for 1 to 7 Years on Growth of 100 Children, with Growth Hormone Deficiency, Low Birthweight, Inherited Smallness, Turner's Syndrome and Other Complaints," which Hintz renamed "Dr. Tanner's Paper of 100 Patients with Everything I Can Think Of." The early studies produced varied results, but additional hGH did seem to make some children who did not test deficient grow faster. Another experiment in the 1970s found that four of ten short normal children increased their growth rates by more than 3.4 cm (1.34 inches) a year. In 1981, a researcher reported that he had given hGH treatment for six months to a small number of extremely short children with normal hormone levels but with a current and predicted adult height below the third percentile—and increased the growth rate in some of them fivefold. It seemed likely that GH treatment could accelerate growth in short children, even if the cause of their small stature remained unknown.

Curiosity drove the early studies. "If you have a new treatment, you're going to explore the boundaries," Hintz explained years later, echoing Bob Blizzard. Hintz acknowledged liking not only a good story but a good gadget—a fascination that he suggested "seems to be a male thing.

"When you have a new tool you want to use it, you're going to see what the limits are. . . . There is a lot of short stature that is not due to growth hormone, so when you have somebody in your clinic that's just short for whatever reason, the temptation is, well, growth hormone works in growth hormone deficiency, why not this? It's not very sophisticated reasoning, but it's very common in medicine."

Such studies now took on more than academic curiosity. Families were seeing news reports. They would be pressing their pediatricians for information and advice on what could be done for their sons who got teased in the locker room or scratched from the varsity squad. They'd seek help not just to make short kids normal but average kids tall.

Most children brought to pediatricians by parents concerned about height were short, but growing at a normal rate; X-rays would reveal a delayed bone age, meaning they literally had more time and room to grow. Without treatment, they would remain short through childhood and adolescence but grow for a longer period than most, and eventually reach a normal height. This pattern of constitutional growth delay often has a family history. For years, doctors had treated some late-blooming boys with a short and inexpensive course of male hormones, which kick-start puberty. Now they might treat them with hGH instead.

Children with familial short stature, on the other hand, did not have retarded bone age. They just had, recorded somewhere in the many genes probably involved with determining height, short ancestors. Height is mostly hereditary—identical twins differ on average only about an inch. Parents who are similar in height tend to produce children close to that height. One tall parent and one short parent tend to produce medium-size children, but with a much larger range of variation. Now there was the possibility of tampering with this genetic destiny.

"The identification of short, otherwise healthy children who may benefit from growth hormone therapy has now become clinically important, since there is no theoretical limit to the amount of biosynthetic human growth hormone that can be produced," explained a pivotal UCSF study published in *The New England Journal of Medicine* in October 1983, which looked at healthy but slowly growing kids who stood at the extreme of short stature for unknown reasons—possibly a combination of familial short stature and constitutional growth delay. Its conclusion: "A dose of growth hormone comparable to that used for the treatment of hypopituitarism increases growth rate in some short normal children" by 2.2 to 4.2 centimeters a year. Almost half grew an inch a year faster than they'd been growing on their own.

This did not prove that hGH made these kids taller adults. They could simply have reached their predetermined adult heights faster. It also didn't answer whether their rate of growth would decelerate to below pretreatment levels when the shots stopped. The study didn't help doctors figure out who would respond and who would not. And it couldn't reveal long-term side effects or tell physicians what dose was safe to use in children already producing normal levels of growth hormone. Excessive GH in acromegalics produces devastating ailments—including diabetes, hypertension, coronary artery and cerebrovascular diseases.

Even so, the results made the editors of *The New England Journal of Medicine* very nervous. They asked the authors to add a caution, which they did: "Until we have more knowledge of its long-term effects and possible adverse actions in these children and more sharply defined criteria for the selection of patients and dosage regimens, the extrapolation of these findings to support indiscriminate treatment of short normal children with this potent hormone is premature and unwarranted." The editors would have liked an even stronger warning.

Alarmed, the American Academy of Pediatrics in 1983 issued a committee report that cautioned against the indiscriminate use of hGH in children not diagnosed with growth hormone deficiency, concluding: "If it ain't broke, don't fix it."

Selna Kaplan, one of the UCSF doctors who had conducted the controversial study, found herself ambivalent about treating nondeficient children in spite of its success, and not only because endocrinologists did not yet know whether therapy would make their patients taller in the long run. Besides the clinical issues, there were economic and ethical ones. If she were justified treating those in the third percentile, would she be justified *not* treating kids in the tenth percentile or the twenty-fifth? She also recalled how, just ten years earlier, doctors dosed tall girls with estrogens at levels known to be dangerous by the mid-eighties. It hadn't been the physicians' change of heart that limited treatment of the tall girls, but a change in culture that made tall stature more acceptable in women and therefore less worrisome to parents. Now some parents wanted their daughters made taller, not shorter. Kaplan—whose parents were 5'2" and 5'3"—stood only 4'11" tall, and though she endured a lot of teasing while growing up, her lack of height had never interfered with what she had wanted to do. She'd become a pediatric endocrinologist and a researcher. But she realized that not all her colleagues shared her views.

"There is a group that feels that no children with short stature who are not hormone deficient should be treated. There are those who feel any child of short stature should be given a trial. Most of us are in the middle. Some feel if the parents have the money, try it," she said in an interview at the time. She noticed that doctors were among the most persistent in seeking treatment for their own children.

THE FUTURE BEGINS NOW

As they debated, the small band of pediatric endocrinologists realized they stood as gatekeepers to what many people regarded as a scary future that went well beyond height. They even marked a coincidence: George Orwell's famous book about a terrifying future was called *1984*, though like many people they tended to confuse it with Aldous Huxley's *Brave New World*, in which scientists crafted test-tube babies to society's order.

In 1984, Hintz put hGH into this context: "It's a first case study, in a way. Here we have what amounts to hormonal plastic surgery. There are likely to be ways developed in the future to alter your genetic makeup or your child's by implanting foreign genetic material. You could make up some *1984*-style scenario of developing people specialized for different functions, by altering the human genome for some social purpose. Should we set up a world where every male who wants to be over six feet tall will be if he has enough money? Or every woman who wants to be under 5'9"?

"If your hair is dark and your husband's hair is dark and you've always wanted a blond child or you want your child to be left-handed instead of right-handed or have a small nose instead of a big nose—some of those capabilities are bound to be developed in the future, knowing what we can do now with embryonic mice."

In November 1983, the National Institute of Child Health and Human Development convened some fifty experts for a two-day conference in Baltimore on the uses and possible abuses of biosynthetic growth hormone. The concern that brought them together, pediatric endocrinologist Louis Underwood wrote later in *The New England Journal of Medicine*, was this: "In a society that values tallness, it is inevitable that enormous pressure will be put on physicians to prescribe growth hormone. Indeed, it is anticipated that much of that pressure will come from parents whose children, although not truly short, are not fulfilling parental expectations in competitive sports, social interactions, and academic achievement. The question that physicians must face is whether to prescribe growth hormone, with its wide spectrum of metabolic actions, to children whose shortness may reflect only genetic variation. Physicians will be forced to decide whether it is appropriate to tamper with a normal child in the hope of making him or her 'better.'"

But the conference established no consensus other than a call for a controlled study of hGH in short, normal, healthy children. Participants could not even agree on a term to use for small kids without growth hormone deficiency, but everyone knew they were discussing Genentech's future market. As Underwood wrote, children with familial short stature and constitutional growth delay represented "by far the largest number of persons with short stature who may benefit from treatment with growth hormone." They did agree that treating such children when so many questions remained would not be appropriate outside a study designed to provide some answers. There were those who questioned whether it would be appropriate even in a study.

Some worried that a child's expectations would be raised too high. Even among the biggest success stories, growth-hormone-deficient children whose growth rate doubled with injections, doctors found feelings of disappointment. Children fantasized and overestimated what the shots would do for them, and felt like failures when their fantasies did not come true. They endured years of painful injections, but still didn't think that they measured up. Some became depressed or acted out in school, and focused more than ever on their size. Boys seemed particularly vulnerable. Fathers and mothers had an especially hard time accepting extreme short stature in a son. While mothers typically became overprotective, fathers more often conveyed disappointment that, however subtle, their sons felt as rejection.

Being evaluated and treated for height could make short kids think of themselves as unacceptable as they were, just as it did among tall girls like Laura. The shots, even if they worked from the standpoint of a chart, did not represent a quick fix for family problems, because the treatment itself was stressful and could exacerbate tensions. There could be a huge distance between what the child wished for, what the parents expected, and what the doctor categorized as therapeutic success. As one researcher who conducted in-depth interviews of such families put it: "The need to perform—to grow biologically, to be a 'big boy' or 'big girl,' and to be grateful for receiving the precious growth hormone—placed insurmountable burdens on these children. They felt unable to resist the painful injections, for which they had wished so much, and they felt impotent to alleviate the disappointments mirrored in the faces of their parents." They could even feel they had failed their doctors.

Among the ethical issues facing pediatric endocrinologists was the fact their patients were children, but those demanding treatment on their behalf were parents. This represented a potential conflict of interest. Should doctors comply with a parent's request to help a healthy child become more competitive at basketball, or help a healthy, average child reach above-average height? Would they be treating the needs of the youngster, or the parents who—as psychologists put it—found having a child who was different both disappointing and "narcissistically frustrating." And wouldn't insistent parents just keep shopping for the physician who would comply with what they wanted for their children? Doctors weren't necessarily more comfortable when it was the child who insisted, who desperately wanted shots to get taller. How much could a child really understand about the risks and benefits?

Not that medical experts understood all the risks or all the benefits, either. All the risks would not be known for a very long time, and the benefit for which there was evidence was an accelerated growth rate in some, but not all, children. Even this depended on pediatricians' equipment and techniques for measuring height; errors of only a few millimeters a year could lead to mistakes in charting growth rates and interpreting success. That came before any attempt to calculate benefits in terms of adjustment, happiness, success.

While pediatric endocrinologists dealt mainly with ethics in the examining room, some did join bioethicists in asking larger questions, including those of social justice. A 1984 Hastings Center report coauthored by bioethicists and a pediatric endocrinologist predicted that recipients would be "mainly children of upper-upper-middle- and upwardly mobile middle-class parents who can afford to pay for what they regard as every possible advantage for their youngsters. Thus if height is somehow correlated with success in certain occupations and pursuits, the ideal of equal opportunity will receive a striking blow, and current differences among social classes will become more deeply entrenched."

Who would look at the social justice aspect, decide the value of using medical resources to add a few centimeters of height to gain advantage for a few when so many children didn't even receive basic medical care? The diagnosis of short stature was not a disease, it was statistical. But there would always be a lowest 3 or 5 or 10 or 25 percent. Even after a doctor figured out where he or she stood on these questions, the Hastings Center report conceded, "the dilemma for the pediatrician who says no is that the insistent parent may simply go elsewhere."

Such debates brought them to the crux of their belief in their roles as physicians. Certainly, specialists treated for reasons other than disease. Orthodontists straightened teeth, plastic surgeons straightened noses. But most pediatric endocrinologists did not seem ready to see themselves as cosmetic pharmacologists. Some argued doctors did alleviate suffering: that was the rationale for treating tall girls. They couldn't yet say with assurance that treatment would turn short kids into taller adults. But they did have accumulating evidence that it might make many grow faster in childhood and adolescence. So the question of treating suffering came down to this: Just how awful, really, was it to be a short kid?

PSYCHOLOGICAL PROBLEM—
OR SOCIETY'S PROBLEM?

There was yet another large gathering. The Psychosocial Aspects of Growth Delay Conference convened in Washington, D.C., from October 19 to 21, 1984, sponsored by the Human Growth Foundation and the pituitary hGH manufacturer Serono. It focused on the question of how disabling short stature was for a child's development, even a child who would ultimately reach normal height.

In the 1960s, and to some extent in the 1970s, studies of children with hypopituitary dwarfism assumed extremely short children experienced more problems—social, psychological, and academic—and suffered from low self-esteem, isolation, withdrawal, immaturity, and poor body image. This literature, which almost unanimously described short stature as a "handicapping condition" associated with a host of pejorative adjectives, spurred doctors to find treatments for height. But more recent studies following up growth-hormone-deficient children concluded, instead, that most of them had achieved normal psychological adjustment. Height was not the determining factor; families were. Kids encouraged to participate in activities at which they could succeed became happier kids.

As one researcher reported in more scientific language: "The child's adaptation to his or her size and the limitations that may impose on his or her life is largely determined by the capacity of parents to come to terms with their own grief and disappointment over the less-than-perfect child, and to promote the child's mastery of age- and phase-appropriate developmental tasks," not by how many inches hGH boosted height.

This conclusion did not pertain only to children with growth hormone deficiency, though they had been studied the most. Investigating late bloomers, one group of researchers at the State University

Hospital in Syracuse, New York, did find such children tended to be shy. But "no more hostile, power-oriented, aggressive, preoccupied with sexual concerns, or less likely to establish affiliation than their normal peers." In fact, the study described them as "comparable to the normal children across the majority of variables" and concluded that "although occasionally there are short children who clearly suffer from serious psychological disorders, they are the exception rather than the rule. Psychological adjustment does not hinge solely upon one's stature." These researchers, too, found that parents and teachers could help short children by offering acceptance and support, and by treating them in a way appropriate to their ages rather than their sizes.

Yet the audience did not seem ready to fully believe that extremely short kids didn't suffer lifelong and devastating damage. The keynote speaker listened to the mounting evidence. He was Leonard P. Sawisch, Ph.D., a clinical psychologist and disability expert with the Michigan Department of Education—and, at 4'4" tall, a member of Little People of America. When he finally took the microphone, Sawisch joked: "I found it refreshing that the researchers reporting at this symposium were very honest in expressing their surprise that we're not as psychologically, socially, or academically screwed up as they originally thought. Of course, as some folks did suggest, it was probably an error in their data!"

He was there to talk about what he called the "dwarf experience," and this was not a medical problem or a physical condition, but sociocultural. If he, or his 3'9" wife, had to climb onto the wet sink in a public restroom so that they could look into the mirror and comb their hair, the problem lay with the height of the mirror, not with them. An exclusive focus on size ignored the fact that Little People, as they called themselves, were a lot of things besides short. They were children and students, brothers and sisters, spouses and parents, and working people. In spite of being told by society all the things he could not do, Sawisch had learned to like himself and to take pride in other Little People; that had led him to accept other human beings with handicaps and, generally, to accept other human beings. This was the era of disability rights. There had never been a better time to be small and proud. Diagnosing short stature as a disease only undermined people's acceptance of differences.

"The irony," Sawisch told the conference, "is that growth-delayed individuals who may eventually reach 'average size' need to accept that being a dwarf is okay, in order to feel that being average sized is also okay. Parents may also need to come to this same conclusion, in order to find the peace that they seek."

But pediatric endocrinologists did not design restrooms, and Genentech was not in the business of selling sinks. Doctors concluded from the symposium that psychologists weren't going to be much help in providing the answers to which patients they should treat, or for how long, especially in the case of kids whose short stature, compared with their peers', would eventually cure itself. No one knew how much happiness a few inches might buy, or at what cost.

to market,
to market . . .

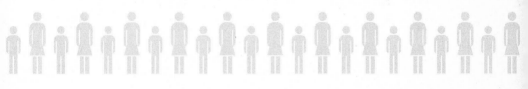

"only genentech is not
in mourning"

TERRIBLE NEWS FOR THE CHILDREN

On Sunday, June 17, 1984, Raymond Hintz received a disturbing phone call at home from the mother of a former patient. Hintz had treated Joey Rodriguez, who suffered from diabetes as well as growth hormone deficiency, with insulin and growth hormone until the boy reached eighteen, then passed him on to an adult endocrinologist. At more than 5'5" tall, Joey was considered a medical success story. In May 1984, the family flew from San Francisco to visit Joey's grandparents in Maine. Changing planes in Atlanta, their son rose from his seat and complained that he was dizzy. He was not a complainer, but an optimistic twenty-year-old man who had endured with stoicism years of treatment for his multiple hormone deficiencies. Thinking that her son's blood sugar was low, Joey's mother gave him some candy. But a few days later, in Maine, the young man mentioned the dizziness again and turned down a ride in his grandfather's motorboat. By the time the family returned to the Bay area, Joey's speech seemed a little different. Their local physician checked him out, found nothing obviously wrong, but suggested he go to the Stanford University Medical

Center in case of a possible middle-ear problem. The family thought of their long relationship with Hintz and phoned him instead.

"She noticed that when he got off the plane he was unsteady on his feet. So she watched for a couple of days and it seemed like he really was unsteady. And this wasn't like him at all—a very healthy, active young man. So she called me up and told me the story. For some reason it really sounded suspicious to me that there was something going on. . . . It sounded like he had a neurological disease and I knew that he had not had neurologic disease when I saw him."

Hintz met them at the emergency room. Joey did indeed have some impairment to his coordination and to his speech, and some involuntary eye movement. Over the next few days, as the family waited for testing at Stanford's neurology clinic, Joey deteriorated so rapidly that they took him up to see a San Francisco doctor who could examine him sooner. At a meeting to discuss the young man's puzzling case, an alert UCSF neurologist ventured that the symptoms looked like Creutzfeldt-Jakob disease, though the disease struck elderly people and, even then, only rarely. It was virtually unheard-of in a man barely out of his teens. Joey now stooped, drooled, and showed signs of dementia. The diagnosis seemed so improbable to the other doctors that they discharged him to a nursing home without a consensus.

Joey Rodriguez died in November, about six months after his parents first noticed his symptoms. A UCSF pathology resident asked the family for permission to transport the brain to San Francisco for a postmortem exam. Hintz advised the family that it was crucial to get a diagnosis if they could, for the sake of everyone receiving growth hormone. If other pediatric endocrinologists remained unaware of transmissible spongiform encephalopathies, Hintz was not. He'd attended an FDA conference in 1982 on standards for insulin, somatotrophins, and thyroid axis hormones, and remembered some informal discussion of slow-virus contamination being difficult to detect in tissue extract. He even remembered turning to a colleague from KABI at the conference who commented that it was pituitary growth hormone they all should be worried about. When the autopsy of Joey Rodriguez's brain revealed the spongy pattern typical of CJD, Hintz suspected that he or another doctor might have infected Joey with a fatal disease. He knew he needed to alert the federal government.

"The horror was even greater because when we first realized this one patient had it, for all we knew half or all of the patients who had gotten pituitary growth hormone in the seventies and the sixties...The feeling was, *Oh my God.*"

On February 25, 1985, Hintz wrote letters to Salvatore Raiti at what had been the National Pituitary Agency but had been renamed the National Hormone and Pituitary Program; to the NIH; and to the FDA. He wanted to make sure he got someone's attention. He described how Joey Rodriguez had been diagnosed with a variety of medical problems, including profound growth hormone deficiency, and started on pituitary hGH before the age of three in Los Angeles. The family moved to northern California, and the boy received daily injections and fairly large doses—so he'd probably had more growth hormone, beginning at an earlier age, than most patients. In case they missed the point, Hintz wrote that CJD was extremely unusual in a twenty-year-old and that slow viruses could be transmitted through contaminated central nervous system tissue. Since the patient had been treated for fourteen years with growth hormone, Hintz stated: "I feel that the possibility that this was a factor in his getting Creutzfeldt-Jakob disease should be considered." He called for a thorough search for other possible cases, and a follow-up of all patients treated with pituitary growth hormone in the previous twenty-five years, looking for any other diagnoses of degenerative neurological diseases. Hintz did not suggest that pituitary hGH be whisked off the shelves. But physicians needed to know about the possible link between CJD and growth hormone treatment. Unlike Joey Rodriguez, whose diabetes required continuing care, most young hGH patients did not get referred to adult endocrinologists once they stopped growing. Who knew how many cases might already have occurred?

"Because at that point people were not alerted," Hintz remembered thinking when he later described the events. "And the other possible complication was, once their patients were done being treated with growth hormone they sort of drifted off the face of the universe. They weren't followed forever."

Dr. Mortimer Lipsett, director of National Institute of Diabetes and Digestive and Kidney Diseases—the institute within the NIH that oversaw the pituitary program—read Hintz's letter and immediately convened a meeting to be held within days, on March 8, 1985. There, it was decided to halt all clinical experiments with pituitary hormones that did not involve therapy, to notify physicians and ask them to search among their patients for possible CJD deaths, and to reconvene six weeks later.

Pediatric endocrinologists did not want to give up hGH, their miracle drug. Leading those who argued that the link between the treatment and CJD had not been established was Bob Blizzard, the doctor who helped launch the federal program in the 1960s. His mantra now remained the same as it had been in the early days when he had seen a single case of growth hormone resistance: "One is a series of nothing." Blizzard, ever the believer in scientific medicine, had begun injecting himself with hGH in 1982 as part of a pilot experiment on how growth hormone affects aging. Two and a half years later, he was still taking it. Nothing had convinced him yet that it was unsafe.

But after hearing about Joey Rodriguez from Hintz at the meeting, Blizzard returned home to find a letter in his mailbox from a Texas family. They wrote to say their son, his former patient, had recently died in Dallas at age thirty-two. Blizzard contacted the family for details. The young man's mother had noticed he staggered a little when he walked and trembled lifting a cup, and a neurologist came up with a variety of possibilities, including multiple sclerosis. Blizzard convinced them to exhume the body and autopsy the brain; it revealed CJD.

In Buffalo, pediatric endocrinologist Margaret MacGillivray mulled over the case of a twenty-two-year-old patient of hers in a nursing home with unusual neurological symptoms. He'd been walking along a street and started veering to the right, then he'd developed double vision and other "funny sensations in his head." Like the Dallas man, her patient had not shown signs of significant mental deterioration and he died with no one suspecting he'd had CJD. It now seemed likely that both these deaths were related to pituitary hGH. Even Blizzard conceded that these two cases plus Joey Rodriguez *was* a series of something. Two others turned up in Britain. In the six short weeks between the two meetings that would determine the future of hGH, the number of confirmed cases of CJD among pituitary hormone recipients had jumped from one to five.

The second meeting, held on April 19, 1985, included scientists from the NIH, the FDA, and the National Hormone and Pituitary Program, along with representatives from KABI, Serono, and Genentech, and pituitary hormone programs in other countries. Raiti wanted the U.S. government to continue distributing hGH until more evidence showed a link to CJD; he suspected the commercial manufacturers of using what he saw as a scare to eliminate his program. Albert Parlow retained faith that his roomful of glass columns and improved processing eliminated any danger of new victims. A reporter quoted Parlow complaining later: "What we have is panic, what we have is jitter, what we have is super caution." Commercial manufacturers, too, stood by the safety and purity of their products. The head of the French program argued this was an American problem. On the other side, the British reported their cases, and American pediatric endocrinologists Hintz, Blizzard, and Selna Kaplan from UCSF united in calling for the withdrawal of pituitary hGH. Experts from Gajdusek's lab warned that eventually, most or even everybody exposed to growth hormone preparation might get Creutzfeldt-Jakob disease. They wouldn't know the toll for decades. It could be total disaster.

The United States ordered an end to distributing pituitary hGH that very day. Canada, which used the Raben method for processing, also ceased. Britain stopped its pituitary program on May 8. KABI agreed to withdraw its product. Serono, unlike its competitor, did not have a biosynthetic version in the works, and kept selling its hGH in

Europe for a few more months, arguing that the U.S. government had acted "much too hastily." Australia cut back, and programs in New Zealand, Hong Kong, Belgium, Finland, Greece, Sweden, Hungary, West Germany, Argentina, and the Netherlands shut down. France continued.

Many pediatric endocrinologists in the United States also thought their government had acted before all the evidence was in. They did not unite to hail Hintz as a hero. "They weren't at that meeting. At that point the majority of pediatric endocrinologists hadn't even heard of this...so there was a kind of skepticism involved: *It's only a few cases,*" Hintz recalled. "And I got some phone calls basically saying, 'Why are you waving this red flag until you know more?'...From the point of view of pediatric endocrinology, that's like taking away one of our legs. Now we were all of a sudden going to be back for an unknown period of time not being able to treat these children." They had current patients whose treatment would be cut off. And they had to phone parents to tell them why.

At UCSF, Selna Kaplan vividly remembers, doctors divvied up the list of 120 patients. "It was the worst time of my whole career to have to call them. We'd been saying, 'Growth hormone is safe,' because we thought it was. Antibodies, okay, but it wasn't deadly. And here we had to say to them... 'We don't know for certain that your child is infected, but...we do know that some preparations of the hormone were infected and we can't be sure. So to be certain, we're going to discontinue distribution.' Some said, 'Okay, if that's the way it is, do you think my child has it?' And I'd say, 'We don't know.' Some panicked and wanted to come immediately to see us, to have a neurologist see their child. We accommodated those that wanted to do that. We tried to reassure them." In fact, there was no reassurance—no test except in brain tissue taken at autopsy. No certainty about the length of incubation—ten years? Twenty years? Thirty? And no cure.

At Stanford, Hintz and two colleagues sat down with their patient list. He spent a Saturday morning dialing families, steeling himself for their reactions. To his surprise, he found that after he delivered the news, parents still did not want to stop injecting hGH into their children. "The most amazing thing to me, I expected people yelling and screaming over the phone: 'What do you mean, you've given my child inferior hormone!' A lot of people said: 'Well, I still have a supply, can I keep giving it to my child?' And there were two people, obviously well off...fathers who traveled a lot [and] actually went to the Zurich airport pharmacy and bought pituitary growth hormone, the Serono brand, so they could keep their children on it.

"Both of these cases had responded well, so their children had evolved from being the shortest not only in the class but in the school, to being close to normal or normal size." When Hintz quizzed one father on why he took the risk of continuing to procure hGH for his son, the man responded that he figured that if growth hormone were contaminated with CJD, his son had probably already been exposed. He didn't want to sacrifice the chance for more growth. Hintz thought this was a strange attitude, as if the father felt: "He's already bought the farm, so..."

GOOD NEWS FOR GENENTECH

On April 19, 1985, growth hormone derived from human pituitaries was "officially executed," according to one dramatic medical journal account of the decision to curtail it in the United States; "among the spectators at graveside, only Genentech was not in mourning."

The sudden unavailability of hGH put enormous pressure on the FDA. The Lawson Wilkins Pediatric Endocrine Society endorsed the decision to stop harvesting cadavers for pituitaries, but noted that it would take one and a half to three years to test stored batches of the federal program's hGH for contamination, and up to a year to test the safety of Parlow's filtration methods using material from scrapie-infected mice. In spite of the fact that in ongoing clinical trials biosynthetic hGH produced a higher incidence of antibodies than pituitary preparations did, the studies also showed it to be "as effective as pituitary GH in promoting growth." The society supported the FDA's effort to gather information and approve biosynthetic hGH to treat growth hormone deficiency "at an early date."

Faced with the sudden absence of pituitary hGH, the FDA approved Genentech's application for Protropin on October 19, 1985—just a few days after the British approved KABI's biosynthetic Somatonorm. It had been only six months since the first FDA meeting about CJD, and doctors believed that an interruption in treatment of more than six months would affect the outcome in final height. The FDA had responded to the pressure, approving Protropin about twice as quickly as usual.

Protropin also received orphan drug status, meaning Genentech got a seven-year monopoly because it produced a drug for a condition affecting fewer than 200,000 people in the United States. Congress had passed the act in 1983 in order to stimulate the development of drugs for rare diseases. Biosynthetic hGH was licensed only for use in children with hypopituitary dwarfism, meaning growth hormone deficiency. Companies legally could not promote hGH for any other condition, though it was not illegal for physicians to prescribe it off-label, like any drug, for any medical purpose they believed suitable. The FDA's role was not to determine who would get hGH, or whether it would be given by any doctor or only pediatric endocrinologists, just that it was safe and effective in growth-deficient children. As an FDA medical officer put it to a reporter: "We cannot regulate who prescribes it or to whom. The FDA doesn't judge whether society needs more six-foot children."

Still, the agency attempted to assert some measure of control by demanding that Genentech design a market survey system, collecting data on each patient about diagnosis, growth rate, and side effects. This was expensive, and the company viewed it as burdensome.

Genentech, already famous for the Friday beer busts that its employees called "HoHos," pitched a giant tent and threw a large party, complete with fireworks. They celebrated the company scientists who had made recombinant hGH possible; Peter Seeburg, the former UCSF postdoc with the disputed test tubes, gave a speech. October 19 was a

Friday. The following Monday, seventy-five sales representatives that Genentech had recruited away from Big Pharma—hiring them on a contingency basis in anticipation of the FDA action—arrived ready to market Protropin. Genentech bragged that these reps formed an elite staff already based in academic hospitals where they had established long-term relationships with physicians on behalf of Merck, Pfizer, Upjohn, Eli Lilly, and other companies. Now Genentech made them the first sales force equipped with their own laptop computers as they set out to sell the first recombinant pharmaceutical product developed, manufactured, and marketed by a biotechnology company.

Genentech had stockpiled Protropin for almost a year; the product was ready to ship. The market was all theirs, at least temporarily, and they moved aggressively to capture market share. Genentech was valued at $2 billion, though it hadn't made a single product of its own until now. Its future, and therefore the future of the biotechnology industry, rode on human growth hormone. In its rambling buildings, spicing up the muted earth-tone carpets and undecorated cubicles, a grease-penciled sign sat on a counter, updated throughout the day, to inform employees of the changing value of the company's stock.

Many pediatric endocrinologists already knew Genentech well. Kaplan, Hintz, Blizzard, and University of North Carolina professor Louis Underwood had all been paid advisors who helped design clinical trials for Protropin. Doctors appreciated that, thanks to Genentech, they had a treatment available to children who needed it, including the hypoglycemic babies who would die without growth hormone and who had been the only group allowed to continue with pituitary hGH. As academic medical researchers, many also appreciated that the company provided a new source of funding outside of NIH. They were exhilarated with the possibility of exploring new applications.

Blizzard had calculated two decades earlier that if pathologists collected a pituitary from every autopsy performed in the United States, there would be enough cadaveric hGH to treat only about 4,000 patients. Even then he'd predicted that growth hormone therapy might work for many more forms of short stature, including Turner syndrome in girls, and that if hGH could ever be made available in abundance, it might become as widely applicable as cortisone.

Now Genentech set out to make a pediatric endocrinologist's dreams come true. The company financed a journal to collect and review published information on growth from all over the world. Genentech not only funded studies but also was happy to fly clinical investigators to meetings to share findings, and to help out with the expenses of providing data for the postmarketing survey the FDA had insisted on at the time of approval. As a specialty, pediatric endo-crinology traditionally did not attract those chasing the big bucks in medicine. These doctors did not perform procedures that made a large profit. Their practices existed almost exclusively within hospital settings, most of them academic. Rather than courting the much larger number of pediatricians, the company was content to keep hGH in the hands of this intimate medical community, and to form a close relationship with it. They would be colleagues in advancing the knowledge of growth.

Among pediatric endocrinologists and the public that knew about it, the CJD tragedy blunted enthusiasm for growth hormone, but only briefly. Protropin came from bacteria that had been altered with a gene to make a specific protein, not from cadavers mined for pituitary glands. There was no risk of CJD from biosynthetic products. While some physicians saw CJD as a cautionary tale, others thought the lesson was that technology had come to the rescue. It was a good thing. The public seemed to agree.

Newspaper and magazine articles about the biosynthetic miracle reached families, touching what one physician called "a pressure point in our society." Doctors reported that their own caution in prescribing treatment sometimes provoked a furious response from parents. A father, told that he should not be concerned about his son, who was growing normally and would probably reach 5'7", roared back: "That's absolutely unacceptable!" Girls, always in a minority at growth clinics, started appearing because they didn't want to be short, not because they were afraid of getting tall. A pediatric endocrinologist commented, "For the first time in my life, I am seeing girls who want to be taller. The social acceptance of tallness in women used to be negative. Now it is positive."

"It really is a Brave New World," lamented James Tanner, the British growth expert who had been one of the first to experiment with the effects of growth hormone on all sorts of conditions, including familial short stature. Now he sounded ambivalent: "All of us in our hearts believe it will work. But in many ways, I rather think it would be better if it did not." He predicted: "We are now moving from an era in which there were too many patients chasing too little growth hormone to an era in which there will be too much growth hormone chasing too few patients."

Extremely short but healthy children were the objects of the chase. Just as it had done before approval, Genentech continued to exploit the blurriness around what was considered normal. The fuzzier the dividing line between deficient and normal, the more room to expand the market without adding a new indication that required clinical trials and FDA authorization. Genentech set out to influence the criteria doctors used to select patients by funding doctors whose research investigated current standards and tests. Sometimes the company tried to exercise its influence on medical opinion more obviously.

For example, at a Genentech-sponsored symposium in 1986, doctors differed widely on which children they should treat. Genentech representatives stoked physicians' uncertainty about their ability to diagnose deficiency, suggesting the best solution when unsure would be to give the hormone a trial run.

Along with the long list of prominent academic pediatric endocrinologists, Genentech's director of clinical research Barry M. Sherman participated, and later coauthored a chapter in the proceedings about controversies in treating short stature. The chapter described the expanding "doubt" about using stimulation tests, and the "growing awareness among pediatric endocrinologists that the capacity to define growth-hormone deficiency is limited and not nearly as good as once thought." Perhaps measuring growth hormone levels was not even worth doing, especially given the studies that showed hGH boosted growth in children who were not deficient: "The accelerated growth of these so-called normal short or constitutional growth delay children raises questions about the value of exhaustive efforts to define a given patient's GH secretory status precisely." The alternative to these "exhaustive efforts" was to give Protropin to short children and see what happened.

Sherman and his coauthor, medical professor Louis Underwood, presented three case studies to leading pediatric endocrinologists and asked for opinions on whether or not to prescribe growth hormone. Again, the message was that physicians who were unsure were not alone in questioning current definitions. To encourage endocrinologists to think about how they might use the hormone in ways they had not before, these case studies also asked them to consider psychological factors in their young patients. No one had needed to evaluate a child's misery before treating for clear-cut growth hormone deficiency. Kids were missing a hormone, doctors supplied it. Psychology was slippery new terrain for pediatric endocrinologists, and many had reservations about prescribing a powerful hormone in hopes of improving a child's social adjustment. Some responses to the case studies revealed as much about a doctor's personal attitude as a patient's. They made interesting reading.

CASE NO. 1: A fifteen-year-old boy who was sexually immature and just over 4'8" (142.8 cm) had become more distressed by his size when he moved from Latin America to the United States. Even though he was predicted to reach close to 5'8" (172 cm), the boy was depressed when he compared himself with North Americans. The doctors asked to comment agreed it was most likely a case of constitutional delay. The boy would be a late bloomer. One recommended a six-month trial of hGH to see if it boosted his growth rate. Another recommended trying testosterone first to start puberty. The third and most cautious was a Canadian named Harvey Guyda. He suggested testosterone coupled with psychological support but flatly ruled out growth hormone. Guyda noted that patients often expressed crushing disappointment with the results of hGH therapy.

As if to contradict this caution, however, a triumphant editor's note in the published proceedings announced that the boy had been treated with *both* growth hormone and testosterone for several months and had gained both physically and psychologically: "His growth rate increased dramatically, to 17 cm/year (6.7 inches). More importantly, he experienced an impressive improvement in his psychological status, seeming to benefit greatly from this treatment." It seemed a rebuke to those who would have denied the unhappy teenager hGH.

CASE NO. 2, a nine-year-old boy below the third percentile whose classmates teased him, provoked especially caustic commentary from one pediatric endocrinologist who opposed medical intervention. He declared the boy's height "a nuisance to him and his family" rather than "a serious handicap." As in the first case, this child was predicted to grow to about 5'8" and taller than his parents, who stood at the twenty-fifth percentile. The pediatric endocrinologist warned that benefits and risks remained uncertain. Knowledge about increasing adult height with hGH was "primitive," and no one knew how much excess hormone led to the premature death of people with acromegaly. Some similar children who had been given pituitary hormone had gained nothing, he pointed out, except possible exposure to CJD.

"Instructions in prickliness and self-preservation and encouragement to learn sports that require skill rather than bulk would bring a better return than would an investment in biosynthetic GH," this pediatric endocrinologist declared. He thought trying an expensive treatment, if it didn't work, "would be a heavy burden for a family that, by history, seems to regard their child as a loser."

CASE NO. 3 struck Selna Kaplan as genetic short stature—an eight-year-old boy below the third percentile, with a 4'9" mother and a 5'2" father, and whose psychological adjustment was good. The boy not only came from a short family, he seemed to be growing normally. She doubted injections would add inches, since her research found that only 5 to 10 percent of children with a delayed bone age but normal growth rate could be accelerated by hGH, compared with 70 percent of those whose delayed bone age was accompanied by slower-than-normal growth. She wouldn't treat this child, even if he did exhibit psychological problems. "We do not resolve the psychological problems if we recommend GH therapy and no benefit is derived," Kaplan wrote.

Bob Blizzard, on the other hand, thought the case more complicated. The boy's adult predicted height differed by more than two inches, depending on which method was used: 148 cm (4'10¼") with the prediction scale developed in Britain, and 154 cm (5'½") with the more commonly used American method. This was exactly the type of child who *should* be enrolled in a study to determine whether or not he responded to treatment, "even in the absence of psychological problems of significant degree" and unless the boy "resists adamantly," according to Blizzard. This youngster might or might not benefit, but medical science could learn something.

IN SPITE OF THESE wide-ranging opinions, some pediatric endocrinologists obviously were ready to give Protropin a generous try. By the end of 1986, as the new relaxed standard for growth hormone deficiency gained general acceptance, the number of U.S. patients doubled to about 6,000. Genentech's sales of hGH soared to $41 million. The brand loyalty Genentech established with the pediatric endocrinologists paid off, given that a patient might be on hGH for ten years or more, especially when the FDA handed the company a rude shock by approving Lilly's recombinant growth hormone product in 1987. Genentech had assumed the Orphan Drug Act protected its monopoly of the American hGH market. But Lilly, too, received orphan drug status, based on the fact that its hGH had 191 amino acids, as in nature, while Genentech's Protropin still contained the extra methionone. Now Genentech was shut out of marketing its own met-less product by Lilly's guaranteed seven-year monopoly. The FDA hoped to bring down the price some by encouraging competition.

But Lilly had trouble wooing pediatric endocrinologists to switch loyalties. Genentech's aggressive campaign had locked doctors into the long-term use of Protropin; physicians didn't usually change brands unless they saw either major problems or advantages to a patient who might be treated for a decade. The price of treating a child remained about $40 per milligram, meaning therapy for a youngster weighing about sixty-six pounds (thirty kilograms) totaled close to $18,700 a year. Treatment could end up costing some families as much as $150,000 or even $200,000.

By 1988, biosynthetic growth hormone, which Genentech had predicted might reach $10 to $30 million in sales, was a worldwide market worth more than $100 million. And the line on the company growth chart headed steadily upward. Genentech hoped the FDA would approve its use for girls with Turner syndrome next and, eventually, for short healthy children.

Yet the doctors still did not know:

- The cause of short stature. Endocrinologists used the term to describe healthy children who grew more slowly than average for their age and were among the shortest 0.6 percent—more than 2.5 standard deviations below average height. Short stature probably represented a combination of inherited height and constitutional delay, but the kids lumped together under the label were a heterogeneous bunch, which is why doctors squabbled even about what to call them. Pediatric endocrinologists generally remained unconvinced that otherwise healthy children had a disease just because they were extremely short or tall compared with others in a population.

- How to tell which children would respond to hGH. They lacked standards for normal hormone secretion levels in boys and girls at each age, since even normal children exhibited wide variation. No tests usefully discriminated between those who would or would not grow faster with treatment. However, there was mounting evidence that most strikingly short children growing at below-normal rates would add at least two centimeters per year more with hGH shots, at least for the first year. Also, doctors now knew that daily injections worked better than injections given only three times a week, and that giving them just under the skin rather than deep into the major muscles worked just as well.

- Whether hGH made kids grow taller, or just got them there sooner. Or even whether the increased velocity lasted as treatment extended over years.

- Whether it was safe in the long term.

- What the best doses and treatment schedules were, and how long therapy should continue. People with pituitary giantism or acromegaly had anywhere from three to one hundred times normal GH levels, so what was the safe upper limit to avoid the devastating effects of excessive growth hormone?

- Who should pay for this treatment? Should anyone who could afford it get it? There were much cheaper alternatives for late bloomers—testosterone for boys, low-dose estrogens for girls— therapies they had used for years to shove kids into puberty and help them mature like other children the same age.

- Even if growth hormone boosted how fast kids grew, did it provide any psychosocial benefit? This was the ultimate reason for treatment. But daily injections could, in themselves, be a psychological burden for a child. And they all had witnessed the disappointment that accompanied unrealistic expectations.

Summarizing all these unknowns in a 1988 letter to *The New England Journal of Medicine* published with the title "Growth Hormone Therapy and the Short End of the Stick," UCSF pediatric endocrinologist Melvin Grumbach urged the FDA to move slowly when considering approval for using hGH beyond growth hormone deficiency: "Before considering its release for the treatment of short healthy children, we need more data on the effects of long-term treatment on growth and final height and any untoward clinical and psychological effects. In considering growth hormone treatment in such children, we should recognize that the problem lies not in their growth hormone profiles but in the role of heightism in our society and the psychosocial disadvantages it confers."

That year, 1988, pediatric endocrinologists still reeling over the CJD tragedy nervously read a Japanese report that a small number of children developed leukemia after receiving treatment for growth hormone deficiency. They rushed to an NIH workshop hastily called in Bethesda to examine the Japanese cases. A closer look convinced them that the children involved had disorders that put them at higher risk for leukemia, and that the chances of a normal child developing cancer of the blood from GH therapy were small to nonexistent. The Lawson Wilkins Pediatric Endocrine Society concluded that that there was insufficient evidence to suspect that GH treatment was responsible. The medical society would continue to monitor all reports of leukemia annually among patients getting growth hormone. The postmarketing survey that Genentech originally found onerous and expensive had turned out to be an excellent marketing tool; the accumulating data quickly reassured doctors about the safety and efficacy of biosynthetic hGH. Such statistics could be an important part of the sales pitch to physicians. Still, the data was not sufficient to reveal the long-term risks of raising hGH levels in healthy short children.

Yet the sales bubble continued to expand. It didn't even pop in

1989, when Grumbach's colleague Selna Kaplan told an international endocrinology meeting in Stockholm that only two of the twelve short normal children she'd been treating for up to a decade had reached an adult height more than two inches above their predicted height before therapy. Others countered that these children had been started on pituitary hGH, and experienced interruptions in their treatment.

In 1990, Protropin sales brought Genentech $157 million, an increase of more than 40 percent from just two years before. Genentech controlled 75 percent of the $200 million market in the United States. And so far, biosynthetic human growth hormone still had been approved to treat only hypopituitary dwarfism.

WHAT ARE THEY TREATING?

Even as hGH sales took off, the debate continued. There were those who insisted that short stature was not a disease but a genetic variation and, for both economic and ethical reasons, should not be medically treated. "We do not usually call prejudice-induced conditions, which confer social disadvantages but have no intrinsic negative health effects, diseases," argued ethicists in the journal *Acta Pædiatrica Scandinavica*. "Which stature is normal in Sweden, Mexico, Nigeria, or Japan? Who does set the standards and define the limits for short stature? The fashion and the furniture branches?" There was no "definitive evidence" that short normal children actually were at risk for psychosocial problems, while there was evidence that treating such children could reinforce their self-perceptions that something was wrong with them.

But in the same issue of the journal, Louis Underwood, one of the American pediatric endocrinologists who had a long affiliation with Genentech, made the opposite case: he argued for the ethical use of hGH in some short healthy children, even if it didn't make them taller adults and even if all the long-term side effects remained unknown. Sure, short stature was a social disadvantage rather than a disease. "However, because societal prejudices about shortness cannot be corrected easily or rapidly, some short individuals may benefit from GH therapy." In other words, nothing as convenient as a series of shots could fix society.

Attempting to boost height in healthy children could be justified, because it "may reduce the severity of the disadvantage and improve psychological adjustment and the capacity for social achievement," Underwood wrote. According to this argument, it didn't matter that the injections might not make kids taller in the long run. Increased adult height was not the best measure of successful treatment. "Rather, improved self-concept and better psychosocial adjustment should be the desired objectives. In some children, these goals might be achieved by improving height centile standing in comparison with peers, even though adult height is not increased." As long as pediatric endocrinologists kept hGH out of the hands of pediatricians and other doctors, and as long as they were clear with parents about realistic outcomes and unknown risks, this was not different than many other medical practices that enhanced well-being: "Although GH therapy is potentially more costly, its use for improving physical attractiveness and self-concept is as justifiable as the correction of physical defects that detract from an individual's attractiveness and impair social functioning."

Cosmetic endocrinology in young children that involved years of injections could be justified, because being the shortest kid in the school could ruin your whole life. Or, as University of North Carolina psychologist Brian Stabler (who was also affiliated with Genentech) liked to say: Being short might not be life-threatening, it just made you *wish* you were dead. Stabler's was the loudest psychological voice for the point of view that even a short-term increase in height velocity could make a big difference in self-image and confidence. It might also reduce "family frustration." Yet even he acknowledged that "there is as yet little empirical evidence that specific psychological benefits are associated with increased growth velocity."

So opponents and proponents agreed that there was no definitive evidence that hGH therapy made children happier or psychologically healthier. But families and doctors intrinsically appeared to believe it was true. Parents willingly shelled out $100,000 or more, children held out their arms or legs, and obviously, given the sales figures, endocrinologists found many more candidates for treatment than even those kids who fit the newly expanded standards for growth hormone deficiency. Powerful cultural social assumptions, as well as powerful marketing strategies, were at work.

That these assumptions had to do with gender was evidenced by who sought treatment for height: just as in the earlier era, and even though there was no reason to believe that growth hormone deficiency did not strike girls and boys equally, two-thirds of the children brought to growth clinics for evaluation were boys. Extreme differences in height are more common among males, as is constitutional growth delay. But more important, height continued to matter more for men. Though gender roles had relaxed in the 1960s and 1970s, knocking down height barriers for police officers and army recruits, and creating a new kind of leading man who was more in touch with his feminine side, the idea stubbornly persisted that short men were not manly.

Doctors in the 1960s had described tall girls as unfeminine, as Amazons, as masculine, and John Money had lectured in the 1970s that men with dwarfism could end up with deviant sexual fantasies; now came even more explicit warnings that one of the psychological consequences of being a short male could be homosexuality. Not just being shorter than normal but even being shorter than average put men at risk. In *Stature and Stigma: The Biopsychosocial Development of Short Males*, published in 1987 and widely cited afterward, psychologists Leslie F. Martel and Henry B. Biller wrote that they had been stimulated by the new availability of hGH and the possibilities of "height control" to call attention to the terrible failure of psychological textbooks, which did not acknowledge the impact of stature on personality development. "A major goal of the present book is to underscore that even more modest stature deficits among adult males well within the normal distribution, such as being relatively

short (e.g., 5'5" or even 5'7" or 5'8") may be associated with a vulner-
ability to certain types of psychological difficulties and personality
adaptations." They spelled out what these certain types of adaptations might be.

"It is almost axiomatic that short males are not attractive, or at
least not as attractive as their taller counterparts," Martel and Biller
wrote. While women wanted to be petite except for their busts, men
wanted to be large and muscular. "The male must have a body that
can offer physical security to self and others." Without that body, men
had difficulty forming a feeling of adequacy; they faced daily trials as
subtle as making eye contact or not submissively yielding their space;
and frequent reminders of their inferiority, like bar stools that were
too high to be comfortable or chairs that left their feet dangling above
the floor (a "particularly poignant experience for the short male"). It
might be an era when the traditional notion of machismo provoked as
much derision as admiration, but these psychologists still agreed with
Alfred Adler's theories from the 1920s that the desire to obtain power
motivated a person's life, and that feeling physically inadequate could
lead to a Napoleon complex. They acknowledged there had been little
research on this.

Martel and Biller's own 1986 study led them to conclude that
males in lower-economic-status groups managed their lack of height
by becoming more aggressive physically, while those in upper-
middle-class groups became more cerebral. Some also used humor,
which they termed "the clowning or mascot-adaptational response."
The outcome might be "quite positive" for a short male with a well-
developed physique who was also smart and had a supportive upper-
middle-class family. "Nevertheless, no matter how successful they
may eventually be, there are very few, if any short men who do not
experience significant stress as they have to cope developmentally
with the reality of their stature deficiency." Women viewed short men
as insecure, immature, and feminine. A very short or very thin boy
might be at such a disadvantage that he gave up on women.

"While no systematic research has been conducted, one potential coping behavior for the stresses of short male stature in adolescence is the choice of homosexuality as a sexual orientation. This allows avoidance of heterosexual competition and accommodates the short boy's admiration for height in taller males. Although this choice of lifestyle does not meet with general societal acceptance, it brings membership in a male group that may provide a strong sense of belonging which the short boy might not otherwise experience." It was Martel and Biller's "strong clinical impression," though they admitted they did not have studies to back them up, that more short boys than tall boys developed emotional, social, and sexual difficulties.

So parents with shorter-than-average sons had reason to worry. While he might become intellectual or artistic, a short boy would have to make a real effort to foster a positive male identity and self-image, since "it almost certainly could not be done through the traditional masculine routes." To Martel and Biller, a boy merely below *average* height for his age stood at risk for psychological difficulties. Modern medical advances would only make this worse. They predicted that widespread use of growth hormone, followed by genetic engineering in the future, could diminish differences in height and make being short even less acceptable.

They were only stating what many parents felt, but cloaked in the academic language that made these fears seem scientifically grounded and with the credentials to justify doctors who prescribed hGH to alleviate the suffering of short boys. Gender roles were changing, but deep insecurities about raising sons who might be less than manly remained. Those fears, along with the desire to do everything they could to help their sons succeed, drove some parents to the growth clinics. It was reminiscent of the mothers who heeded warnings that tall girls would never find mates and gave their daughters estrogens.

The relationship between physicians and patients had changed since that earlier era. The days when Laura's parents did what the doctor ordered because they believed the doctor always knew best, when Bob Blizzard could promise other endocrinologists that a parent organization could be kept under control—when physicians wore white coats and their diagnoses and prescriptions went unquestioned—had passed. Patients increasingly were seen—and saw themselves—as customers. They could shop around for a doctor just as easily as for a car dealership where the price was right. Only it was not price but prescriptions they sought. If one pediatric endocrinologist squirmed at the idea of giving hGH to a healthy child who was shorter than average but in the normal range, or who might spurt up later anyway, there would always be another more sympathetic who found the idea perfectly justifiable for psychosocial reasons. Doctors told themselves that even if they said no, parents would just find another physician who said yes. And quite a few therefore thought, especially given the uncertainties of diagnosis and the unclear ethical guidelines and the opportunity to discover more about what growth hormone could do, they might as well go along and prescribe hGH if parents insisted.

HOW MANY ARE INFECTED?

Even as they pioneered expanding uses for growth hormone in new patients, no one could predict how many of their old, pituitary-era patients would die of CJD. Gajdusek's laboratory warned that none of the filtration methods might have been safe. The cases uncovered in 1985 might be the "burst" marking the peak of the epidemic, or the blip that signaled the beginning of a vast outbreak.

Cases slowly accumulated. In 1986, a thirty-one-year-old New Zealand woman whose doctor had received hGH from Wilhelmi's lab at Emory University was diagnosed with CJD. In New York, reexamination of slides taken of the brain of a former hGH patient who died from pneumonia in 1979 at age nineteen revealed telltale signs of CJD. In March 1987, a Pennsylvania neurologist reported the CJD death of a thirty-seven-year-old. The average incubation seemed to be about fifteen years, meaning the vast majority of pituitary hGH recipients had not yet reached the end of the period when symptoms might appear.

Meanwhile, the federal government searched National Hormone

and Pituitary Program records from the previous twenty-five years, and cross-referenced them with the files of hundreds of physicians and treatment centers across the country. Some doctors kept poor records; patients had moved; no one tracked a child who reached adult height or who had stopped the injections for some other reason. Epidemiologists painstakingly came up with a list of 6,284 people who had been enrolled in the program and began the massive effort of contacting them with questions about their health, reaching about 84 percent. Those most difficult to locate were also those probably most at risk based on the emerging cases—patients who started treatment before 1970. An additional 2,000 to 3,000 Americans who bought commercial pituitary hGH were not on any lists, unless they'd also used some of the government-supplied hormone. About 10,000 in all were believed to have received pituitary GH in the United States from some source or other.

Alfred Wilhelmi brought his laboratory notebooks to the NIH. He was, according to the researcher in charge of the epidemiological study, devastated that the hormone he had processed might have sown the seeds of death. The mood among the officials who oversaw the National Pituitary Agency and then the National Hormone and Pituitary Program, which had distributed hGH free to thousands of children, also was grim. They had liked to brag they'd made these children grow a combined total of eleven miles. They'd taken pride in how they made their miracle available to people who needed it, regardless of cost, even when commercial manufacturers pressured the government to step aside. Now they braced themselves for the possibility that their patients might die, one by one, over the next twenty years or longer, from the medicine only meant to make kids grow.

At the beginning of 1988, the National Institute of Diabetes and Digestive and Kidney Diseases (NIDDK) sent out a letter and a five-page fact sheet, beginning: "Dear Growth Hormone Recipient." It informed former patients that five out of the approximately 7,000 people treated under the government program had died with a confirmed diagnosis of "a rare, fatal brain disorder called Creutzfeldt-

Jakob disease," and that "we believe some of the growth hormone derived from human pituitary tissue was contaminated by the CJD agent." Because there was no way to detect the infection, the government recommended that they not donate blood or tissue in order to ensure the safety of the blood supply.

The enclosed fact sheet, in question-and-answer format, anticipated what families might ask. The answers were straightforward and terrifying. There was no cure or way to slow CJD. It was virtually certain that hGH had been a source of infection. Since only nine patients younger than thirty years old had been diagnosed with CJD before this cluster, the odds that these cases among hGH recipients represented a mere coincidence were less than one in a trillion, "vanishingly small" in the government's own words. Those processing pituitaries ground hundreds or thousands of glands for each batch; it was likely that one or more of these glands could have come from someone with undetected CJD, or even from someone "known to have died of the disease." Though the program had attempted to prohibit collection of pituitaries from cadavers with infectious brain diseases like encephalitis and meningitis, "CJD was not a specific criterion for exclusion."

The government believed that the hormone produced since 1977, when Albert Parlow took over, was more than 95 percent pure. Yet the fact sheet acknowledged that "there is no certainty that the modern preparation is safer." CJD was extremely difficult to inactivate. Even 95 percent might not be good enough. Without mentioning the Scottish veterinarian whose midnight revelation had driven him to warn the British Medical Council more than ten years earlier, the NIDDK did report that a British Medical Council experiment into the safety of the modern processing methods in 1980 had proven encouraging. That was the year Dickinson and colleagues finally published the reassuring results of testing scrapie-infected tissue; word that they had succeeded in eliminating scrapie with processing similar to Parlow's column chromatography had circulated even before publication. But some American CJD experts continued to worry that Dickinson's evidence was not conclusive.

A revolutionary new theory about what causes diseases like CJD had slowly gained acceptance in the 1980s. Stanley Prusiner, a molecular biologist at UCSF, was considered heretical when he first began to argue that the transmissible spongiform encephalopathies, though also called slow viruses, were not viruses at all. He gradually won over most in the field, and earned a Nobel Prize, with his idea that the infectious agent was a type previously unknown, something he called a prion. Unlike any other source of disease, bacterial or viral, prions do not contain DNA. This might explain why methods that reliably sterilize instruments and tissue from infectious organisms do not protect against diseases like CJD. It also means that a single prion might cause disease and that the study done in Dickinson's laboratory, which had injected only some samples of purified hormone into test animals, might have missed a lone infectious particle.

Even if one vial of hGH did not contain a prion, another vial in the same batch might. Samples of all the available lots of NHPP hormone were injected into animals that had been watched for two and a half years in 1988, but would be watched for five more. Yet even if the animals continued to live symptom-free, their survival would not be conclusive about any other vials. Pituitary hGH recipients were told to stay in touch with their physicians.

The federal government no longer distributed hGH for human use—but some former recipients undoubtedly had turned to Genentech and Lilly's recombinant products and the government vouched for their safety, on the basis of the brief history of the postmarketing database. The fact sheet ended with reassurances that there was no chance of contamination of biosynthetic hGH with CJD. Biosynthetic hGH might produce antibodies, but those rarely interfered with growth. It posed its own question, in bold print: "We were told that pituitary hGH was safe, too. How can we be sure that biosynthetic hGH is safe?"

"Unfortunately, it is not possible to guarantee that any medication will be 100 percent safe," the fact sheet answered, adding that six years of records offered "no reason to believe that biosynthetic hGH will cause serious or long-term health problems."

The NIDDK wrote again at the end of 1989, to report that interviewing for the epidemiological follow-up study was now complete, and that two new cases of CJD among hGH recipients in the United States had been discovered. Seven cases out of the nearly 6,300 known to have been treated with NHPP hormone struck the head of the agency as "reassuring." The attached update also reported four cases outside the United States, and an additional case associated with a different pituitary hormone. Because of the mingling of various batches of pituitaries, and the fact that no single lot had been shared by all those who had developed CJD so far, there was no way to tell whether any particular recipient had received a contaminated batch, let alone a vial that contained the infectious agent. There also had been no cluster at any single treatment center. The incubation time still could not be determined. Worldwide, the interval between the end of therapy and the onset of CJD ranged from two years to nineteen. The interval from starting treatment to developing symptoms ranged from twelve to twenty-eight years.

The Public Health Service that conducted the study had better luck locating parents than their grown children. This led to a problem. Not all parents decided to tell their children about the risk. The government agreed to respect their wishes. But the NIDDK argued in its 1989 letter that unless a child was "mentally or emotionally impaired," he or she should be informed. "Understandably, parents may hesitate to give their children information that will alarm them. Parents making the decision to withhold this information might consider how they themselves would feel if they were not told about a condition that could affect their health." Blood banks had been asked to exclude all potential donors who'd received pituitary hGH. Some recipients had learned about their possible exposure to CJD for the first time when they went to donate blood and were turned away.

Linda Sluder, who had been a beautiful blond "doll" as a child on Long Island; the two Mahler children; Tony Grossenburg, who had suffered through high school in South Dakota and gone off to Creighton University in Nebraska—all heard about the letters from their parents. Patsy Grossenburg felt sick to her stomach at the news. The sick feeling returned when she gave blood and was asked whether or not she'd ever been given pituitary human growth hormone. The Grossenburgs debated about withholding the information from their son at college, but they decided he was an adult. There were only a handful of cases. Tony Grossenburg chose not to think much about it. He had his Catholic faith, and a disposition not to dwell on potential tragedy.

Fred Mahler had taken shots, too, as part of Blizzard's small experiment on the role of growth hormone on aging. Still a pilot, now he only ferried passengers rather than pituitaries across the country. He had found it inconvenient to be questioned frequently about why he was traveling through airports with syringes, so he'd stopped injecting pituitary hGH sooner than Blizzard. When Fred and Gwen Mahler heard about CJD, for some reason they believed it was a European rather than an American problem.

A young man named David Davis was at home when his parents called him into the dining room shortly after his college graduation and handed him the letter they'd received from the government. He also did not worry about it at the time. There were too many other things going on in his life—decisions about what career to follow, where to live, when to settle down—to think about the minuscule chance that he was infected with an obscure deadly disease that might strike him in twenty years. He had been diagnosed with growth hormone deficiency as a child, and the shots that he received from his mother, a pediatrician, had granted him the gift of normal height, though below average. As a child, Davis hated the injections deep into the muscle of his upper arm, and would retreat to his room to rub the sore spot and dream of becoming tall enough to play professional basketball. The results left him, at 5'4", far below his hoop dreams, and disappointed. He appreciated being treated, but thought of himself as a short man, and minded it. Only gradually did it sink in that because of those treatments, he was living with the biological equivalent of a ticking bomb: a terrible, undetectable, and always fatal disease that might have been planted in his brain. The ticks could get louder or softer, depending on what the epidemiologists and biologists found and reported in the coming years. But it didn't seem as if anyone would be able to call the all clear for decades yet, if ever. This began to bother David Davis a lot.

CHAPTER 8

dear parent...

THE GOVERNMENT
EXPERIMENTS ON CHILDREN

Wanted: Healthy girls and boys not yet in early puberty, extremely short and willing to get shots. For an experiment.

Entering the 1990s, doctors didn't know whether or not they could increase the final height of short children who didn't have any growth hormone deficiency. They knew only that they could make almost any short child grow faster. Or, as Ray Hintz and others liked to say, enough hGH would "make a stone grow." It couldn't help a short adult, however, whose epiphyses had closed and whose growing days had ended. When fielding an inquiry from a man or woman who wanted to be taller, Hintz would joke, "I can only uglify you," referring to how an excess of growth hormone in acromegaly enlarges a person's jaw and nose and lips, as well as hands and feet.

In short children whose bodies produce normal levels of growth hormone, the question remained whether extra hGH would only speed them up to the height they would have reached anyway. Or might it even accelerate them into puberty so that they ended up shorter than if untreated? And was it safe, given the serious heart and other problems of people with acromegaly? When they'd convened at the National Institute of Child Health and Human Development in the early 1980s to discuss uses and abuses of growth hormone, pediatric endocrinologists had agreed on the need for a definitive study. That meant enrolling short normal children in an experiment; dividing them randomly into two groups; giving some hGH injections while the control group received placebo shots; and measuring them all at final height. Called a randomized controlled blind study—blind because neither the families nor the doctors would know which children received hormone and which got syringes full of saline solution— this type of trial is the gold standard in research.

Gordon B. Cutler, a pediatric endocrinologist at the NIH, had set out in the early 1980s to conduct such an experiment, but the CJD scare sidelined his plans. Now, in the biosynthetic hGH era, manufacturers had as much interest as scientists in the answers. Eli Lilly wanted to seek FDA approval to market its growth hormone product for potentially millions of short children diagnosed with idiopathic short stature—kids in the lowest percentiles for unknown reasons— not just those with hypopituitary dwarfism. With Lilly underwriting the government study and supplying the recombinant hGH, Cutler was back in business. He argued that only this type of clinical trial, conducted over a dozen years and following the subjects to their final heights, would show which children became taller adults, or even whether medical attention and placebo injections alone stimulated growth.

In the early 1990s, orphan drug protection was set to expire soon on both Genentech's Protropin and Lilly's Humatrope. They would lose their monopoly on the American market; more manufacturers would enter and compete; the prohibitive price of growth hormone treatment might plummet. Pediatricians anticipated parents dragging their short offspring to medical offices in droves. Whether or not they personally believed in treating idiopathic short stature, a lot of doctors wanted the medical issues settled so they could answer questions from families about risks versus benefits. The federal government also argued that it was important to investigate whether growth hormone therapy was either effective or safe for short normal kids, because it was already being widely prescribed: about half the American youngsters receiving biosynthetic hGH did not have abnormal growth hormone levels.

But not everyone was comfortable with the idea of subjecting a group of healthy children to years of shots that might or might not be helpful and would certainly pose at least some risks. Besides the shots three times a week through childhood and adolescence, adding up to more than a thousand injections for some, the young volunteers would be examined; photographed nude against a grid; hospitalized; X-rayed; subjected to magnetic resonance imaging, and blood and urine tests; and psychologically evaluated. All of them would go through this in hopes of getting taller, but half would receive placebo injections. They were being recruited for an experiment only because they were extremely short. Through human history up to that point, height had been considered a human characteristic that, at its extremes, was sometimes a disadvantage, but not a disease.

In fact, critics argued the government had reasoned backward. They called on the medical profession to decide first whether or not short stature was a condition that required medical treatment. If not, then the government had no business experimenting on children, labeling a social problem as a disease, and helping industry inflate stigma for profit.

The argument over the NIH experiment illustrated a wider debate over the potential use of new technologies to enhance inheritance. Bioethicists described hGH as the perfect case study, a harbinger of other possibly imminent technologies. The first gene therapy attempt was made in 1990. A Harris Poll in 1992 reported that 43 percent of Americans "would approve using gene therapy to improve babies' physical characteristics." Given the importance attached to size, height was an obvious early candidate for such tinkering once scientists fingered the genes and perfected the method. It seemed a matter of time before it would not only be possible to make such alterations—to give a baby blue eyes, perfect pitch, and a five-inch advantage over his father—but to someday engineer these improvements into the genes that could pass these desirable traits on to future generations. This raised fears of a new eugenics, an attempt to improve the human race rather than embrace its variations. The fact that the manipulation of inherited physical characteristics might be done first with a drug like human growth hormone, rather than by altering the genes themselves, did not make it less ethically troubling for some critics.

In 1992, two groups petitioned to stop the experiment. The Physicians Committee for Responsible Medicine, which claimed about 3,400 doctors as members, along with the Foundation on Economic Trends, an organization that questioned the expansion of biotechnology, joined forces to charge that the government violated federal regulations covering research on children. Jeremy Rifkin, the activist who led the Foundation on Economic Trends, focused on the issue of genetic engineering. In his view, short children were getting medical treatment because they were victims of discrimination, not of disease, and future technologies could head the same way in an ominous drive for perfection:

"What about fat people? What about people with different skin pigmentation? What about young girls whose breasts won't grow to the size that society desires? This experiment moves us onto a very, very dangerous journey that starts with 'enhancement' and ends up with eugenics," Rifkin told the press. "There is nothing wrong with these children. What is wrong is society, the biases, the discrimination. But don't address the biases of society by changing the physiology of the individual." Rifkin also charged that experimenting on children who did not have a disease was "exploitative and abusive."

In response to the criticism, the scientific director of the National Institute of Child Health and Human Development, Arthur S. Levine, echoed John Crawford's rationale for treating tall girls thirty years earlier, agreeing short stature was not exactly a disease: "But in our society, height is generally seen as a positive characteristic, and extremely short stature is seen as a negative characteristic. If a child becomes so disabled by anxiety and worry about his short stature, it becomes tantamount to a disease." One of the study's scientists recited a litany of handicaps short people faced: they had difficulty driving cars, finding clothing, sitting in standard-size chairs; very short kids faced lower expectations and ended up working below capacity. An NIH spokesperson objected to press descriptions of the experimental subjects as normal: "These kids are not normal. They are short in a society that looks at that unfavorably."

The Physicians Committee for Responsible Medicine, for its part, condemned the federal trial as needlessly endangering the physical and psychological safety of children. The group worried that young volunteers risked disappointment and an increased negative self-image if they didn't gain inches and, even if they did, there was no evidence this would by itself improve their social adjustment. Height is only one way teenagers differ from each other, and only one possible factor in low self-esteem, the group pointed out. But years of injections and examinations reinforced a child's sense that he or she was unacceptable and needed fixing.

In terms of physical risks, the physician's group compiled a list of theoretical side effects that began with cancer and fatal renal failure and ended with the possibility that the hormone's effect on metabolism might make some children unusually lean and "inappropriately muscular." Against this list, the benefits seemed unclear, given the lack of hard evidence that kids who were extremely short but not growth hormone deficient had either more intellectual or academic problems than those of average height. Sure, some kids passionately hated being small. Even so, not every U.S. family would have the money to attempt to change that. If treatment could make them taller, which boys and girls would get the chance? The Physicians Committee for Responsible Medicine thought it would be more responsible—both cheaper and more effective—to spend the money to invent ways to help short kids cope with stigma without resorting to drugs.

In the face of these public challenges, the NIH suspended recruiting research subjects and convened a panel to speedily review its protocol. Experiments on children must meet certain ethical standards derived from recommendations of the National Commission for the Protection of Human Subjects. These boil down to the requirement that youngsters not be placed at more than minimal risk if they do not have the potential to benefit directly from the outcome of the trial. The appointed panel—made up of pediatric endocrinologists, bioethicists, and others—deliberated, then concluded that the hGH study did, indeed, place its child subjects at somewhat greater than minimal risk. It also agreed that the individual boys and girls would not necessarily benefit. However, the panel decided the experiment should proceed because it did meet one other requirement for children enrolled in research: it could answer vital medical questions about their disorder or condition.

The rules governing experimentation had been written to protect sick children. The panel did not question the underlying value judgment that being very short was equivalent to being sick, and that medical treatment was appropriate. It called extreme short stature a pathological condition. Nor did it dispute that the study's measure for successful treatment should be height.

In 1993, the outgoing head of the NIH allowed recruiting to resume.

UCSF pediatric endocrinologist Melvin Grumbach, who served on the review panel, was happy to see the experiment move forward. He praised the "incredible" parents who allowed their sons and daughters to participate for the advancement of science, without knowing whether or not their children would benefit from the shots. But finding volunteers remained difficult. At the time that the study was suspended, investigators had only managed to enroll thirty-six patients, fewer than half their goal, and two subjects had already dropped out. According to the NIH website, they were still seeking volunteers years later: girls ages nine to fifteen and boys ten to sixteen. A nine-year-old girl needed to measure no more than 3'10" to participate, a ten-year-old boy no more than 4' tall. At age fifteen, girls had to be 4'9½" or less; sixteen-year-old boys no more than 5'1".

Parents understandably hesitated to take the fifty-fifty chance
their child would be among those assigned to years of placebo shots.
Especially since, as one newspaper reported, a significant number of
families who inquired and decided not to enroll still found a physician
willing to give them hGH. At the same time the scientific director of
the National Institute of Child Health and Human Development justified the experiment precisely because it was possible that "growth
hormone doesn't work" and that it "could be dangerous" if it was given
to short healthy kids, pediatric endocrinologists were prescribing it
to short healthy kids. The largest experiment was taking place not at
the NIH but in doctors' offices around the country. Marketing departments helped make it happen.

SCREENING FOR DISEASE OR
SCROUNGING FOR CUSTOMERS?

In Charlotte, North Carolina, in the early 1990s, John and Terri
Trowle brought their eleven-year-old son, Brodie, to a pediatric endocrinologist for evaluation. On the one hand, Brodie was the shortest
in his class—a small boy with a big personality. On the other, both
his parents had been late bloomers. John was a skinny 5'7" senior in
high school who filled out and grew an additional three or four inches
taller in college, a late spurt that he jokingly credited to all the beer
he drank there. The couple expected Brodie also would eventually
reach at least 5'6" or 5'8", which was fine. However, they followed
their pediatrician's recommendation to consult a specialist, just to
eliminate the possibility that any underlying medical problem could
be slowing their son's growth.

Pediatric endocrinologist Mark W. Parker examined Brodie, and
suggested more tests. Parker didn't recommend treatment with biosynthetic hGH, though the couple felt that must be where the tests
were heading. The Trowles harbored doubts about the benefits and
qualms about the long-term risks of hGH therapy; John had a background in both bacteriology and chemical engineering, and had read

about side effects, including the alarm raised over potential links to leukemia. Drawing from their own experiences, they felt equipped to deal with any psychological aspects of Brodie's being short through adolescence. A pediatric endocrinologist was not an expert in psychology, and certainly not an expert on their three children, who all measured below the twenty-fifth percentile. Being short might sometimes cause stress, but the couple didn't think it automatically needed to be psychologically damaging or a deterrent to ultimate success. They had proof of that in Charlotte, which boasted not only the smallest guard in the NBA but the shortest chairman of the board of any major bank in the country. So, although the Trowles wanted to do the best for their son, even to give him advantages they never had, they also kept returning to their belief that, as John summed up later: "Stature is relative. We felt it was not a life-or-death matter."

As the doctor talked, however, the couple felt he assumed they would proceed with treatment. They attempted to express some of their beliefs in Parker's office, but thought the endocrinologist brushed their concerns aside and pressured them to change their views. John Trowle testified before a congressional hearing in 1994 that Parker asked how they would feel when Brodie reached a final height of 5'6" or 5'8" at age eighteen and then demanded to know: "Mom and Dad, you could have put me on growth hormone when I was eight or nine, why didn't you do that to make me 5'10"?"

The Trowles never brought Brodie back to Parker, fearing more tests might only cause their son psychological trauma. John Trowle did write a letter to the Foundation on Economic Trends, Jeremy Rifkin's biotechnology watchdog group; it had lost its fight against the government hGH experiment, but had a standing interest in the drug's misuse, along with a good grasp of how to attract publicity.

The $217 million annual sales of Protropin represented more than one-third of Genentech's total revenue in 1994. The growth spurt in the use of hGH had to be based on more than hypopituitary dwarfism. There were still only a few thousand children in the country each year diagnosed with growth hormone deficiency (GHD) and a study of elementary school children found that, even though the disorder occurred more often than it was diagnosed, it affected only an estimated one in 3,000 to 5,000 American kids a year. Besides GHD, the only other approved use was for chronic kidney disease in children until they were large enough to receive a transplant. This indication, which the FDA added to the label in 1993, included perhaps 2,000 children in the entire country.

Nevertheless, by 1994, some 20,000 children in the United States had received prescriptions for biosynthetic hGH. While physicians could legally order drugs for any medical reason they judged fit, it was illegal for companies to promote their products for off-label use. Industry critics believed companies *were* covertly marketing hGH to short healthy kids and their families.

Critics pointed to height screening programs in elementary schools, which looked like dragnets for tiny customers. In 1993, the Human Growth Foundation received $100,000 from Genentech to organize a screening program in Atlanta's grade schools, measuring about 35,000 students. The foundation trained gym teachers to take the measurements using devices that Genentech supplied. If their child turned up in the lowest five percent for age, parents received a letter urging them to contact either the foundation or a doctor if the family had concerns. That year, Eli Lilly, whose Humatrope had captured about one-third of the U.S. market, was the second-largest donor to the foundation, contributing $45,000. Executives from both companies had sat on the charity's executive board, and at the time of the schools' program remained members of its advisory board.

The Human Growth Foundation still viewed itself as a charitable group of parents reaching out to other parents, just as in the days when Bob Blizzard gathered them together to help publicize the need for pituitaries. But by 1991 it reportedly received some 60 percent of its budget from pharmaceutical companies. The companies described themselves as good citizens who contributed to help educate the public about growth disorders.

In some areas, community screening programs cosponsored by

charity, industry, and health centers bought billboards or newspaper advertisements that boldly asked the public: "Is your child the right size for his age?" or "Are you concerned that your child is too small for his age?" Describing a boy as the "right size," as if all other sizes were wrong, seemed intended to trigger anxiety and a trip to the doctor. Yet only a tiny fraction of children brought to a pediatric endocrinologist have a diagnosable condition and even fewer have a serious illness.

In North Carolina, where the Trowles had been directed to Mark Parker by their pediatrician, other parents received letters directly from Charlotte-Mecklenburg district schools informing them that their sons or daughters had measured in the lowest percentiles of height. As in Georgia, the letter urged parents to contact a physician with their concerns, and included a form to be filled out by a doctor and returned. Pediatric nurse Susan Parker initiated and ran the Charlotte-Mecklenburg School District screening program. She was Mark Parker's wife, and he was the only pediatric endocrinologist serving the region. The letter mailed to parents did not mention this relationship. It also didn't reveal the fact that Genentech supplied the equipment and paid for her salary. When newspaper articles on the program raised questions about this industry connection, the school district announced that it would no longer participate in the screening. A spokesman said that school officials had made a mistake and felt they had been used by Genentech.

CONGRESS HOLDS A HEARING

On October 12, 1994, Congressman Ron Wyden (D-Oregon), armed with documents supplied by the Foundation on Economic Trends, staged a one-day hearing in Washington, D.C., on "Questionable Sales Practices in the Drug Industry." In spite of the broad title, he focused on Genentech's alleged veiled promotion of Protropin. The company had managed to retain two-thirds of the U.S. market in hGH, even though Eli Lilly's product was cheaper. Convening the

Subcommittee on Regulation, Business Opportunities and Technology, Wyden charged that the growth screening project in the North Carolina schools smacked of a "marketing effort." Though he could see the value of screening to identify health problems, he grew suspicious when it was paid for by companies "with a direct interest in identifying potential patients," especially when the company also appeared to have links to the prescribing physician.

Even before the hearing doors opened, Genentech issued a statement that it would cease supporting such programs, though it argued the company had meant to perform a public good, not to promote its products. It would also stop issuing research grants directly to clinicians or paying for such costs as nurses or office equipment.

At the hearing, Mark Parker testified that it had been his wife who designed the North Carolina program for research purposes and that she had approached Genentech to fund it. He defended her motives, describing how she sought to discover whether in-school screening would detect children who weren't growing at a normal rate, and find previously undiagnosed cases of underlying diseases. Parker insisted he had received no patients from the letters home. He told a somewhat different story from the one John Trowle related to the subcommittee. Specifically, Parker denied ever asking the Trowles what they would say if Brodie demanded to know why he hadn't been allowed to grow to 5'10". In fact, Parker emphasized that he did not recommend hGH for Brodie or ever finish his testing and diagnosis. Parker did not consider himself an aggressive prescriber of hGH. He said he spent a considerable amount of time arguing parents out of using it.

Representative Wyden also had his sights set on other industry practices. These included funding doctors' research into unapproved drug uses; offering financial inducements to doctors or hospitals to prescribe specific drugs; and paying doctors who collected information for post-marketing databases, like the follow-up surveillance the FDA demanded of Genentech. The drug industry in the 1990s had become one of the most profitable in the world, largely because of its increasingly creative and aggressive courting of the medical profession. Company marketers showered much more on physicians than pens and prescription pads—money, golf weekends, airline tickets, office overhead expenses. They handsomely paid doctors who delivered papers about the results of trying drugs for unapproved indications and flew other doctors to plush resorts to hear them. (Genentech favored Palm Springs, Pharmacia the Caribbean.) But these studies might be based on a handful of patients, and never undergo the rigorous peer review required for publication in a reputable medical journal. Critics charged this amounted to a financial incentive to prescribe off-label and then use anecdotal evidence to sway other physicians to prescribe off-label, too.

The FDA intended postmarketing databases to monitor the side effects of drugs that had been prescribed for FDA-approved reasons, not as an industry tool to show the positive effects of a drug used in untested ways. A doctor and bioethicist from the University of Minnesota, Steven Miles, told Wyden he worried postmarketing surveys were being turned into "an unregulated form of drug advertising," especially if the surveys became a cheap substitute for expensive and more scientifically valuable controlled trials, and circumvented patient protections for research subjects. Corporate marketing had been thoroughly "integrated" into the training doctors received, Miles complained, as well as into their continuing education when they became practicing physicians. The companies also used "intermediaries" that the public trusted, like the Human Growth Foundation in the North Carolina schools, in ways he thought might "improperly, needlessly, and destructively fan anxieties and fears about social stigmatization from normal physical conditions." If marketing departments peddled stigma and banked on fear, height might be only the beginning.

The American Medical Association had kicked off the 1990s by issuing voluntary guidelines on drug company gifts to physicians. Yet Wyden heard testimony that the Department of Health and Human Services surveyed physicians in 1992 and found 82 percent of those who responded reported pharmaceutical houses had offered them gifts or payments. Moreover, the most frequent prescribers of a drug were the likeliest to receive such offers.

The pediatric endocrinologists were represented, too, and they attempted to give Wyden a quick course in the complicated science of growth. The two who spoke at the hearing on behalf of their professional societies said that while company salespeople, or detailers, visited their offices frequently, neither had witnessed any inappropriate marketing. They believed that school screening of growth rates was a good idea because normal growth is the most important indicator that a child is healthy. They explained that there was a gray area—children without growth hormone deficiency who were both exceptionally small and growing unusually slowly—where doctors exercised their individual judgments about prescribing hGH off-label. But they didn't feel undue pressure to treat short stature as a disease. To the contrary, the physician representing the Endocrine Society, University of Virginia professor Alan D. Rogol, testified that he considered treating short but normally growing children with the hope of improving on their genetic heritage "cosmetic endocrinology" and "unethical." He pointed with some humor to the fact that he himself grew at a normal rate and yet never made even the lowest percentiles, because both his parents had been shorter than five feet. Or as he put it to the committee, "Scottie dogs have Scottie dog puppies and Great Danes have Great Dane puppies."

But FDA Deputy Commissioner Mary Pendergast bluntly questioned whether pediatric endocrinologists did make independent medical judgments, or whether they'd been co-opted. She reminded the committee that doctors had no scientific evidence yet that proved growth hormone treatment worked to make short healthy kids into taller adults. In her view, drug manufacturers were "driving a truck through" a loophole in federal regulations that allowed a doctor to exercise some medical judgment on behalf of a patient—say, trying a cancer drug found effective against one type of solid tumor on a patient with a solid tumor of a different type—"to simply bypass the entire approval process and do a widespread promotion of unapproved uses." Pendergast testified that manufacturers were financing "bogus" scientific seminars and journals to legitimize off-label use, as well as buying the allegiance of doctors, pharmacists, and charities, so that "what we are seeing is that the person or entities that we thought were independent, that we thought cared about us...are really just agents of the drug companies and are being paid to take the positions that they're taking."

These points hit home for the Dobrins, who came from Minneapolis to tell their story in Washington. The Dobrins had made the difficult decision to treat their two sons with hGH. A dozen years later, after spending more than $300,000, the family believed the therapy had done little to no good, especially for their younger son, Benjy.

Benjamin Dobrin, now a young man about 5'10" tall, appeared before the hearing himself and confessed that he never felt he needed medical treatment for height; therefore, he'd secretly skipped many injections after being put on Genentech's Protropin in seventh grade. At monthly checkups, however, nurses still told him, "You're doing great." In the fall semester of his freshman year at high school, when he was about 5'7", he decided to quit taking the hormone. Then he continued to grow three more inches on his own, and gained about thirty pounds.

His father, Stanley Dobrin, picked up the story: The family had been referred to pediatric endocrinologist David R. Brown in the early 1980s, when their older son, Jon, measured two or three standard deviations below the norm for his age. After stimulation tests, Brown diagnosed Jon as having minimal growth hormone output and prescribed Crescorum, pituitary hGH manufactured by Pharmacia, a Swedish company for which Brown consulted. Carol and Stanley Dobrin had been skeptical because, like the Trowles, they had both been small and matured late. Stan grew five inches his freshman year in college, when he was eighteen. They asked why their children wouldn't follow the same pattern. Brown assured them there were no side effects, and while he made no firm prediction of Jon's ultimate height if left untreated, Stan Dobrin recalled, Brown threw out numbers of less than five feet and warned them it would be too late if they waited until the growth plates solidified in puberty. Jon was ten or eleven. "Carol and I basically felt we had little choice. As a responsible parent, I felt we had to do something."

When the CJD outbreak shut down the pituitary hGH supply, Jon went a few months without shots, then began Protropin. The family had known about Brown's relationship to Pharmacia—they had even allowed Jon to be in a film for the company—but they said they were not told about Brown's relationship with Genentech and its distributor, Caremark. Or that Eli Lilly made a significantly cheaper product.

Stan Dobrin was co-owner of a small business, and the medical expenses for his two sons grew so large that insurance premiums for the company soared; eventually, to spare his business partner, he pulled out of the company plan. Jon grew to 5'8" and 130 pounds. They thought he might have benefited by at least a few inches from his treatment, but remained "reasonably convinced" that Benjy had never needed it. They'd been pressured by hearing that, if they were going to act, they had to do it before it was too late. Stanley Dobrin told the hearing: "It's the guilt thing that he did, and I'm told other doctors do the same thing."

Like other parents he had met, Stan Dobrin realized he brought his own childhood experiences as a late bloomer into the consulting room with him: "It was always a little bit difficult, it was never harmful, because I was a reasonably good athlete, and I could always do everything that the other kids could do and I was smart enough to keep up with them in most things." Still. "There was always that problem of being the littlest guy in the class. If there was somebody that was going to get picked on, it was you. You think about that in terms of your own kid, and you say, hey, if you save them that, maybe that's worth it...."

A CRIMINAL TRIAL IN MINNESOTA

The Dobrins' pediatric endocrinologist, David R. Brown, was one of the country's largest prescribers of human growth hormone in the early 1990s, with a reported two hundred to three hundred fifty patients. He was unusual as well, given the rarity of childhood endocrine diseases, in that he had a thriving private practice rather than a position within an academic medical center. He caught the attention of federal investigators.

Just a few months before the Wyden hearing, the government accused Brown of receiving some $1.1 million from Genentech and Caremark "in return for prescribing Protropin." A federal grand jury also indicted Genentech's vice president for sales and marketing for the alleged kickback scheme, as well as Caremark and three of its executives. Caremark, an Illinois-based home health care company, held exclusive rights to distribute Protropin outside of hospitals. Brown, who had established his own consulting company, received money from Caremark and Genentech; but he stated these were research grants and consulting fees, not kickbacks for prescribing.

When a child got Protropin, which was not made available to local pharmacies, the prescription went to Caremark, which delivered the supply to the patient's home, then billed insurance. The government accused Brown of having solicited and received payments from Caremark in exchange for the large number of patients for whom he prescribed Genentech's product. Since Caremark then billed Medicaid for some of these patients, this was a potential violation of the Medicaid/Medicare anti-kickback statute. On the basis of a document summarized in the indictment, the government argued that from January 1, 1989, through April 4, 1990, Caremark gave Brown a $100,000 research grant and received a return of $4,372,000 in revenue from his patient referrals.

About a month before going to trial, Caremark agreed to plead guilty to mail fraud in relation to the case and to pay a $161 million fine. But its officials, as well as the Genentech executive, moved for acquittal, which a federal judge granted after hearing the government's evidence. Brown alone went before a jury. He pleaded innocent.

Brown said the $1.1 million covered the cost of research he'd presented at meetings and consulting he'd done for Genentech. Entering data into the postmarketing survey on two to three hundred patients consumed a lot of time, and so some of the money enabled him to contribute information to the database and to pay his nurse's salary.

During the Minneapolis trial in the late summer and early fall of 1995, a Genentech official testified for Brown's defense that the company did not offer a standard rate to cover costs of filling out paperwork for the database. Instead, doctors individually negotiated such payments. The company didn't follow up on how much money was actually used for the purpose. The prosecution questioned whether this qualified as research, since Brown did not publish results in any peer-reviewed journal. Also, why did the money come from Genentech's marketing and sales division, not its research arm? Sometimes Genentech's detailers did the actual work of entering the data onto the forms.

A central question was whether Brown, in order to boost his payment, prescribed hGH to children who should not have received it. The government brought in only one physician to testify against Brown's prescription practices, a retired endocrinologist from the University of Minnesota who was not a growth hormone expert. Prosecutors had trouble finding any experts who did not have some sort of relationship with hGH manufacturers. But doctors who testified for the defense said they also sometimes prescribed hGH for short normal children and other unapproved uses. In fact, the defense introduced a survey that reported that four out of five pediatric endocrinologists had recommended hGH for children with a variety of diagnoses other than growth hormone deficiency. A Genentech witness stressed the inadequacy of laboratory testing for GHD, and the importance of physician judgment, including the judgment of "how psychologically affected the child is, how many problems they are having in school, how many problems they are having with their peer group."

Brown was convicted of taking kickbacks. However, the judge in the case set aside the verdict after learning that a juror, against the court's orders, had shared the prejudicial knowledge of Caremark's fine with the rest of the jury. The judge ordered a new trial, but federal prosecutors did not pursue the case.

Asked about his case years after the trial, Brown complained bitterly that he'd been singled out for prosecution. He thought the University of Minnesota doctor who testified against him had resented mainly the fact that Brown had opened a private, competitive practice. His entire subspecialty, Brown said, had been somewhat "naïve," and a "captive audience" for the drug industry that had courted them monetarily in ways they had never seen before. He described a meeting in which he and other endocrinologists learned they could be compensated as much as $7,500 for each patient they wrote up for the postmarketing survey, and said he watched as "jaws dropped" among his colleagues while they did the multiplication. Even if that money did not go directly into a doctor's pocket, it could be used by a medical practice to cover a nurse's salary, or by a university medical center to fund a student pediatric endocrinologist.

Though the federal government didn't resume its case against Brown, it did not back off the criminal investigation into Genentech's marketing. The FDA and the FBI interviewed hundreds of people, including detailers and doctors, about how Protropin was sold. They asked pediatric endocrinologists about financial incentives they received for prescribing Protropin "in the name of studying the drug's effectiveness," seeking to determine whether the company's grant programs served as cover for illegal kickbacks. But the government decided to shift its focus from doctors to the marketing department, and from potential kickbacks to Genentech's off-label promotion. The FDA calculated that the company made $20 million from illegally peddling Protropin for use in short normal kids, beginning almost as soon as biosynthetic human growth hormone hit the market in 1985 and continuing until 1994.

Genentech was a different company in 1994 than in years past, the government was willing to concede that. Swiss-based Roche Holdings had obtained a majority interest in Genentech in 1990, bringing in a CEO, G. Kirk Raab, who was a former pharmaceutical salesman. Raab adopted the strategy that there should be no salary limit on what a detailer could make: he rewarded detailers with gold Rolexes, cut bonus checks as large as $380,000, and distributed so much money for cars that his marketers became known as the sales force driving BMWs. Raab told his detailers they did not have to fill out call reports on up to eight doctors a day, like the Big Pharma companies, they could just see one and then maybe take another to play golf. Growth hormone sales reflected his bold marketeering. Genentech's second-quarter results in 1993 reported that sales of Protropin climbed by $3.3 million in that quarter alone, because of "an increased number of patients diagnosed with growth hormone inadequacy."

Raab was ousted over accusations of financial impropriety in 1994, and the man who took over was a scientist, not a salesman. The new CEO, Arthur D. Levinson, called employees together and made what was described as an emotional plea that Genentech should never again face criminal accusations. He established some controls over marketing, including requiring that the legal staff review all sales materials. Growth hormone no longer featured so prominently in the company's portfolio. Genentech was betting on new areas of research and new products, especially cancer drugs.

But that didn't stop other companies from aggressively competing for hGH sales. Pharmacia's former vice president of marketing for Endocrine Care, Peter Rost, discovered after he was hired in 2001 to oversee the company's growth hormone Genotropin, that 25 percent of Genotropin's pediatric sales since 1997 had been for unapproved uses. Pharmacia offered its product for free while patients sought insurance company coverage, a charitable practice Rost noted could be abused to increase off-label prescribing. Especially since detailers were paid cash incentives for each new Genotropin patient, even when the medical condition was an unapproved use—including attempts to reverse aging or to make short normal kids grow.

Rost eventually filed a whistle-blower suit, which he lost. He also wrote a book, *The Whistleblower: Confessions of a Healthcare Hitman*, in which he described how in the late 1990s Pharmacia "paid for many hundreds of physicians to go to wonderful locations in the Caribbean and Mexico," subsidizing their spouses as well. American Medical

Association guidelines prohibited physicians from accepting pharmaceutical industry gifts, but these were research meetings and the doctors were called investigators. An enterprising endocrinologist who prescribed growth hormone from more than one manufacturer might enjoy the incentives, including the resorts, offered by each company.

"Needless to say, few of them did any real studies," wrote Rost, who is also an M.D. "To become an investigator was all too simple: fill out a form with information about how much Genotropin they had given a particular patient, write down a few patient measurements, send it to Pharmacia and—voilà—you're an 'investigator.'"

The cash changed pediatric endocrinology. One pediatric endocrinologist uses the word "seduction" when describing how wine and dollars flowed into the subspecialty, especially in the late 1980s and early 1990s, admitting: "It was too easy to make money." As a group, these were not men and women who went into medicine with visions of huge salaries; they left that to the cardiologists and neurosurgeons. This didn't make them immune—perhaps it even made them more vulnerable—to the sudden influx of money and attention to their work. Like wallflowers who came to the ball with low expectations, they found themselves enjoying the attention of slick partners.

A visible example of this new generosity appeared at the joint meeting held by LWPES and the European Society of Pediatric Endocrinologists in San Francisco in 1993. Pediatric endocrinologists had long complained they couldn't afford travel to international conferences. The chairman that year, UCSF's Melvin Grumbach, remembers he planned for a little more than a thousand doctors to attend and ordered meeting programs accordingly. But with pharmaceutical firms paying travel expenses, that number almost doubled overnight, throwing him into panic when "all of a sudden...these 747s arrive from Europe with these Italian and German and Scandinavian participants."

Each time a company sponsored a symposium for investigators, checkbooks opened. "I gave a talk at one of these meetings, and the next thing you know, you got $2,000 for an hour and a half, and for showing up," Grumbach recalled. Once, when he turned down an expenses-paid invitation to a weekend meeting, the sponsoring company contacted him to ask: "Huh? Wasn't it enough? Do you want more money?" Grumbach explained that he had family events scheduled and hadn't been angling for an additional thousand dollars.

Another pediatric endocrinologist remembers getting a phone call from a friend at one of the companies just to say they hadn't done anything for her in a while, to inquire what she would like, and to offer to write out a check.

Drug houses could also be generous to academic departments that, without their support, wouldn't have had money to train fellows, as the doctors learning a specialty are called. If a university clinic prescribed the company's hGH to enough patients, a detailer might nudge his or her company to throw some money at that school in return. The marketing people would ask the departments what they needed to support a fellow, and offer to pick up the tab. Before being taken over by Pfizer in 2002, Pharmacia liked to brag on its website that it had been "training pediatric endocrinologists since 1993." The cooperative arrangement benefited universities and young physicians in training, certainly, but it also ingrained industry into medical education where it could put its drugs in a positive light, and gave academic clinics the incentive to keep prescribing a company's product.

This influx of money made it unnecessary for younger researchers to endure the same ordeal-by-funding as their academic predecessors. They no longer had to go through the rigorous process of designing a study and competing for NIH grants. Perhaps that change contributed to how few large-scale, long-term studies got done.

A little more than ten years after the introduction of biosynthetic hGH, there were seven major manufacturers competing to market it around the world. There were two large databases compiled from voluntary reporting by doctors—Genentech's Collaborative Growth Study and the survey of European patients begun as the KABI International Growth Study, or KIGS. These two databases alone included more than 40,000 patients who had received treatment with hGH.

Physicians were attempting to modulate growth with a growing arsenal of strategies that included other hormones and peptides with complicated names known by strings of initials: growth hormone-releasing peptide (GHRP), recombinant insulinlike growth factor 1 (IGF-1), anabolic steroids, gonadotropin-releasing hormone agonists (GnRHa). They were identifying other substances, too, that affected bone growth and metabolism, as well as genes linked to short stature. Biotechnology had made that all possible.

Yet with all this experimentation and tens of thousands of patients, a 1999 review of growth hormone research found only eleven randomly controlled studies, the definitive measure of whether something works and is safe. As the authors of that overview wrote in *Clinical and Investigative Medicine*: "The more common strategy has been to rely on donations of drugs from pharmaceutical manufacturers, and to offer treatment to all patients meeting entry criteria or as many patients as the donated resources permit, and sometimes follow the 'refusers' as a parallel comparison group." This could bias the research and make the outcome look more positive, depending on who enrolled and who chose not to, and on who stuck with it or dropped out. Patients getting the best results also seemed likeliest to remain to the end.

When it came to treating kids who did not have GHD, the positive conclusions were not based on following these patients to final adult height, let alone on measuring changes to a young person's quality of life. Doctors assumed hGH worked when it increased growth rate or when a patient grew taller than predicted. But additional hGH gave almost all kids an initial spurt. Also, height prediction methods were based on how people normally grow, and weren't terribly precise even when applied to healthy children. Who knew how accurate they were in a child with Turner syndrome? Height prediction accuracy for the many different conditions now being treated with hGH remained largely uninvestigated.

The authors of the review, Canadian researchers Shane Taback, Guy Van Vliet, and Harvey Guyda, wrote that they could not trace the direct influence of the pharmaceutical companies. They noted there might be other reasons why better and long-term studies were not being done, including the variation in how doctors diagnosed growth disorders and discomfort with the idea of assigning children to a placebo, or fake treatment, group. There was also the history of endocrinology itself, its practitioners' historic faith in their ability to work miracles without needing a scientific study to tell them they'd succeeded. With insulin and cortisone and other treatments from the early part of the century, doctors relied on the evidence of their eyes: dying patients got out of bed and lived.

It seemed as if commercial interests and physicians and anxious families all stood on the same side: the side of using new technology immediately rather than waiting ten or fifteen years for evidence. "Physicians, advocacy groups, and corporations may be impatient with the additional years of study required to follow children until they reach adult height, delaying approval of the drug for prescription, marketing or reimbursement," the Canadian researchers wrote. "As a result, many children may be receiving treatment that will not be ultimately effective."

THE DECADE ENDS FOR GENENTECH

The year 1999 proved an expensive postscript to Genentech's headiest days.

In the spring of that year, the company admitted that from 1985 to 1994, it had aggressively marketed Protropin for short normal kids; it pleaded guilty to one criminal violation of the FDA's rules against promoting a drug for unapproved uses. Genentech and the flagship product that launched an industry made new kinds of history: this was the FDA's first criminal prosecution of a drug company for promoting off-label, and one of the largest penalties a drug company had ever paid. Some of the $50 million settlement was a criminal fine; the rest, a civil penalty to reimburse Medicaid and the federal military insurance program that had footed some of the growth hormone bills.

As part of the plea agreement, the FDA accepted that this criminal behavior ended in 1994, noting that Genentech had new management and had reeducated its sales force on what was legal.

There was still a bit of hGH history, however, that remained to be settled—the dispute over whether Genentech stole the growth hormone gene material that it inserted into bacteria to make Protropin. Genentech had paid the University of California $2 million back in 1979 to deal with allegations that one of its scientists, Peter Seeburg, had swiped patented DNA from a UCSF lab, and then used it at Genentech. But as the profits from biosynthetic growth hormone mounted up, the University of California sued Genentech for patent infringement, seeking billions rather than millions. In 1999, the case finally went to trial in federal court.

No one disputed there had been a raid on a university laboratory. Seeburg described how he and another Genentech employee drove to San Francisco on New Year's Eve, 1978, arriving just shy of midnight, and rode an elevator up to the lab where, as a postdoctoral student a short time before, he had helped isolate the gene for human growth hormone. They took some vials containing the DNA, and raced back down the highway to Genentech. But Genentech argued that the filched material had never been used to make Protropin. Another former Genentech researcher testified that he had succeeded on his own in sequencing the gene that triggered bacteria to churn out recombinant hGH.

Seeburg also was no longer at Genentech, and since his name was on the UCSF patent, he stood to gain more if the university won than if it lost. He testified that they had repeatedly failed in the Genentech laboratory, until they used the stolen DNA. If the jury found that UCSF's patented material lay at the center of Genentech's first product, the university would be entitled to royalties on the sales of Protropin since the beginning. Genentech's accumulated recombinant hGH sales by 1999 had amounted to some $2 billion.

The jury deadlocked over whether Genentech had infringed UCSF's patent. In November 1999, the two parties reached an agreement, one of the largest patent settlements in U.S. history at the time. Genentech paid $200 million, a quarter of it dedicated toward building a new research facility at UCSF. The university general fund received $30 million in cash, and the five scientists who discovered the hGH gene while at UCSF—including Peter Seeburg—split $85 million. Both sides agreed this was not an admission of guilt.

In fact, the relationship between the University of California and Genentech was chummy. The UCLA student newspaper reported that Genentech would be allowed to name the new research building "as a sign of goodwill" and that the company and the university already cooperated in about a dozen joint programs. There was no more ivory tower, at least in the sciences. The colleagues who scorned biologist Herbert Boyer for defecting to industry when he knocked on their doors about his start-up venture by now either took corporate grants, worked in buildings named after corporate donors, or had established companies of their own. Genentech Hall is the edifice that growth hormone built.

CHAPTER 9

"never before in the
history of medicine"

TOO IMPATIENT FOR EVIDENCE

Most doctors weren't waiting for the federal experiment that would take a decade or more to answer the question: Could biosynthetic hGH make a taller adult out of just about any kid who was short? Not when the world had all the human growth hormone it could possibly need, and families wanted to try it.

The availability of recombinant growth hormone changed most things about the way physicians used what had once been rationed. In the 1990s, pediatric endocrinologists prescribed growth hormone not only for more conditions—including idiopathic short stature, constitutional growth delay, and a string of inherited disorders that stunt height—but also at double the dose and frequency as in pituitary-GH days. Those prescribing it were no longer primarily academics conducting growth hormone research. They gave it to patients for longer periods of time. Some routinely bumped up the dose at puberty, though studies hadn't been completed showing the benefit or safety, and it remained unclear what impact hGH therapy had on either the beginning or the duration of puberty.

Each physician developed a personal formula for deciding who should get hGH and how much and for how long, with a lot of instinct and not a lot of scientific evidence to go by. Answering a survey in 1995, 82 percent of the sizable number of pediatric endocrinologists in the United States who responded said they prescribed hGH for short, poorly growing children regardless of the results of stimulation tests used to diagnose growth hormone deficiency. Ten percent gave it to short children who not only passed the tests but were growing normally. Some would prescribe if the child was short enough, others if the child seemed unhappy enough, still others if the child's growth slowed enough, and some if the parents pushed hard enough, or a combination of those factors.

When it came to determining who should be treated, most pediatric endocrinologists continued to order stimulation tests only because their patients' insurance companies required them. They didn't have faith that the tests diagnosed deficiency, which was especially difficult to measure in obese children and those who had short parents; or that the results forecast who would respond to therapy. Besides, they knew they could make kids grow who did not have unequivocal growth hormone deficiency.

The expanding list of patients added up to the fact that, for the first time ever, a lot of children whose bodies produced growth hormone received even more growth hormone by prescription. Pediatric endocrinologists acknowledged that 42 percent of their current patients did not have a deficiency, according to a study of physician recommendation patterns published in 1996, and that about 9 percent of the children had been diagnosed with familial, constitutional, or unknown causes of short stature. They were prescribing hGH to almost half their patients off-label, which meant in cases where its safety and efficacy remained scientifically untested.

Late bloomers, typically boys, with constitutional growth delay were increasingly likely to get medicine. In the pituitary era, physicians would take a family history and look for delayed bone age to make the diagnosis. Delayed bone age meant more time to grow, and doctors would tell parents that almost all these youngsters would reach a normal height in their own good time. Usually, that would be that. In the biosynthetic era, there still were pediatric endocrinologists who avoided treating boys with constitutional delay, seeing their growth patterns as harmless variations of normal puberty.

Many physicians believed these boys suffered more from their sexual immaturity than they did from being short. They would treat late bloomers as they had for decades, not with hGH, but with low doses of testosterone—cheap, well studied, and short-term—to kick off puberty and its growth spurt, whatever the impact on final height. Even then, they applied their own standards. Douglas Frasier at UCLA, for example, did not believe in giving medicine to healthy kids. But he did soften occasionally and give a late-blooming boy testosterone according to his own guidelines: the boy had to be at least fourteen and cry when he described his problems.

However, testosterone, at best, just made a boy reach his final height sooner and, at worst, if it advanced bone age too much, might even cost him some final inches. With growth hormone plentiful, some pediatric endocrinologists felt compelled to do more than wait and see. They could hear the clock ticking even louder than the parents.

"My advice to any family that wants to say, I am a later bloomer, therefore my child is a late bloomer, is to take the growth records of the parents, and compare them [with] the growth record of the patient. If the growth of the father was very, very different from the growth of his son, he has a serious question to answer, and that is: Will my child reach my height?" University of Buffalo pediatric endocrinologist Margaret MacGillivray commented to Congress after listening to the Dobrins and the Trowles complain they'd felt pressured to treat their late-blooming sons. "I'm not worried about a youngster who is 5'4" as an adult if he's not worried about himself being 5'4" as an adult," MacGillivray added.

But now doctors could aim higher. With hGH therapy, late bloomers might make up some of the ground lost in prepuberty when other children their age grew faster, and end up taller than if nature took its slow and unpredictable course. More and more endocrinologists hoped to get these youngsters to target height, according to a formula calculated from the heights of both parents. They called this a child's "genetic potential."

Doctors also experimented with going beyond genetic potential, by increasingly prescribing hGH for children with a variety of genetic disorders, even when there was no hard evidence that it would improve either height or well-being. The 1995 survey of physician practices found that the responding pediatric endocrinologists treated a median of six "therapeutic indications beyond proven efficacy"; in other words, they ordered hGH for half a dozen uses without knowing that it would work. Some of these conditions caused far more disabling effects than retarding growth, which made other medical experts question why doctors would expose these children to risk just to add a few inches.

The experimental use of growth hormone in children with Down syndrome drew especially scathing reactions from some physicians, who questioned the benefit of trying to make such children taller given all the other cognitive and physical disabilities associated with the chromosomal condition. When a study of Down-syndrome children who received growth hormone appeared in the *Journal of Pediatrics* in 1992, one pediatric endocrinologist wrote to condemn the hazards of giving hGH to these children, who not only produce normal amounts of growth hormone, but also have a predisposition to leukemia. He asked acidly whether parents assumed that increased head circumference could somehow be equated with increased intelligence.

It was enormously satisfying to make a kid grow. So satisfying that some did not stop trying with growth hormone alone. For a while, doctors also experimented with growth hormone–releasing hormone (GHrH), which is made in the hypothalamus of the brain and stimulates the pituitary gland to manufacture growth hormone. But giving extra GHrH did not produce the expected boost. They had more success manipulating another hormone, one that delayed puberty.

MANIPULATING PUBERTY

Paradoxically, at the same time pediatric endocrinologists prescribed recombinant hGH to late-blooming boys because they expressed sympathy for a teenager who still looked like a child, they also sometimes artificially kept other patients childlike to increase final height. They called this "managing puberty."

The idea of controlling the timing of puberty for the purpose of making kids taller occurred to pediatric endocrinologists who noticed what happened when they treated children with precocious puberty: typically, girls younger than eight who started developing breasts or younger than ten who began menstruating, or boys below the age of nine whose genitals matured. Endocrinologists could stop this premature sexual development, or even reverse it, by giving patients something to suppress sex hormones. Gonadotropin-releasing hormone agonists (GnRHa), marketed most widely as Lupron, halted puberty in its tracks; doctors discovered the longer they waited before letting it start up again, the taller the kids grew. With Lupron, doctors could artificially prop open the growth plates that maturation closes.

Unfortunately, when they tried it on kids with normally timed puberty, suppressing their sex steroids also slowed their growth, and offset the advantage of delaying bone age. They might still be only four feet tall at age sixteen, even if they kept growing till they were twenty. But endocrinologists could add hGH to the equation. GnRHa to extend growing time, plus hGH to boost growth rate, should equal added height.

Like everything about altering height—except for the consensus that true growth hormone deficiency should be treated—delaying puberty sparked controversy among doctors themselves. As one pediatric endocrinologist put it: "Adolescence is hard enough when everything's going right," let alone when a boy is the only one in the locker room without pubic hair. And there were questions about whether a medication that delayed puberty might lead to weakened bones or have a long-term effect on reproduction. Lupron added another

$10,000 or so a year on top of the already hefty cost of growth hormone. Still, some families would pay just about anything.

Bioethicists didn't sit in those medical offices where the decision to try growth hormone in a case that was not clear-cut turned into a negotiation between doctors, parents, and insurance companies. Pediatric endocrinologists found themselves pushing unfamiliar ethical boundaries. At several conferences called in the 1990s and in medical journals they debated: Who besides kids with growth hormone deficiency should get growth hormone therapy? When should treatment stop? Should they keep going until patients reached the bottom of the normal range—about 5'3" for a male and 4'11" for a female in the United States? Or should they continue as long as a child was still growing, as parents typically wanted? Who should decide, physicians or families? Within families, children or parents? Was it fair to give hormone to one youngster diagnosed with growth hormone deficiency, but not to another who was just as short? Wasn't that penalizing someone because medical science didn't know all the answers about growth? What were the risks of giving growth hormone to a normal child, especially long-term, and were they worth it?

The drug manufacturers had a stake in these philosophical debates as well, of course.

TURNER SYNDROME OPENS A DOOR

In the early days, when Genentech had a product in search of a market, the company asked the two Stanford University pediatric endocrinologists who had helped them with their first trials of recombinant hGH, Raymond Hintz and Ron Rosenfeld, what group of patients should be the next target. Turner syndrome girls, they replied, and ticked off the reasons: the condition affects about one in every 2,000 females—by their estimation, 150,000 girls and women in the United States alone. Almost all of them end up with significant short stature, an average adult height of about 4'8". Unlike growth hormone deficiency, Turner syndrome could be definitively diagnosed with a chromosome study.

"So they were a great group to go after," Rosenfeld said, recalling the discussion. "That was our recommendation." Genentech began studying biosynthetic growth hormone's potential in Turner syndrome practically from the day its bacteria started churning.

Unlike patients with hypopituitary dwarfism, girls with Turner syndrome have normal levels of growth hormone. An important line was about to be crossed.

In the 1980s, pediatric endocrinology clinics saw few girls with the condition, which arises when a female baby is born missing all or part of one of the two X chromosomes that are normal to women. "A lot of the patients weren't diagnosed. Nobody was really concerned about short girls. Teachers weren't worried, parents weren't worried, doctors would say, 'She's a girl, so she'll be cute,'" according to Rosenfeld. Besides, medicine couldn't change the abnormality, which occurs randomly and causes a lack of ovarian development and other effects besides short stature. Girls could be put on estrogen in adolescence so they would develop breasts and other secondary sexual characteristics, though that would not make them fertile.

Then along came biosynthetic growth hormone, which could not give these girls the ability to reproduce, but might make them taller so they would stand out less: "It doesn't cure the condition, but these families were so desperate for anything that could help them. Suddenly these patients came out of the woodwork," Rosenfeld said.

With Genentech's backing, Rosenfeld and Hintz organized the first Turner syndrome support group at Stanford; it expanded to become a national organization. The pharmaceutical companies were pleased to finance international Turner syndrome symposia as well. The industry attention and funding that led to educational material, parent support groups, and even special clinics all benefited the girls and their families, according to Rosenfeld. He "can name a hundred other pediatric conditions that have never gotten this kind of attention." It also created a potential lobby to work for FDA approval.

A late-1980s study authored by Rosenfeld, Hintz, and a Genentech researcher found that growth hormone treatment made girls with Turner syndrome grow. Even before a well-controlled trial had been completed, a spate of small industry-sponsored studies spread the impression that hGH boosted these girls to above five feet. Still, there were major questions.

It wasn't only that girls with Turner syndrome do not have abnormal levels of natural growth hormone. To accelerate their growth, doctors had to inject them with doses two to three times higher than they gave children with growth hormone deficiency. Giving them more meant they would have above-normal levels—in essence, a touch of acromegaly. In fact, one of the first things mothers of these girls typically noticed when their daughters began hGH treatment was the increasing size of their feet and hands. The girls did not seem to mind.

When the FDA approved biosynthetic hGH for use in kids with chronic kidney disease, another group who make enough growth hormone, the agency argued it was helpful for children who would have been normal height if their disease had not interfered to stunt their growth. A child could grow to a better size to get a kidney transplant. So hGH could be looked at as part of the treatment of the disease.

But the FDA balked at adding Turner syndrome. The agency asked for data, not just on whether this would make these patients grow faster, but also on whether it would improve final height. It did not ask for proof that the therapy helped girls psychologically, but families seemed convinced that it did. Genentech and Lilly combined their data and went to the FDA together, with support from the family groups.

Some pediatric endocrinologists who opposed hGH for short normal boys supported efforts to gain a little extra height for Turner syndrome girls, arguing the aim in this instance was more than cosmetic: it might allow a woman to work at a desk, reach cabinets in a kitchen, drive a car, and generally function better in the adult world. If those were appropriate goals for short males, those should also be appropriate goals for females.

In 1997, the FDA, satisfied that most evidence showed the therapy could make these girls taller women, approved biosynthetic hGH for the treatment of short stature in Turner syndrome. Afterward, the Turner Syndrome Society complained that it received just as many phone calls from parents with stories about insurance company denials. The society argued that treatment was important because it meant "lessening the chief visual cue that sets these individuals apart." But insurance companies could see into the future: the FDA approval opened a door that could assume much larger—and more costly—importance later. Biosynthetic hGH had been approved for the sole purpose of increasing final height in children who produce normal levels of growth hormone.

While most studies showed better final height compared with predicted height in cases of Turner syndrome, the improvement was modest and variable. Height prediction, imprecise even in normal children, was especially uncertain in a syndrome that sometimes produces skeletal disorders. Some women remained significantly short even with therapy, their expectations raised higher than their final measurements.

There also had been no evaluation of the psychological benefits of treatment, even if it did add height. The best strategy for increasing final height depended on holding off puberty by giving the girls estrogen later. But some asked whether the trade-off, delaying breast development, was worth it psychologically and socially for a teenager who wants to look like other teenagers, and who also has to deal with the knowledge that she probably cannot have her own child. This led some to wonder what the rationale was for giving the girls years of expensive injections. Nonetheless, by 1998, U.S. doctors prescribed growth hormone in about 96 percent of Turner syndrome cases they saw.

More than half of the pediatric endocrinologists in the United States—58 percent—also acknowledged that they recommended growth hormone for at least some children with idiopathic short stature, though that remained unapproved by the FDA.

IF THE FAMILIES PUSH HARD ENOUGH

The decision to prescribe hGH, even in cases where it posed risks and the benefits remained unclear, was not being made on medical grounds alone. There were cultural factors at work, too. When doctors answered questions in the mid-1990s about why they prescribed hGH, psychosocial reasons led the list. Almost all the pediatric endocrinologists agreed that "short stature matters" and that it had a negative impact emotionally in children and later, when the kids became adults. Few thought that youngsters between the third and fifth percentile were never emotionally impaired by their height, and barely any thought that this was true for those below the third percentile.

Many, almost a third, also believed that hGH helped kids emotionally, even if it didn't finally turn them into taller adults. Not unexpectedly, the more they saw short stature as an emotional handicap and hGH as a positive antidote, whether or not it added final inches, the more likely pediatric endocrinologists were to prescribe.

They were more likely to recommend treatment for boys than girls. Other nonmedical factors influenced their decision making as well, including price and what the families wanted. If it cost less, and if families pushed hard, they would pull out their prescription pads even more often. If the price ever fell radically to only a hundred dollars a year, doctors said, they would prescribe it in twice as many cases. If families strongly wanted treatment, recommendations grew almost one and a half times.

Obviously, it paid off for manufacturers to try to influence the attitudes of both families and physicians: the difference between the 14,000 American kids with GHD eligible for treatment and all 1.7 million children with short stature was the difference between an annual growth hormone bill of about $182 million and one of $22 billion. While they couldn't legally promote growth hormone to short normal kids, they could peddle the idea that being short condemned youngsters to misery.

Eli Lilly's pamphlet "Short Stature Due to Growth Hormone

Deficiency" reassured parents that children tease each other about all kinds of personal characteristics "that do not meet the normal standard," from glasses to braces to hair color. "Stature is no different; both very tall and very short children become the object of other children's attention and sometimes their jokes." But it turned out that being short *was* different: "Short stature is the more troubling because Western society values tallness and tends to view shortness as an inadequacy."

In their material for parents, other manufacturers talked about growth hormone deficiency, but made clear that many short nondeficient youngsters also received hGH. By implication, all "slow growers" and those with "abnormal stature" were at risk: playmates and teachers might treat them as younger, and "teasing and name-calling may lead to insecurity and behavioral problems." On the other hand, "even transitory increases in height" could boost self-confidence at a critical period such as entering school. In a typical testimonial on a pharmaceutical website, a mother gushed that hGH could help her daughter achieve the goal of becoming a Hollywood actress, because the girl would be depressed and lack confidence without it. According to the flashy brochures and websites, biosynthetic hGH had helped children become more socially successful and made them feel better about themselves. The frequent mention of the sports teams children joined after they began therapy seemed to suggest that hGH even turned kids into athletes.

But the evidence that short stature caused significant psychological and social problems, or that treatment made life better, did not add up to anything as definitive as a slam dunk. Brian Stabler, the University of North Carolina psychologist who was a Genentech consultant, wrote the studies that companies especially liked to cite. He consistently found that kids diagnosed either with GHD or idiopathic short stature had problems with adjustment (in 1991), problems with academic achievement (in 1994), and problems with behavior (in 1998). He also found that, though hGH therapy didn't improve either academic performance or social competence, it did help behavioral problems. "Study: Behavioral Problems Can Follow Shortness, Growth Hormones Could Help," the university press office announced, and news outlets around the world translated this into headlines reading "Short Kids Likely to Be Misfits" and "Very Short Children Prone to Bad Behavior."

Beginning in the late 1980s and extending into the 1990s, the British attempted to look at the wider population, not just those brought to growth clinics by worried parents. The Wessex Growth Study set out to investigate how most short kids got along out in the community. The researchers concluded that they seemed to function fine in childhood. There was little increase in the risk of psychiatric disease "simply as a result of being very short."

As Linda Voss, a lead investigator in the Wessex Growth Study, wrote, no empirical study captured the everyday experiences of short and tall stature, and trying to differentiate between slight and serious stress, or between stress and poor adjustment, was especially difficult when dealing with children. Even being at risk of poor body image and lower self-esteem did not mean worse quality of life. There is more to someone than height. She reminded those who believed that height should be treated that short stature, usually defined as the lowest three percentiles, was only a statistical category; "in our haste to correct the 'abnormality' we could be in danger of paying too little attention to the whole person or child whose body we were seeking to modify."

Similarly, in the Netherlands, when researchers looked at kids around the third percentile who came to clinics versus those who did not, they found growth clinics drew children who blamed their problems on height and whose parents also had negative experiences being short. Extremely short youngsters who never saw the inside of a clinic found height something of a practical problem and wanted to be taller, but either didn't see it as medical problem or had found ways to cope—the chief strategy being "acceptance."

Short kids got teased. Studies confirmed teasing was common. But multiple pieces of research found short kids well adjusted in terms of social skills and self-esteem. They were not handicapped academically or socially, but normal. They not only were accepted by their peer group but had a relatively positive self-perception. Kids who were just short remained difficult to differentiate from average kids in how they went about their lives.

Not only did it remain unproven that short stature caused significant emotional problems, but also it was far from clear that treatment made life better. Looking at those with idiopathic short stature who did get hGH, the Dutch didn't find it had made a difference in quality of life. They did discover, however, that patients greatly overestimated the height they gained from the years of injections.

Summary after summary of the psychosocial data toward the end of the 1990s reached the same conclusion: There was little evidence that short stature led to lower self-esteem or lower quality of life for kids. And little or conflicting evidence that it led to lower quality of life for adults.

This did not mean that society did not greatly value height. A 1990 study of salaries among MBAs found that taller men had "marginally greater" annual starting salaries and, more significant, that height became more important later in their careers when each additional inch tended to increase salary by $600 a year. This supported earlier work on power and height. Perhaps tall men suggested dominance, even unconsciously, and their powerful image won them financial rewards. The $600-per-inch finding spread like gospel. But the same study found short men did not feel discriminated against. And overweight men suffered even larger financial penalties.

Frustrated by research that looked at different populations, asked different questions, used different measurements, and came up with different answers, pediatric endocrinologists relied on their own assumptions. Their subspecialty didn't teach them how to treat behavior problems. They tended to believe their own experiences, and the experience of a pediatric endocrinologist rarely brought him or her into contact with an extremely short child who did not have difficulties, who did not suffer.

In their clinics they saw kids with physical problems beyond height, like patients with Turner syndrome or short-limbed dwarfism. Also, patients who came to clinics came because they had concerns, or at least their parents did. The shortest kids in growth clinics did not necessarily exhibit the most behavior problems. Those who did demonstrate the most emotional difficulties tended to belong to families, especially from upper socioeconomic groups, who had higher expectations and worried about psychological problems. Parents preferred to bring their children in with a physical disorder rather than seek out mental health services for family problems. Frequently these parents remained dissatisfied with their own heights.

Even parents with unhappy memories of adolescence, though, thought twice when given the information about what hGH therapy really accomplished in most cases. One study explored whether parents who had been unusually short kids themselves would consider trying to make their children taller. The parents generally responded that they wished their offspring could be tall. They remembered how they had been teased and treated like babies, that they had problems finding age-appropriate clothes and getting dates. Being short had often been painful. But the study found these adults had turned out to be well adjusted and functioning. When asked if they would consider treating their own youngsters for height, just under half said yes. That number dropped dramatically—to only 14 percent—when they were told the gain would be two inches.

A MODEST BUMP TO FINAL HEIGHT?

In spite of the lack of clear evidence coming from psychologists, the medical professional societies in the United States cited children's emotional health when they weighed in with guidelines in the late 1990s, cautiously endorsing hGH for short normal kids in certain circumstances, while acknowledging that it remained experimental and carried potential side effects. Though the Lawson Wilkins Pediatric Endocrine Society continued to advocate against hGH for idiopathic short stature outside a clinical trial, the society's 1995 guidelines instructed members to consider how a family viewed shortness before deciding whether or not to prescribe. In 1998, both the American

Association of Clinical Endocrinologists and the American College of Endocrinology issued guidelines for clinical practice, referring to the "handicap of short stature," and suggesting growth hormone could be considered for reasons other than hormone deficiency. The Endocrinology Society in Britain commented that physical stature correlated with social status, and noted that those late bloomers with slow growth and psychosocial problems might benefit from hGH.

The American Academy of Pediatrics stated that GH was recommended for extremely short children whose size "keeps them from participating in basic activities of daily living and who have a condition for which the efficacy of GH therapy has been demonstrated." Even when offering the advice that it might be better in most cases to help kids develop pride in themselves and their accomplishments, the academy noted in its discussion that being tall in our culture brought indisputable benefits, from income to academic achievement to self-esteem and social status.

But was treatment effective? Was it safe? Even at the end of a decade of experimentation, no one could say for sure.

Two major studies drew opposite conclusions about whether hGH therapy worked to make short normal kids taller adults: French research published in the *British Medical Journal* and headlined on the front page of *The New York Times* in 1997 declared that biosynthetic hGH not only had proven ineffective in adding final height but could even stunt ultimate growth in children without growth hormone deficiency. The *British Medical Journal* editorialized in September 1997 that on the basis of these findings, hGH should not be used for short normal children. In Japan, some research also found cases where GH therapy accelerated bone maturation and therefore might be counterproductive.

On the other hand, Raymond Hintz, lead author on a Genentech-sponsored study published in early 1999, summarized his results with the flat statement that hGH could increase adult height in children with idiopathic short stature. Treatment boosted some kids beyond their predicted heights. It did not make them tall; on average, it added about two inches. Two inches, critics pointed out, was about the margin of error for the standard American method of height prediction, Bayley-Pinneau; they questioned how even that modest bump could be attributed to the hormone.

Some kids grew more than two inches, some got no benefit; most did not reach target height. Even if some children did end up incrementally taller, there was no way to tell before investing in years of shots which ones those would be. Hintz himself said he found the results "somewhat disappointing." Headlines reflected this "good news, bad news" aspect, ranging from "Hormone Boosts Height for Some Kids" to "Study Questions Growth Hormone Use in Children."

Reviewing four decades of GH therapy for short children, Canadian expert Harvey Guyda concluded in 1999 that the results *had* been disappointing, except in cases of growth hormone deficiency. Hintz's study remained much more positive than others, but Guyda argued that its high dropout rate made it suspect.

Given what was known at the end of the decade, if the injections worked at all, a short healthy child typically gained about an inch and a half or two (3 to 5 cm), which added up to about $18,000 a centimeter and some twenty-five hundred shots. No significant psychosocial benefits had been demonstrated. The assumptions from the 1980s—that short, normal height was a disadvantage both in childhood and adulthood—had not been proven. Constitutionally delayed boys typically seemed more concerned about late puberty. For kids in general, height represented only one concern in their daily lives. Psychological intervention made more sense to one prominent member of the British Pediatric Endocrinology Society, at least, who concluded: "The case for intervention with growth hormone seems to be rather thin."

OTHER UNSETTLED QUESTIONS

Against this rather modest possible benefit, parents needed to weigh the still unknown long-term risk. The databases seemed to indicate hGH was safe in the short term. According to Genentech's postmarketing surveillance, reports of what are termed "adverse events" had been rare in GH treatment; even those that had been reported were difficult to attribute to the GH shots, because of the variety of patients and their diagnoses. These events included cases of intracranial hypertension (also called benign pseudotumor cerebri), pressure in the fluid around the brain that can cause severe headaches and, if ignored, threaten eyesight, but which typically disappeared if shots were suspended. Also, dark moles grew larger; there were reports of tumors, inflammation of the pancreas, and breast enlargement in boys, though the link to hGH had not been proven. Earlier suspicions that the therapy caused leukemia in the absence of other risk factors had not been substantiated. Neither had its relationship to the curvature of the spine called scoliosis, but scoliosis can occur whenever there is fast growth, as can a painful hip condition that was also reported among children taking growth hormone. Called slipped capital femoral epiphysis, or SCFE, it occurs when the ball-shaped head slips backward off the thighbone.

Of course, these conclusions about risks depended on whether the reporting was accurate and whether it continued. Databases tend to underreport adverse events. Doctors who enroll patients in them are asked to report those occurrences they believe are associated with the medication. If a physician didn't believe that a side effect had been caused by hGH, the case wouldn't necessarily be reported; and the largest prescribers of any drug are those who believe in its safety.

Attempts to look at safety outside databases remained few. For example, only two or three studies directly examined the effects on blood pressure and the heart. Among those, one European study showed that children dependent on GH therapy who withdrew from it not only grew significantly more slowly than they had before they began treatment but also developed reduced cardiac output—leading to questions of permanent changes. Because of that, in 1997, the *Journal of Pediatrics* asked whether GH was good or bad for the heart, and called for a long-term investigation, especially among patients who were not growth hormone deficient.

Just as there was consensus that hGH was largely safe in the short term, there was also consensus that long-term safety remained unknown. There were theoretical causes of concern: malignancies can take decades to develop, and growth hormone is potentially carcinogenic; it signals the liver to produce insulinlike growth factor, or IGF-1, which has been found to stimulate breast cell growth in the laboratory. Slightly elevated hGH might explain the finding that women taller than 5'6" have twice the risk of breast cancer, particularly before menopause, than women under 5'3". The degree of cancer risk involved in giving additional hGH to children whose bodies already manufacture a normal amount remained unknown.

Diabetes, hypertension, and joint problems are common in people whose pituitaries overproduce growth hormone and cause acromegaly. So those illnesses also remained possible hazards. Diabetes bore monitoring, especially in Turner syndrome, where it has a high natural occurrence.

Then there was potentially worrisome evidence on longevity: short people live longer. In 1997, scientists who had implanted either human or bovine growth genes into mice reported that the mice doubled in size but also aged prematurely, surviving half as long as their non-engineered relatives.

At the end of the decade, safety had not been firmly established and many other questions remained unsettled, starting with the definition and diagnosis of short stature. The standard definition of growth hormone deficiency had expanded, so that compared with a child in the pituitary era, a child in the 1990s could produce twice as much hormone naturally and be diagnosed with GHD. Even so, as children who had previously been diagnosed with GHD became adults and were retested, as many as 60 to 70 percent responded with normal levels, meaning that their deficiency either had gone away or had never existed. This raised suspicion of widespread overdiagnosis.

Evidence favored "very early and prolonged treatment"—starting children younger than five to get the best possible long-term results and, because its effect lessened over time, using it as long as possible.

Yet studies showed more hormone might lead to better results or, to the contrary, might unduly advance bone age and stunt final height. Higher doses also increased the likelihood of side effects. Increased doses at puberty might add height in the short term but accelerate and shorten puberty. Artificially delaying puberty improved final stature, but if it also prolonged the sexual immaturity that children minded even more than being short, any psychological benefits might be lost. There remained no agreement on when to stop. Even though Hintz's study confirmed what many pediatric endocrinologists already suspected, and what some had liked to say for years—use enough hGH and you can make even a stone grow—the question remained whether or not it was worth it.

But plenty of parents still wanted it. Kids would rejoice to see the new inch marks on the kitchen wall. There was always the chance that a child might hit the hGH jackpot and gain a lot of height, or at least catch up to his friends faster and get picked on less. Patients tended to be very satisfied with the results, even though no increased quality of life after therapy had been proven.

The insurance industry in the United States, especially in the era of increased managed care, attempted to apply the brakes, although different insurers held different policies. Some would allow experimental use on a case-by-case basis. Some stated flatly that they didn't consider giving growth hormone to children with idiopathic short stature a medically necessary treatment of disease. Insurers had more at stake than the considerable expense of tampering with height; they worried about other technologies that might be down the road as well, and felt pressure to draw the line between treatment and enhancement.

Many medical experts, too, felt uneasy. One doctor noted the large percentage of American youngsters getting hGH who were not growth hormone deficient, and that in cases like Turner syndrome they were being pushed beyond genetic potential. He concluded, in the journal *Growth, Genetics & Hormones*: "Never before in the history of medicine has a biologic agent been used in an attempt to produce such widespread and permanent physical changes." He warned that even without considering psychology, the benefits to final height and the ultimate safety for short normal kids remained unknown. The experiment continued, at the NIH and outside it.

At the same time, in Australia, some women who had been tall girls were learning that they'd been part of a different experiment.

reckonings

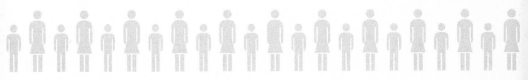

CHAPTER 10

absence of evidence is

not evidence of absence

WETTENHALL MAKES HEADLINES AGAIN

On Friday, June 27, 1997, Janet Cregan-Wood, then forty-three and a health care worker with two sons, spotted a headline in a Melbourne newspaper that transported her back to a year of her childhood she'd tried hard to forget. "Hormone Tests on Teenage Girls Referred to Inquiry," read the headline in *The Age*. According to the article, Australia's federal health department was reviewing a medical trial in which DES was given to more than 160 girls from the state of Victoria between 1959 and the mid-1970s in an attempt to reduce their adult height. "One of the researchers, Dr. Norman Wettenhall . . . yesterday refused to comment."

Janet was dumbstruck. She remembered her visits to Wettenhall during those years; she must have been one of the girls. She had stayed with the therapy for less than a year before the side effects had sidelined her. Her predicted height had been 5'11". Her final height was 5'10". Had she been part of a medical trial when she was a child and never realized it? Had her mother, Peg, knowingly enrolled her in an experiment—one that had transformed Janet from a tall, slender girl to an unhappy, overweight young woman? One that may have pushed her into a serious depression that required hospitalization? One that caused Peg to burn all the photographs taken of Janet during this period because they brought back such painful memories? Surely her mother would not have agreed to a treatment that was not a proven therapy.

Over the weekend, Janet called her mother and told her about the article, and another that appeared the next day in *The Herald-Sun*, which reported that Wettenhall would be happy to speak to an official inquiry and that his conscience was clear about the treatment. Peg said she was sure the pills Janet took had not been part of a trial or experiment; Janet had been a private patient and nobody had ever said anything about a study.

On Monday, Janet screwed up her courage and called one of the reporters who had broken the story in *The Age*. She explained that she had been one of the tall girls treated by Wettenhall, and asked if he could send copies of the research papers he had unearthed for the article. Then she called *The Herald-Sun*, which reported that several worried tall women who had been treated had contacted a support group for DES daughters and mothers looking for information. Janet called as well and was told the DES group had information about the effects of diethylstilbestrol on the offspring of pregnant women who had received the drug, but nothing on the long-term effects of DES given to young girls. They could, however, give Janet the phone numbers of the other concerned tall women who had also telephoned looking for information.

Finally, Janet telephoned the University of Melbourne. Remembering the basement in the red brick building where she had stood naked on a brightly lit platform for what seemed hours while men in white coats measured and photographed her, Janet hoped her records, including the photographs that had been so embarrassing, could shed light on the type of study or experiment in which she'd unknowingly been involved. The university suggested she write a formal letter requesting the information.

As Janet read through the research papers authored by Wettenhall and supplied by the newspaper reporters, her fear that she'd been part of some sort of experiment seemed justified. "It was not known at the outset that treatment would be effective, but oestrogen was considered worthy of trial," she read. "Stilboestrol was chosen as it had been in use for many years and its effects were well known."

But they hadn't been well known. Janet remembered the stir that had been caused when stilboestrol, or DES, was found in the 1970s to cause cancer and reproductive difficulties in young women whose mothers had been given the drug during pregnancy.

On July 3, after reading and rereading the research papers, Janet turned to the list of telephone numbers she'd been given by the DES support group, and with hesitation began to call the other women who'd sought information about the treatment. Janet had confided in only a few people about what she'd undergone as a child, and she found it difficult to initiate a conversation with a complete stranger about something that had been emotionally painful and personal. But the first few conversations went well. In fact, Janet felt an instant rapport with the women whose stories turned out to be so similar to her own. They talked about how tall they were and how tall they were predicted to be. They discussed the doctors who had treated them. None of them thought they were taking part in a medical trial; all assumed the pills were standard therapy. And all had suffered medical problems that they believed might be related to what they'd been given for their height. They agreed to meet.

On July 9, *The Age* published a letter to the editor from the scientific director at Royal Children's Hospital Research Foundation. He defended Wettenhall's meticulous recordkeeping, and argued that medical advances could not be made without clinical trials. "Benefits are enjoyed today as a result of past contributions by public-spirited individuals who volunteered," he wrote. But Janet hadn't volunteered, nor had any of the other women she'd been talking to. Three days later, eight women—five tall women and three of their mothers— gathered at Janet's home for the first time. Although they were strangers, the ice broke easily as the women, all tall, found themselves in the unusual situation of facing one another eye to eye.

When comparing medical histories, the women learned they had more than their height in common. "Of that original group," recalled Janet, who speaks carefully and thoughtfully, "none of us were exactly the same, but of the five women two had never been able to conceive, all of us had required surgical intervention for ovarian cysts. We had endometriosis. Depression had been a big problem for all of us. So we asked the question: Is it just coincidence? Or is it related to this thing we all shared in our lives?"

After listening to one another's experiences, daughters and mothers got to work. They agreed that what they wanted was an investigation by the government that would explain fully what had happened, how it had happened, and what sorts of long-term effects on their health the treatment may have caused. They also drafted a letter to the editor in response to the scientific director's assertion that they had been "public-spirited volunteers."

"Neither we, nor our parents, ever knew that we were part of an ongoing experiment," they declared. Furthermore, in light of the health problems resulting from stilboestrol exposure, they asked for a "properly conducted epidemiological follow-up, not paternalistic reassurance that the treatment given to us was without fault, ethically and medically."

They called themselves the DES Tall Girls. Each put ten dollars into a kitty to cover postal and copying expenses and sent off the letter with Janet's phone number as a contact. They agreed to reconvene in three weeks.

On July 15, the letter appeared under the headline "Tall Girls Require More Real Research." Janet's phone began ringing and didn't stop. Newspapers and radio stations called to set up interviews, and suddenly, after more than thirty years, the treatment of tall girls was back in Australia's newspapers. But unlike the chirpy testimony from young teens happy with their curvy new figures, these articles listed a catalog of bitter complaints from women now in their thirties and forties who feared the therapy had injured them physically and emotionally.

GOING PUBLIC

Janet was no stranger to political activism; she and her longtime partner, Ed Wolf, had marched and spoken out about government decisions or inaction on a number of occasions. But agreeing to be interviewed about something so personal was different. It meant airing in public very private experiences: her past problems with obesity and severe depression, her three miscarriages, her surgery for ruptured ovarian cysts, and the year of wearing rubber pants to school. She wasn't eager to do it, but knew it could serve at least two useful purposes. First, she hoped media coverage of the story would pressure the government to fund a follow-up study to determine if these health problems were, in fact, related to the treatment. Since the federal government's health department had provided funding for the experiments decades earlier, it seemed reasonable that it should undertake a follow-up study to see if this group of women who had been treated in childhood were suffering a disproportionate number of problems.

Second, the media was the only way to reach other women who had been treated, and so far, it was achieving this purpose. The publicity over the next few weeks brought calls from dozens of Tall Girls all over Australia. Janet kept careful notes, looking for similarities and patterns. Her ironing board became her office, and she purchased an answering machine to help with the calls she missed when she was at work. School was out, and Ed, a teacher, found himself taking long, sometimes heartbreaking messages from women who had been treated years earlier. Janet returned calls when she got home from work, but each conversation could take an hour or more. Women who had never talked about the therapy with anyone else finally had a sympathetic ear, and they had a lot to say about an assortment of physical and psychological problems. Some had been unable to conceive; others, like Janet, had suffered miscarriages. Some, like Janet, had developed ovarian cysts, many complained of severe endometriosis. Some recalled a surge in libido at an inappropriately young age. Mood swings, eating disorders, and depression plagued others. Some complained they were given frequent internal pelvic exams as part of the treatment that were unnecessary, even abusive. One mother told Janet that a physician in Tasmania had treated her daughter when she was only eight years old. The girl, who was suddenly pushed into puberty, ended up only 5'3"—a foot shorter than her predicted height of 6'3". The girl's mother wondered if her daughter's muscle and skeletal problems were related to this.

Often, Janet was moved to tears by the women's stories: some mothers expressed profound guilt for having permitted their daughters to be treated, blaming themselves for their daughters' infertility and their own lack of grandchildren. The most Janet could do was listen and then mail copies of the early research papers she'd acquired. Peg stepped in to help around the house and transport the couple's younger son to and from school now that Janet was tethered to her telephone and the growing pile of notes and messages on the ironing board. By the first of August, Janet had heard from nearly seventy tall girls. She'd also heard back from the University of Melbourne: none of the documents and photographs related to Janet's medical history could be located. Decades earlier, Alex Roche, the anatomist who had been responsible for the measurement and height prediction of hundreds of girls, had taken a job in the United States. The university had asked that he take only copies of the research he had done in Melbourne, but a representative told Janet the originals were nowhere to be found.

In early August, three days of prime afternoon radio talk time was given over to the Tall Girls story. The discussion centered on the difference between medical trials and established therapy. Although Wettenhall, eighty-one, declined to participate, saying he would talk only to an official inquiry, pediatric endocrinologist George Werther, who had worked closely with him, said that many of the health problems the women had reported were common in the population. Ross Pagano, a gynecologist and DES expert at the Royal Women's Hospital, stressed that there were no reports of long-term side effects of the use of DES in tall girls, although he admitted there had been little in the way of follow-up.

Initially, it seemed unlikely that anybody within Australia's federal health department would take the women's fears seriously. And in fact, two months later, the federal health minister announced that a review of the evidence surrounding the treatment of tall girls revealed "no evidence for concern." Janet believed the "evidence" examined was nothing more than several studies Wettenhall himself had authored decades earlier, including a survey of his own patients who claimed to be happy with the treatment. She and Ed agreed that absence of evidence is not evidence of absence.

But the Tall Girls had found an unlikely ally in Werther, the pediatric endocrinologist who had worked with Wettenhall in the later years of the latter's long career. While the story was bouncing around the media, Werther persuaded the Joint Council of the Endocrine Society of Australia and the Australasian Paediatric Endocrine Group to support an application for funding to the National Health and Medical Research Council (NHMRC), which is similar to the National Institutes of Health in the United States, for a tall-girls follow-up study. Janet was pleased, but concerned that Werther's interests were not the same as those of the Tall Girls. After all, Wettenhall had been Werther's mentor. How impartial could he be? Janet and the Tall Girls insisted they play an advisory role in the design of the study to be certain that issues important to them were represented. As far as anyone knew, a consumer group had never had this kind of influence in the design of a medical study. It was an odd and often uneasy alliance: George Werther had been Wettenhall's protégé, Janet his dissatisfied patient.

BEYOND AUSTRALIA

By this time, Janet and the other women in the fledgling organization had used the Internet to track down medical journal articles on subjects ranging from the use of DES in farm animals to the little-understood but potentially disastrous effects of endocrine disruption in the environment. As Janet saw it, the tall girls were like the proverbial canaries in the mine; if somebody cared to look, the experiment in which they'd played an unwitting part might tell scientists a great deal about what kinds of damage chemicals that mimic estrogen play in causing disease in those exposed to them.

Moreover, Janet's research revealed that the practice of stunting tall girls was not confined to the United States and Australia: thousands of girls in Europe—including Russia, Czechoslovakia, and Turkey—had been treated, and were continuing to be treated, despite published fears that the long-term side effects remained unknown. Beginning in the 1960s, papers by German and Swiss pediatric endocrinologists were published, each referring to dozens of girls they had given estrogens. The author of one paper noted that girls living in northern Germany tended to be taller than those in southern Germany and Switzerland, so in an effort to help a youngster feel more normal, the height at which growth suppression would be considered was adjusted downward according to geography.

Doctors in the Netherlands—where the average girl and boy are taller than anywhere else on earth—and Scandinavian countries have also treated girls (and some tall boys) for decades. In 1986, a paper published in a Scandinavian medical journal referred to 680 tall Norwegian girls between 1980 and 1985 given high doses of estrogen. The author noted that the girls were not followed up systematically after completion, although, he added, "some have become mothers and, as far as we know, none has developed infertility problems or malignant disease. This is too early to ascertain breast and genital carcinoma."

Massachusetts General's John Crawford estimated the number of girls treated in the United States to be between one and five thousand, but admitted the actual number is unknown. The use of hormones to stunt a girl's growth was considered the province of pediatric endocrinologists, but that did not stop pediatricians, gynecologists, and internists from prescribing, particularly in out-of-the-way areas where pediatric endocrinologists were few and far between. Crawford alone had treated several hundred, including the tall daughters of mothers he'd treated a generation earlier.

The revelation that so many girls had been prescribed estrogens for height, and were still being treated despite published warnings that long-term side effects were unknown, flabbergasted Janet and members of the fledgling organization. The women were more determined than ever to have a say in the design of the study and what it set out to learn. They wanted not only girls who had been given DES to be included but also girls who received ethinyl estradiol—as that had become in Europe and Canada, at least, the estrogen of choice for doctors who treated tall girls. "We really needed this study to be world-class, because we felt it would be looked at closely in North America and northern Europe, where tall-girl treatment was continuing," Janet explained.

On November 17, Tall Girls was incorporated. The organization began publishing a newsletter and eventually designed its own Website. Six months after the tall girls' story first made headlines, Werther's draft proposal for funding the follow-up study arrived in Janet's mailbox. She was disappointed. It failed to incorporate the range of issues—from physical to psychological problems—that were important to the tall girls. Janet and the tall girls had already acquired a good deal of information about the treatment via the Internet, as well as from the detailed questionnaires they'd sent to tall girls who had contacted them. They felt they owned their histories and had a vital stake in the outcome of any follow-up study. They'd discovered that they, in fact, knew more about this particular therapy than most of the medical community. They responded with a counterproposal.

A few days later, Werther called with news that would ultimately—if not quickly—guarantee the success of the project. The Center for the Study of Mothers' and Children's Health at La Trobe University in Melbourne indicated that one of its researchers, Alison Venn, was interested in researching the Tall Girls. Venn, who was born and educated in Britain, received a bachelor of science with honors from the University of London, a Ph.D. in immunology from the National Institute for Medical Research in London, and a graduate diploma in epidemiology from the University of Melbourne. She is acting director of the Menzies Research Institute at the University of Tasmania in Hobart. Her previous epidemiological research focused on female fertility and IVF treatment. Most important, when Janet reached Venn on the phone, she sounded sympathetic to the wide range of topics—particularly the psychosocial ones—that Tall Girls insisted be included. "She was like a breath of fresh air. She really understood what concerned us," Janet recalled.

Venn committed to a three-year project and came to a general meeting of Tall Girls to explain how epidemiological studies work: she would be unable to answer an individual woman's questions about her own health problems, but the study would show whether there were indications of specific health problems among the group of tall girls that did not afflict a group of tall women who had been assessed for treatment but not given medication. The research project would also attempt to determine whether those treated benefited psychologically from the therapy, which was, after all, the only reason doctors had treated girls in the first place.

LAURA FINDS JANET

While Janet was waging a public battle for an investigation in Australia, Laura was searching for answers, too. In 1995 she turned forty, and after years of using no birth control, she became pregnant for the fourth and last time. Her surprise and happiness lasted only a few months. Given her history of miscarriage, her doctor prescribed progesterone in the belief it might help her maintain the pregnancy, but the longed-for baby went the way of the previous three. She miscarried at three months, and this time she asked to have her tubes tied. A few years later she noticed a lump in her left breast. A benign cyst was removed in a lumpectomy, but surrounding tissue showed a small, noninvasive cancer.

In 1998, Laura called the public library in Boston and asked for a copy of The Boston Globe article that her mother's aunt had sent Shirley thirty years before. She had been unable to find Gertrud

Reyersbach after all these years, so she wrote to Crawford, who was still practicing at Massachusetts General. In her letter she described her reproductive history and asked if he'd encountered similar problems in the girls he treated.

"I do not know of reproductive problems that have been clearly associated with prior treatment with DES or any other form of estrogen in the context of curtailing tall stature," he wrote to Laura. "I have looked at the data on my series of treated girls comparing them with girls who were brought to me for the same problem but who decided against treatment.... In studying what had become of these two groups of girls, I found that they could not be compared because they were so different. Larger numbers of the treated girls went on to college, graduate school, and interesting careers. They put off having families largely because of the requirements of their careers rather than because of infertility. Obesity was much more common among girls who had decided against the treatment."

Laura had not put off childbearing for graduate school or an interesting career. She wanted little more than to be a wife and mother, to raise a family with her husband. The girl who happily sewed elaborate clothing for her collection of dolls was now a woman who still sewed—Halloween costumes and velvet capes, skirts and bathrobes—for her nieces and nephews. But it was not the same. Her cats helped fill the void, and she devoted hours to her garden.

After Laura's correspondence with Crawford, her sister, Cathy, discovered Janet's Tall Girls Inc. website. Laura was one of the first American tall girls to contact the Australian organization. Like so many Australian women, Laura wrote to Janet and detailed her experiences. Janet replied that other women in the group had suffered similar problems and passed along the e-mail of someone in California who had contacted her. She also told Laura that plans were under way for a rigorous study that would help elucidate the medical and psychological problems of the treated girls more clearly.

Laura's health problems, she found, were similar to those of many of the Australian girls. Not long afterward, Laura took her mother for an outing and lunch. "We were walking on the beach, [and] I said, 'You know, I have to tell you something, and I know you're not going to like hearing it, because it's very difficult and I know you've always had fears about it.'"

"She knew exactly what it was when I said that," Laura recalled. "I told her I'd come into contact with a whole group of women over in Australia that were treated along the same lines that I had been, and that they were having many of the same problems I had. 'I just wanted you to know about it because it's going to become public at some time, and I rather you hear it from me first,'" Laura said.

Shirley wept. For years she'd worried that the pills that Laura didn't want but that doctors assured her were safe were to blame for Laura's miscarriages and depression. But she'd told herself over and over that doctors had been treating girls for years and no problems had ever come of it.

TRACKING DOWN TALL GIRLS

In Australia, it took nearly three years before the study was funded. Many in the Australian medical community questioned spending limited funds to examine a practice that they believed was no longer fashionable—despite anecdotal evidence that some parents were still seeking treatment for their tall daughters. But even before the project was given a green light, Tall Girls could chalk up one victory: the Australian Health Ethics Committee within the National Health and Medical Research Council revised the rules for consent in research involving humans, particularly young people. Researchers were required to keep records of clinical significance so they could carry out follow-up studies.

In September 2000, the study finally got under way. Venn assembled a team of researchers who, working out of an old brick building only a few blocks from the University of Melbourne anatomy and physiology building, where so many of the girls had been measured and photographed decades earlier, began the arduous task of trying to find them. More than twelve hundred girls had consulted Wettenhall about their height.

Wettenhall agreed to open his files to the researchers so they could find the names and begin to track them down. Eventually Venn's researchers identified another twenty-six clinicians in Australia who had also treated tall girls, but those doctors yielded little information: some had died, others had disposed of their records years earlier, the rest refused to make their records available. None had the meticulously detailed medical records on note cards that Wettenhall had preserved all these years, in cabinets in a ballroom of his large home in Toorak. Armed with laptops, the researchers sat in the ballroom copying medical details from the tattered and taped cards. The excuse physicians have frequently cited for not following up with the girls they had seen was difficulty in tracking them down: girls grow up, move away, and often change their last names when they marry. If a woman developed uterine or breast cancer in her thirties, forties, or fifties, it would be unlikely that she would contact the pediatrician or pediatric endocrinologist who treated her when she was a child; she would consult with her gynecologist or oncologist.

"We had a major task tracing women for the study, some up to forty-two years after they first presented for a medical assessment for their stature," recalled Venn. She and her small team of researchers-turned-detectives tackled the problem in ingenious ways. Australians do not have Social Security numbers, nor is it legal to use driver's license information to locate residents. But voting is compulsory in Australia, so the researchers turned to electoral rolls and old telephone listings for clues to the whereabouts of their potential study subjects. Then they traced them forward in time.

The researchers also placed notices in catalogs for tall women's clothing, and contacted private girls' schools in Melbourne where some of the women had been students. They searched death records to see if a parent had died, and if so whether an obituary named surviving children. They tracked women to the United States, Britain, Europe, and Asia. The hardest to trace were those who had married several times, changing their names to those of new husbands. Research-ers also notified the professional medical societies of gynecologists, obstetricians, and general practitioners in hopes they had come across female patients in their practices who had histories of height reduc-tion therapy. "Of course, what happened is, some of the doctors were the girls we were looking for," said Venn. "Given the demographics of this group, we shouldn't have been surprised, but we were."

Most of the former patients and parents were also surprised—and concerned—when they were contacted. Some feared the researchers had already discovered long-term health problems with the treatment. In a small number of cases, some parents were unwilling to inform daughters about the study because they were still intent on controlling their adult daughters. "They were only a small proportion of parents, but they stood out," said Venn. More often, parents were reluctant to contact their daughters about the study because they feared stirring up uncomfortable memories: the letters and phone calls tapped into com-plicated, unresolved family discord around the treatment. Jo Rayner, a nurse and one of the researchers, recalled one woman who phoned after reading an article about the study. Years earlier, her daughter had left home angry at age fourteen and never returned. The mother begged Rayner to let her know if her daughter called.

Some women didn't want to participate in the study because it dredged up painful memories. "It was not a good time in their lives, it was a time they felt very different from others," said Rayner. "One daughter we called just said she was so angry about the treatment that she couldn't talk about it." Others felt protective of their parents and didn't want them to feel guilty about the decision they'd made on their behalf years before. Although fathers appeared to play a much smaller role in the decision to treat, the researchers talked to them, too. "I had one father who called and said he would kill that doctor if he could." Some conversations were so emotionally draining that Rayner would hang up and cry.

On the other hand, many women were pleased with the results. They firmly believed they were shorter than they might have been, and were grateful for the medical intervention. Many said their parents had acted with the best of intentions. A few said they would have their tall daughters treated as well. Some were angry about the publicity and what they considered the impugning of Wettenhall's reputation.

After eighteen months of detective work, the researchers had found 1,243 girls, or 87 percent of those who had been identified—mostly from Wettenhall's records. Of this group, 63 percent agreed to participate in the study, including 371 women who had been treated. The 409 controls had been assessed—they had been X-rayed, measured, and their mature height estimated—but not given hormones, for a variety of reasons. In many cases treatment was deemed unnecessary because a girl's predicted adult height did not warrant it, or because it was too late—she had too little remaining growth potential, according to her height prediction, for additional estrogen to make any difference. The two groups were similar in terms of age, sexual history, and socioeconomic background. All had been treated or assessed between 1959 and 1993. The treated women had received either DES or ethinyl estradiol.

Unlike most epidemiological studies, Venn and her research team began the project with a series of focus groups to better understand the psychosocial issues that affected tall women in general and those who were assessed and treated in particular. A health sociologist, Priscilla Pyett, worked with the group, and Venn consulted a psychiatric epidemiologist with a special interest in adolescent mental health. From those sessions, the researchers gleaned much about the attitudes of tall women toward their height.

Some women recalled being the tallest in the school photograph year after year, and feeling "like a tree in a field of grass," according to Pyett. Some were left out of certain school activities because of their height; one remembered a schoolteacher telling her she couldn't participate in a school play because she was "too tall and would spoil it." As tall girls, they were expected to be more mature, as they looked older, because of their height and the adult clothing they wore once they'd outgrown children's sizes.

Their height affected how they dressed and how they acted. They didn't wear their hair short because people might confuse them with a man, but they dared not wear high heels, a symbol of femininity, because it increased their height. Bikinis were off-limits, too, because they seemed to accentuate longer-than-average midsections. Pink or frilly clothing was avoided because they thought it looked ridiculous on a tall woman. Many reported that they felt uncomfortable going out with shorter men.

Not only did they choose hairstyles, shoes, and clothing with care, they also altered their personalities. One woman said, "No matter how gentle you are, people find you intimidating. I always try to compensate and be very sweet."

"We did notice, however, a definite difference in attitude between the older women and those still in their twenties, who were much less self-conscious about their height," said Pyett.

The medicalization of their problem, however, added another dimension to their anxiety about their height. Now a doctor was telling them that they were already quite tall—taller than almost all other girls of their age as well as the boys—and could grow even taller. The examinations, too, provoked deep embarrassment at an age when girls are already anxious about their bodies.

For those who began taking the synthetic estrogen, the additional weight gain compounded their anxiety. "It was not unusual for mothers to say, 'You know, you have an appointment coming up and you've gained a bit of weight. Perhaps you should cut back until you see the doctor,'" said Venn. Then there was embarrassment over their sudden puberty—having breasts and periods before their friends—and in the older group of women, heavy, almost uncontrollable bleeding until doctors began prescribing synthetic progesterone for five days each month to stimulate the uterus to shed its lining.

Once the two groups of treated and untreated girls were established, the researchers mailed them detailed questionnaires, then followed up with lengthy telephone interviews with questions about gynecological disorders, reproductive history, time to pregnancy, menstrual characteristics, menopausal status, sexuality, sexual history, and mental health.

As the researchers discovered, tall girls ended up in doctors' offices from a variety of referrals. Some were sent by pediatricians who knew of Wettenhall's work. In some cases, a nurse visiting the mother of a new baby commented on the height of an older child and suggested the mother might want to have the girl—even one who was only four years old at the time—assessed. Sometimes mothers heard about Wettenhall from other mothers who were having their daughters treated, or read about the therapy in the newspapers. Parents frequently were notified by school nurses or principals: notes went home suggesting their girls were growing tall and they should consider getting an assessment. "In some cases, these were tall, happy girls from tall, happy families where no one had ever given a thought about their height," said Venn. "Now, suddenly, there's a letter from the school. The girl's height is a problem—and a problem that required medical intervention." It made the whole family anxious.

IMPAIRED FERTILITY AND DISSATISFACTION

Three years after Venn and her researchers began sorting through Wettenhall's medical records, and nearly three years after his death, at age eighty-five, Venn traveled to the National Institute for Environmental Health Studies in North Carolina, the only one of the National Institutes of Health located outside the Washington, D.C., area. Early on, Venn had sought the advice of several scientists at the NIEHS on ways to strengthen the design of the study, and on June 5, 2003, she came to relay her preliminary findings. Before she announced the results in Australia, she wanted to be absolutely certain there was no design flaw in the research that could account for what the group had discovered.

About twenty-five researchers and epidemiologists were invited to a first-floor meeting room to hear Venn's presentation. Most were unaware that estrogens had ever been administered to girls to stunt their height, and interrupted Venn's presentation frequently to ask questions about it and why it was done. Standing behind a lectern with charts and graphs on a screen behind her, Venn provided a quick summary of the history of the treatment as well as the approach she and her researchers had taken to gathering data and comparing the two cohorts of women.

What they had chosen to study first, she said, was fertility, and what they had found was that the therapy had significantly affected a woman's ability to become pregnant. "The treated women were more likely to have failed to get pregnant within twelve months of trying, they were more likely to have seen a doctor because of difficulty getting pregnant, and they were more likely to have consulted fertility specialists to help them become pregnant," she said. In fact, in any given menstrual cycle of unprotected intercourse, the women who had been treated were 40 percent less likely to conceive than those who had not.

Venn could not point to a reason for the increased infertility, although she theorized that endometriosis, which was more prevalent in the treated girls, might have something to do with it. This condition, where tissue that lines the uterus grows, escapes, and spreads to other areas, can inhibit the functioning of the ovaries and fallopian tubes. She would have to look to reproductive endocrinologists for answers.

While many scientists in the audience were surprised by the information Venn conveyed, one was not. Since 1980, Retha Newbold, one of the country's leading researchers into the effects of DES on the children of women given it during pregnancy, has conducted experiments on mice that have confirmed and predicted the long-term adverse effects of the drug in the pregnant women who took it and their approximately five million daughters and sons. By injecting laboratory mice with DES during their pregnancies, she has been able to duplicate in the reproductive tracts of daughter mice tumors and structural abnormalities that appear in the human daughters of mothers given the drug. Worse, she told a group of DES daughters in

Washington, D.C., in 2001, if her mice were any indication, even the daughters of DES daughters—the granddaughters of women given the drug when pregnant—would have more reproductive tract cancers than the granddaughters of unexposed mothers. Other researchers have found that mothers who took DES and their daughters have a greater risk of breast cancer than women not exposed to the compound.

Venn's findings that girls, not fetuses, pumped full of synthetic estrogen to reduce their adult height later had reproduction difficulties, were not so different from Newbold's findings with laboratory mice.

In experiments with female mice exposed to low levels of estrogens shortly after they were born, Newbold has seen what she called sub-fertility as the mice approach an age similar to that of puberty in humans. "For a mouse, that means it breeds fine the first time. You can't tell the difference between the treated mouse and the untreated mouse. But fertility begins to fall off with subsequent breedings. And as they age, their ovaries poop out altogether before those of the untreated mice," Newbold told Venn after the presentation.

Venn's findings about the tall girls, and her own research with mice, bolstered Newbold's view that that exposure to synthetic estrogens or chemicals that mimic estrogen during critical windows of development—pregnancy, puberty, menopause—can somehow blow the fuse of the delicate hormone messaging system. When those messages become scrambled during a period of development or change in the body, such as puberty, tissues and organs such as the uterus and breast may respond abnormally to estrogen later in life.

DES mothers and their daughters are at higher risk for breast cancer, and as Newbold pointed out, "We know estrogen affects us later in life. After all, look what they found out about hormone replacement therapy." The tall-girls study added more evidence to Newbold's theory that estrogen acts in ways that are not yet understood, and not only on the development of a fetus. And for tall girls treated with hormones it raised questions and fears. If mothers who received DES while pregnant have a higher risk of breast cancer due to their exposure, what about young girls given high doses for longer periods during the time their breasts and reproductive systems are developing?

North Carolina was a test run for a bigger presentation in Melbourne at the annual Endocrine Society of Australia conference in September 2003. The conference took place over three days at the city's convention center near Flinders Station, close to Melbourne's Yarra River and a short tram ride from the offices where the late Norman Wettenhall had practiced for so many years.

After Venn reported her findings about infertility, Pyett told the audience of her psychosocial findings—that the primary reason for the treatment, which was to make the girls happy with their height as women—had not worked very well. While 99.1 percent of the untreated women were happy they had not been given the pills, no matter how tall they became, 42.1 percent of the treated women were dissatisfied with the decision that was made to intervene with estrogen.

Their dissatisfaction, said Pyett, stemmed from many causes: the side effects they suffered during treatment, the examinations they endured—which they described as "scary," "painful," and "intrusive"— fear about future adverse effects, difficulties in becoming pregnant, and, in some cases, their failure to end up shorter. Responses from some of these women, which Pyett reported, included the following:

> "I wish I had not had the treatment as it worries me that I took drugs, especially as I had to take more to start a family with IVF."
>
> "I feel very strongly about medical intervention and the long-term effects it has. Given the choice now I would not even consider it."
>
> "The choice was to go ahead because you were made to feel that it was highly necessary because being tall wasn't appropriate."
>
> "I went along with it as I was frightened I would be lots taller than the norm, and because I had to see a doctor that (meant) there must be something wrong with me."
>
> "I am horrified that I was put at such a risk for one inch of height."

"Because I still grew to 5'11¾", not the 5'10" he predicted, so it wasn't worth the effort."

Of the 57.9 percent of treated women who were satisfied, most were convinced they would have been far taller without the treatment. "I am very happy about my choice and I'm glad I am NOT 6 feet 5 inches," said one. "I am grateful to my doctor every day that I am 6' and not 6'5".

But the question the researchers had was: Would they have really grown that tall? On average, the treatment could trim only one to two inches off a girl's height, according to Wettenhall himself. Yet some parents and girls remember vividly being told they would grow to 6'3" or 6'5". Venn points out that many girls had multiple predictions but remember only one—usually the highest.

"Some girls had multiple X-ray assessments and estimates of their mature heights, and most of those estimates varied with each time they were made. Which is interesting because many women have very clear memories of being told they were going to be 6'3" without treatment, and now they're 5'11." So they're happy. But if you look at the medical records, often there might be four, five, or six estimated mature height measures—all different," she said.

That afternoon in Melbourne, Venn, Pyett, Werther, Bruinsma, Janet Cregan-Wood and her partner, Ed, all gathered in a hotel bar next door to the convention center. Venn popped a bottle of champagne and the group toasted the years of hard work and the mutual respect that had developed over those years. Werther, who had once treated tall girls, optimistically announced that he thought the research would stop the practice cold, particularly in Europe. He was warm and gracious in his praise for Janet, declaring the study would never have happened without her persistence. As for Janet, the results were bittersweet. "I guess it validated our position and what we set out to do," she said later. But it couldn't erase the past or reassure the treated women about what medical problems might lie ahead for them.

Over the next two years, Venn's study concluding that estrogens given tall girls diminished their fertility was published by *The Lancet*, and Pyett's research that found most women dissatisfied with what Wettenhall did appeared in *Social Science & Medicine*.

GROWTH SUPPRESSION CONTINUES

When Janet began her odyssey to learn all she could about estrogens and growth suppression, she contacted an organization in Washington, D.C., the Physicians Committee for Responsible Medicine, the same group that had fought and failed to stop the NIH study of short stature. Dr. Neal Barnard, a psychiatrist who headed the PCRM, learned about the estrogen treatment from both the Australian Tall Girls and DES Action, and set out to discover how widespread it continued to be in the United States. "It was shocking to learn that estrogens would ever be used for suppression of growth, and more shocking to learn that it was still going on," recalled Barnard.

In November 1999, Barnard and his research team mailed a questionnaire to all U.S. members of the Lawson Wilkins Pediatric Endocrine Society, which includes about 80 percent of the country's pediatric endocrinologists. The questionnaire asked how many girls each doctor had treated for tall stature during the previous five years, whether or not the doctor still offered this therapy, why the doctors offered or refused to offer it, how they decided when to begin and end medication, what type of estrogen they used and in what dosage, as well as the duration of treatment and side effects. The questionnaire was sent to 715 clinicians, and 411 responded. The results, published in the *Journal of Pediatric and Adolescent Gynecology* in 2002, were surprising. More than fifty years after the practice had begun, and the same year the Stanford University's women's basketball and volleyball team players were averaging six feet tall or taller, estrogen treatment for tall stature was still offered by 33 percent, or 137, of those responding to the survey.

Barnard commented: "My gripe is that nobody knows if it's safe or not. Kids have been treated since the 1950s. Why has there been no monitoring? In the absence of more complete knowledge regarding the long-term fate of these young girls, the estrogen treatment is questionable. It is important to provide details that allow informed consent." Barnard's study created a flurry of media coverage and several women, including Laura, stepped up to the cameras to tell their stories. They echoed the complaints of the Australian Tall Girls.

In addition to releasing the survey results, the organization petitioned the FDA to change the language in the prescribing information that goes to doctors and patients so it is clear to all that growth suppression is not an approved use of estrogen. Their petition was turned down.

CHAPTER 11

friendly fire

A HOPEFUL SIGN AT FIRST

As the Tall Girls sought answers, so did some of those living with the knowledge that they might have been infected with Creutzfeldt-Jakob disease by the pituitary human growth hormone they took as children. There was no test that could tell them whether or not they were among the unlucky ones whose injections amounted to a death sentence. They could only watch the numbers climb and try to figure out their own personal odds.

As of 1991, there had been sixteen reported CJD deaths world-wide among former pituitary hGH patients, and the odds did not look too bad. In fact, the Public Health Service's February 13 "Dear Growth Hormone Recipient" letter reported no new American cases since 1988; the number still stood at seven. "It is reassuring that there have been no new cases of CJD reported in the U.S.," the government told parents. "Although we cannot predict the total number of cases of CJD that will occur in growth hormone recipients, each year that passes without additional cases is a very hopeful sign."

But the letter did add that there had been two CJD deaths abroad, one in Brazil and one in New Zealand, of people who received hGH processed in the United States at the same laboratories that supplied the National Hormone and Pituitary Program. The small number of cases—considering the large number of people who received multiple lots of hormone—seemed to suggest either that there was "low infectivity" in the contaminated batches or that some people were genetically more susceptible to CJD than others. The major risk factor among Americans, though this didn't hold true elsewhere, appeared to be the length of time someone had been treated. Those who, like Joey Rodriguez, had taken pituitary hormone more than twice as long as the average child, seemed more likely to develop CJD. Other than that, no single batch of hormone or particular treatment center stood out.

Publishing the original results of the Public Health Service study in 1991 in *JAMA*, the *Journal of the American Medical Association*, the endocrinologist Judith Fradkin was somewhat less reassuring. As the doctor in charge of the epidemiological survey, she predicted what everyone investigating the epidemic understood: others had almost certainly been infected. The disease was incubating. There would be more deaths. How many, she wrote, depended on whether or not Albert Parlow's fastidious processing had eliminated CJD beginning in 1977.

Parlow was certain that it had, just as sure as he'd been in 1985 when he argued against stopping the distribution of pituitary hGH and blamed commercial manufacturers for seizing the opportunity to kill the federal program. When he heard about Joey Rodriguez, Parlow remembered, he'd felt "considerable concern, but the kid obviously had not been using my product. . . . It wasn't an overwhelming concern. I would have been devastated if the kid had been treated with my product." Instead, he and the program's director, Salvatore Raiti, had discussed the death as "a severe setback" to the program. Raiti recalls that Parlow even offered to scrub his hormone preparation with chemicals, as an added precaution.

They had lost their argument in 1985. The processing of pituitaries continued afterward, but not for use in humans. In his Harbor-UCLA

Medical Center laboratory, Parlow extracted pituitary hormones from a variety of species for researchers to use in laboratory experiments. He fumed over the scientific work that had been stopped when the federal program shut down. In particular, he'd been on the verge of working with Choh Li, the world-famous chemist at UCSF. More than that, Parlow wanted it known that the CJD debacle was due not to pituitary hGH but to Alfred Wilhelmi's lack of interest in using safer processing methods and the NIH's failed oversight in not insisting. Basically, for taking Wilhelmi's word over Parlow's.

Parlow nursed his grudge against Wilhelmi, the person he held most responsible. He recalled arguing that Wilhelmi "could have produced a higher purification" but wasn't skilled enough to do so. "I let a lot of people know that," Parlow said, including G. Donald Whedon, who officially oversaw the hormone distribution program for NIH as head of what was then called the National Institute of Arthritis and Diabetes, Digestive and Kidney Diseases. But the complaints were delivered in person, rather than in writing, according to Parlow, and he received the impression no changes would be made until Wilhelmi retired.

Parlow likes to turn the discussion away from when the risk of CJD should have been recognized: "The issue is the product, which was intended for human use, should have been brought to maximal purity for that reason. Irrespective of whether one knew about Creutzfeldt-Jakob disease as a potential contaminant of a pituitary product, the issue was there could be any number of contaminants that could be harmful, and if the product were pure then the likelihood of harboring a harmful contaminant is less." The pituitary agency's product wasn't pure before 1977 and the processors knew it. "The oversight failed."

That didn't mean people should have known about the potential for transmitting CJD in particular. "Nobody ignored a warning. They simply weren't aware of it....The scientific community is vast, with many divisions, and the divisions do not speak to each other." Parlow is adamant he took over the processing in 1977 "totally unaware" of CJD but just determined "to produce the best product that was producible."

The experts on transmissible spongiform encephalopathies, however, refused to conclude that Parlow's methods eliminated all danger. The French had used a form of column chromatography, and they had victims. There was still the possibility that a single prion had slipped through Parlow's filtered columns and into a single vial.

Indeed, in the late 1980s, disease experts thought they might have identified two CJD cases among those who began treatment with U.S. pituitary hGH after Wilhelmi retired. But neither patient turned out to have Creutzfeldt-Jakob disease. Parlow wanted a retraction. He chafed at the cautious refusal to endorse the safety of his procedures. He told the disease experts all the careful steps besides gel filtration taken in his lab: the washing, heating, scrubbing, the gowns and masks. Unlike his predecessor's murky preparations, the pituitary hGH he turned out was clear as water, with no particles floating in it that a prion might latch on to. He considered those two to three thousand children who received what he liked to call "Parlow's product" as a long-term clinical trial of his methods, with an outcome he could predict. It was clear to him he would ultimately be able to say his preparations had made no one sick. Did he have any moments of doubt? "None."

He even calculated the date when he could declare he was "absolutely sure in every instance." With a thirty-year incubation period, that would be 2015. But he was impatient. He was ready to rejoice twenty-five years after the last child took his product. "If there's no disease within that time frame, 2010 to 2015, if there are no occurrences during that time frame, then sound the all clear!" That would be when the world would know that Al Parlow had never infected anyone, and had potentially saved thousands from being infected. The date when people could acknowledge he was the hero of the CJD story, not one of its villains.

DECADES TO WAIT

Tension ratcheted up year by year. By 1992, twenty-three CJD cases had been reported worldwide among pituitary hGH recipients. The

French, who had been so dismissive of the "American problem" that they had continued to process pituitaries for three years after the United States and most other countries stopped, reeled with their mounting toll, the highest in the world. In 1993, French authorities notified two doctors in charge of the hormone treatment program in that country that they were under investigation for possible manslaughter charges. A government inquiry found that the program had collected many glands through the 1980s from Bulgaria and Hungary, paying operating room orderlies to mine corpses: six to nine dollars per pituitary, including those from neurological and infectious wards. This in spite of a reported 1980 warning from the French scientist Luc Montagnier, co-discoverer of the AIDS virus, that pituitary hGH could transmit Creutzfeldt-Jakob disease. Montagnier had advised special care when buying glands. It was a second medical tragedy for the French people; a scandal over HIV/AIDS-contaminated blood products had just resulted in jail sentences for four former senior health officials.

No one disputed any longer that doctors had infected their patients by prescribing what turned out to be contaminated growth hormone. These cases were labeled iatrogenic CJD, meaning CJD spread by medical accident, to distinguish them from those that arose sporadically in the general population, mostly in the elderly, or those that ran in some families. Physicians might prefer to use the term "therapeutic misadventure," noted a group of disease experts who preferred the military term for unintentionally causing casualties among your own troops: these patients were victims of "friendly fire." People who had been treated with pituitary human growth hormone worldwide had a one-in-two-hundred chance of eventually dying of CJD. Based on the cases so far, the incubation period had been raised to as long as thirty-five years.

Publishing again in a medical journal in 1993, Judith Fradkin wrote that all the American victims to date began treatment before 1970. Even if only those earliest patients had been exposed, they still had years to worry. The families desperately wanted to know whether their children had received hormone from any infected batches. Frad-kin remembers Wilhelmi "meticulously" searching for some common denominator among the known cases, paging through his detailed notebooks. "Dr. Wilhelmi was tremendously sorry...to find he had inadvertently caused harm was terribly upsetting." But "ultimately we weren't able to identify any preparation" that "enabled us to go back to the actual pituitary." Wilhelmi "did everything in his power to try to shine a light on this. It was a tremendous shock." At least France was able to pinpoint just a couple of years within which everybody who developed CJD had received cadaveric growth hormone. In the United States, it seemed likely that multiple Wilhelmi preparations were infected, and everyone was getting some of every preparation, which had been shipped out every three months.

On March 23, 1995, the U.S. government sent another mailing to the families of former patients with more bad news. There had now been a total of twelve CJD cases among American growth hormone recipients. Still, they had all been treated before Parlow's processing began. At this point the government believed there had been 8,000 federal program patients, and the outbreak had averaged about one case a year since 1985.

The epidemiological survey hadn't been able to track about 2,000 people whose doctors had applied to the government for hormone but either kept no records on whether the patients actually had been treated or could give no contact information. Three of the CJD cases belonged to that untracked group. There was really no way people could figure out their personal odds of survival. The disease had appeared, on average, seventeen years after hormone treatment among the Americans. But it had also occurred as soon as four years after stopping therapy, and as many as thirty since starting it. Once more, the agency cautiously raised the hope that the "chromatogra-phy purification step" introduced by Parlow "markedly reduces any CJD infectious material": "Each year that goes by without occur-rence of CJD in patients who started treatment after the newer hor-mone was introduced provides encouragement about the safety of these preparations." But the long incubation period meant more time needed to pass "before we can draw definite conclusions about the safety of hormone produced for the NHPP after 1977," the 1995 letter warned.

The same letter reported that one of the animals injected with stored NHPP preparations developed CJD after five and a half years. Though this proved that a vial of government growth hormone was indeed infectious, none of the humans who had the disease were known to have received that particular preparation. To confuse the matter even more, two other animals injected with the same batch of hormone showed no signs of illness. As for those humans who had taken hGH from the same lot, but not yet become sick, the letter attempted to reassure families their children were probably not at any increased risk compared with other recipients. That was because experts believed that many preparations contained "very low level contamination," such low levels that "most vials from these preparations would not transmit CJD." You had to be especially unlucky, then. Like finding a prion in a haystack.

One possibility was that people might have varying levels of susceptibility, based on genetic variation in the structure of the brain protein that CJD turns lethal. In any case, the government had no way of confidently knowing which patient took which preparation, because many doctors did not record that information. Whatever information the agency did have about particular batches it wasn't going to share. Former patients were told they could ask their physicians.

By then the number of cases in England totaled fifteen, and there were four cases in Australian women who had taken a different pituitary hormone. France, by contrast, had thirty-two, some in children as young as ten or eleven. It was a cluster linked to 1984–1985, and the quicker onset of symptoms suggested the French preparations contained a much higher level of infectious material. Parlow remained confident; the French chromatography method differed from his, and he regarded it with derision.

The survey established to track former U.S. patients produced one unexpected benefit. In the absence of a centralized health care system, no one had ever followed this group of mostly hypopituitary youngsters into adulthood. After the Japanese reported increased leukemia among children treated with growth hormone, the United States was able to look back at its arduously gathered database of pituitary hGH recipients and conclude there had been no increased leukemia incidence, except among those whose growth hormone deficiency had been caused by either brain tumors or radiation treatment. This additional evidence confirmed what pediatric endocrinologists had decided in the wake of the Japanese report.

The 1995 letter to U.S. recipients ended: "We would like to offer as much support for your concerns as we are able." It included a response card and reiterated the importance of staying in touch. "We would particularly like you or your physician to contact us about any new or worsening neurologic symptoms or any diagnosis of leukemia."

They would soon hear from Lucille Sluder.

PRAYING FOR THE LORD TO TAKE HER

Lucille and Roland Sluder had long lost contact with the Human Growth Foundation in which they had been so active, back when Roland played Santa Claus every Christmas to help raise funds for the dwarfed children. They had moved from Long Island to Greenville, South Carolina. Linda, their doll-like little girl, grew into an attractive young woman who, at less than five feet, always found boyfriends six feet tall. Linda moved to Florida, where she worked as a mortgage loan processor, and bought a small house in Deltona. She had some medical emergencies during which her parents rushed to Florida to nurse her. But in January 1994, she married, and for a brief while things went well.

In October, Linda and her husband drove to Greenville for a visit. Her mother recorded the details: "Linda seemed very depressed and shaky. She was cold all the time. She mentioned that she had several falls in recent months." Over the next few months, her daughter continued to sound depressed on the telephone, complained of feeling dizzy, described more falls. When, in February 1995, Linda mentioned to her mother that a friend had brought her a walker and a wheelchair, Lucille and Roland became more than alarmed. "We packed our suitcases that evening and were in Florida the next day."

The Sluders remembered the letters from the Public Health Service. It was Lucille who mentioned to the endocrinologist and neurologist who saw Linda that her daughter received pituitary hGH in childhood, and that she might have CJD. At this point neurologists had a test that enabled them to diagnose the disease once there were symptoms, by looking at spinal fluid, rather than waiting to biopsy the brain after death. Only a spinal tap would confirm CJD, but Linda rejected the procedure. Lucille's written account of her daughter's downhill slide is almost unbearable in its detail. Stuttering, falls even with the walker, the commode next to the bed. Linda's ballooning weight—226 pounds—made the situation even more difficult.

In April, they could no longer manage at home, and Linda Sluder entered Central Florida Regional Hospital in Sanford, where she consented to the spinal tap, and then went to a rehabilitation hospital eighty-three miles from her home. Her parents visited her daily. She could not speak, and did not improve with physical and speech therapy. A week after the Sluders brought Linda back to the Deltona house, along with a hospital bed, a lift and other equipment, and a nurse's aide in the mornings (Lucille slept next to Linda's bed at night), a CJD expert from the National Institutes of Health phoned with the news: The spinal tap "definitely indicated that Linda had CJD."

"Her hands had become rigid and she could no longer communicate by blinking her eyes or putting out her tongue to indicate yes or no. She had more difficulty swallowing.... Things got really bad when the seizures started. Some were very violent and mild ones became almost continuous. We fed her with a syringe and then with an eye dropper.... When she could no longer swallow a drop of water, we knew the end was near and we prayed for the Lord to take her to heaven soon. Linda passed away in her sleep on Sunday morning, July 23, 1995, at approximately 5:40 a.m." She was thirty-eight. Lucille Sluder notified the NIH. She was told that Linda was the thirteenth death among U.S. hGH recipients and that a fourteenth case had already been reported. A few months after they returned to their South Carolina home, the Sluders learned that Linda's husband had died in a motorcycle accident.

MORE LETTERS, WORSE ODDS

Linda Sluder's name and the details of her death weren't included in the Public Health Service letters, of course. But she was now among the statistics. "Dear Growth Hormone Recipient," another letter, dated April 30, 1996, began. "Since I last wrote to you in early 1994, I have been sorry to learn of four additional American recipients of human growth hormone who developed Creutzfeldt-Jakob disease." Yet another one had turned up from the group of patients they had not been able to track. All had begun treatment before 1977. Among Americans, that meant about one for every 530 people who'd been treated. Once again, the message expressed "concern for your well-being."

The letters never mentioned Al Parlow by name, though they always described his product as the growth hormone "produced in a laboratory using a chromatography purification step that markedly reduces any CJD infectious material contaminating the pituitaries." Gradually, the statements about his method were getting stronger and more optimistic. "As each year goes by without CJD occurring in patients who began treatment after the purer hormone was introduced, we are more encouraged about the safety of these preparations." But this would always be followed with the caution that more time needed to pass. The reassuring news was that most of those who did get CJD had been treated for more than nine and a half years on average, while most recipients in the United States had received it for three years or less.

The letters also moved closer to blaming Wilhelmi's lab, though never mentioning him by name. By 1996, New Zealand had reported a startling cluster of five hGH-related CJD cases, and all of them had been people who received hormone from "a U.S. laboratory that was the major supplier of NHPP growth hormone prior to 1977." This was Wilhelmi's Emory University laboratory. The New Zealand patients had been treated in different years, meaning that there probably had been more than one contaminated preparation: "Hormone preparations from this laboratory were composed of a combination of many separate hormone-rich fragments derived from processing many separate batches of pituitaries. Fractions from the same pituitaries often were included in multiple hormone preparations." The lab sent preparations to the NHHP and to New Zealand that probably contained "some common components." Meaning some of those reading the letter might have injected medicine derived from the same infected pituitaries that killed people in New Zealand.

The private tragedy looming over this small group of people who'd been treated for their height as children merged with a much more public one by the mid-1990s, a different form of CJD, which the press called "mad cow disease." Bovine spongiform encephalopathy (BSE) in England was all over the news, with grim details of young people dying. The 1996 Public Health Service update to U.S. growth hormone recipients discussed the connection, noting that this was a different, or variant, form of CJD probably arising from feeding ground-up sheep or other livestock to cattle. People became infected by eating infected beef. These were separate from the deaths caused by growth hormone, though the diseases were related, both caused by prions. This was followed by an explanation of prions and how, unlike bacteria or viruses, they consist of protein without any genetic material. A prion *is* a brain protein, but in an abnormal and infectious form. Its abnormal shape sets off a chain reaction, at least in some people, and causes the healthy protein in their brains to form abnormally, too. There was now a test to detect this odd-shaped protein in spinal fluid, the test that had been performed on Linda Sluder, so a diagnosis could be made without a brain biopsy. Unfortunately, it was useful only after a patient developed symptoms. It could not identify those who would later develop CJD. Because there was no test to detect infection that was still incubating, blood banks continued to refuse blood from anyone who had received pituitary hGH.

There also was another disease garnering headlines, HIV/AIDS, but it had not been linked to any hGH patients. HIV was more susceptible to destruction, and the agency seemed confident in stating that "HIV would be destroyed by the methods used to process pituitaries and make growth hormone."

Once again the survey proved the value of tracking patients from childhood into adulthood, and the hazards of an American health care system in which records did not follow patients. While investigating CJD deaths, Judith Fradkin discovered that some of those children on her list who had been treated with pituitary hGH later died unexpectedly of an adrenal crisis. This had nothing to do with receiving growth hormone or with CJD. It turned out that a significant number of the patients diagnosed with hypopituitary dwarfism as children had also been deficient in other pituitary hormones, including the one that stimulates the adrenal glands to produce cortisol. Without cortisol, the body can't respond normally to infections, trauma, surgery, or other stress. Preventable deaths had occurred because the patients' adrenal problems had gone undiagnosed and untreated once they became adults. Now the NIH alerted people who had multiple pituitary hormone deficiencies as children that they should be aware of the symptoms of chronic adrenal insufficiency. Fradkin hoped to save lives. Instead, the alert seemed to cause confusion. Some of those who read the warning mistakenly thought that their childhood shots had put them at risk of yet another lethal illness.

March 31, 1997. This letter put the CJD death toll in the United States at sixteen. There was a sense that the epidemic emergency that endocrinologists had set in motion was waning, or at least holding steady. But it was too soon to relax.

In June 1999, the Public Health Service wrote: "We have been

saddened to learn of six new cases of Creutzfeldt-Jakob disease" since
the previous update. There were now twenty-two cases, and the pace
was picking up. The rate had increased to 1.7 cases a year between
1990 and 1998.

Even after all these years of mailings, the Public Health Service
pleaded with parents to share the situation with any adult children
who had not received the letters and to talk about the risk of CJD with
their sons and daughters. "This is a painful situation for all concerned,
but it can be more upsetting to learn of the risk from the media or
other sources." Parents sometimes phoned and confessed they kept
the letters secret because they feared that their grown children would
be angry with them for having given the potentially deadly shots. Six
overseas patients, aside from the twenty-two in the United States,
had been linked to the labs that produced NHHP hormone. One of
these, in Brazil, was a person who had received some Raben product.
Al Parlow did not believe that would turn out to be a case of CJD. He
thought Maurice Raben's method with its harsh acid had probably
worked. All the rest had been infected by Wilhelmi.

No one knew why the U.S.-processed hormone had been so lethal
in New Zealand, where patients had become ill much sooner. Debra
McKenzie was a New Zealand victim whose death produced the first
lawsuit in the world arising from this "friendly fire."

Debra McKenzie had taken the hormone from age sixteen to
age nineteen, beginning in 1970. It had been sent from Wilhelmi at
Emory University in Georgia to her endocrinologist in New Zealand.
McKenzie died at the age of thirty-two in 1987, and her parents sued
in U.S. courts in December 1992. Their attorneys alleged that all
pituitary human growth hormone manufacturers should have been
aware of the potential for CJD contamination by 1969, but failed to
warn potential users.

It was a tough case to pursue, requiring proof the U.S. government
had been negligent, the product defective; and because of CJD's long
incubation, Georgia's statute of limitations had run out. The family's
American lawyers switched the case to Mississippi, which had a lon-

ger limit, and unsuccessfully argued that some of the pituitary glands might have been collected at the University of Mississippi. The case was transferred one more time before being dismissed in 1995, the same year that both Linda Sluder and Alfred E. Wilhelmi died. The McKenzies' attorney had considered interviewing Wilhelmi, but had heard that the chemist was suffering from terminal cancer. Emory University quietly reached an out-of-court settlement with the New Zealand family.

Wilhelmi's papers went to Emory, which restricted them from public view. There were no trials or public inquiries. Few families got as far as court in the United States. Lawyers discouraged them from attempts to sue the federal government. Many were neither well off nor well educated. Some persisted and their cases failed, including the Sluders'. A few were settled for small amounts, like one against Harbor UCLA, where Parlow did his processing; a family received $35,000 in compensation without having to prove that his product had anything to do with their daughter's death.

The NIH updated information on its website, and provided a phone number for people to call with questions. Links were provided to existing organizations for people or families with growth disorders. But some of those groups charged membership fees, and were not an especially good match for people who found themselves in a uniquely frightening situation. When former patients called the NIH concerned about neurological symptoms, Judith Fradkin said, the government had doctors lined up willing to see them. But NIH did not provide support groups, though some former patients asked. It did not help people living with the threat of CJD contact each other, though some asked for that, too. According to Fradkin, who became director of the Division of Diabetes, Endocrinology, and Metabolic Diseases in 2001, it's "very complex information—you don't want them to be giving each other false information."

Though the United States government was widely praised for having halted pituitary hGH distribution after the first CJD cases, and for immediately notifying doctors, assiduously tracking down former patients, and keeping everyone informed of the latest science, it escaped the public exposure and investigation that took place in other countries. Why had this tragedy happened? Should someone have known sooner? Who should help those living with the terrifying threat of CJD?

DAVID DAVIS STARTS TO WORRY

In southern California, nearing forty years old, David Davis would have liked an apology, at least. Davis had never forgotten the years of injections, when he used to rub his arm and dream of playing basketball, and though he didn't wake up every morning thinking about the prion that might be seeded in his brain, he did think of it sometimes, especially as he got older. Before that he was "being young and dumb and a guy and I'm going to kick ass and I'm going to try everything once and just live life."

Davis was a staff writer at *LA Weekly* when something happened to his vision in one eye. He had just recently received one of those letters from the federal government, the ones that kept him up to date on the toll among pituitary growth hormone recipients. The eye doctor who examined Davis was not exactly sure what was wrong at first; he thought that Davis should go see a specialist. In the twenty minutes before he was diagnosed with a detached retina, CJD was very much on David Davis's mind. He was "freaking out."

As he went through emergency eye surgery, Davis also realized no one had asked him whether or not he'd had pituitary growth hormone treatment as a child. He had told the eye doctor, who didn't know what to make of it, though people who received pit-hGH were excluded from giving blood in case they harbored the infection without yet showing symptoms. No one knew whether or not CJD could be transmitted through blood transfusions. Clearly the eye surgeon did not understand that he might have to take special precautions with his instruments so that they would not infect any other patients later. Which made Davis remember that a corneal transplant patient had died of CJD. "I was acutely aware of: 'Oh shit, I could be dead in a year,' in the back of my mind, and that's when that issue came to the fore and I ended up writing about it for the first time."

Davis's first story, which ran in *LA Weekly* in March 1997, began with a scene of himself in 1973 as "a slight ten-year-old boy with light red hair and freckles" waiting in the kitchen for his mother to come in and inject his upper arm. "I dreaded the shots, but I endured them: I was going to grow taller." He described reaching 5'4", not tall "but not abnormal either," and going off to college; coming home for a while after graduation, preparing to travel through Australia. He was twenty-two years old. One night, his parents called him into the dining room and grimly handed him the first letter from NIH. Davis asked them what they thought about his odds of getting Creutzfeldt-Jakob disease, and they recited the numbers from the letter: about one in twenty-five hundred recipients had died. That didn't sound too bad. "I'll take those odds," he said, and went off to live his life.

Then Davis described how with each letter over the years, he would recalculate. In 1987, with five more cases, that was one in 1,600. In 1989, one in 1,150. In 1994, about one in 725. The letter that precipitated his first article meant his odds were down to about one in 500. He didn't like the direction they were heading, or the way his life was going. He'd had some failed relationships, some broken bones, the emergency eye surgery. He wanted to meet other people who had shared the same experiences and lived with the same oppressive knowledge.

In that first story, Davis wrote eloquently, alternating between anger and understanding. His mother, after all, was a pediatrician, and she'd given him the shots herself. "The hGH crisis, like many in medicine was born not of malice, but of unchecked enthusiasm. The physicians who prescribed the hormone believed, with an almost religious fervor, in what it could do for their patients with hypopituitary dwarfism," Davis wrote. He credited pediatric endocrinologists' good intentions. No one meant to do him harm. Yet he also thought that history showed doctors were more likely to experiment on some groups of people than on others, and he did feel experimented on. "Hypopituitary dwarfs don't lead normal lives, and thus were perfect candidates for a virtually untested drug," the article read. "The hGH injections were experiments under the banner of therapy, and physicians used their own patients as subjects."

Davis would have liked to be taller than 5'4", but he certainly appreciated that he hadn't ended up under five feet. He'd dwelt on his height and his treatment for it throughout his life, not just on the possibility he might die of Creutzfeldt-Jakob disease. When he did find a few other people who'd also been diagnosed with hypopituitary dwarfism as children, he was amazed how quickly they connected and discovered their commonalities: "It was clear from talking to the others that the inches we gained didn't necessarily translate into 'normal' lives. Rather, the treatment underscored our pervasive sense of being abnormal and raised expectations (perhaps unattainable) about the outcome."

He discovered they shared something else as well, a sense that they had been handed this potential death sentence and left to deal with it as best they could while the medical profession went on pursuing a new round of miracles. When he met people who received the letters that always began, "Dear Growth Hormone Recipient," they would agree: "The people who got us into this mess have completely abandoned us. Once a year—tops—they send us an update." The doctors and organizations had made their reputations giving hypopituitary dwarfs hGH from cadavers, and then moved on without looking back. NIH did the survey and sent out the scientific information, but had not arranged for counseling or helped hormone recipients find one another to talk about their struggles with the aftermath of treatment.

Writing about it all made Davis feel better. He learned a lot, and met some of those doctors and scientists who made the decisions that changed his life. He talked with Al Parlow. He reached Robert Blizzard. Davis also would have liked to talk with more people in his situation; he asked the NIH to mail a letter at his expense to all pituitary hGH recipients. Judith Fradkin explained that they didn't want to upset people. He understood that reasoning, but he also believed that if he were diagnosed with any other potentially devastating disease a doctor would give him a phone number for a support group along with medical treatment. He didn't think the NIH wanted former patients to get together: "I think there's a paternalism aspect to this. Even Parlow will venture into these realms of, 'Oh, we know what's best for you,' and that really pisses me off. And it may piss me off, because I think it in some ways reflects how we've been treated in the past: 'Here are these little kids, we'll send you the letter when we think it's right to send you the letters. We'll withhold information because we think it's right. We won't let you guys get together and talk.' It doesn't seem like I'm asking for a whole lot."

As his articles appeared, more former hormone recipients contacted Davis.

In 1998, he wrote about a Long Island mother the survey missed until she developed CJD and died; she'd never gotten the word that her childhood growth hormone treatments had put her at risk. In 2000, Davis wrote about how another man lived with the threat of CJD. These connections felt deep. Whenever he found someone who'd been given pituitary hGH, and they talked over a cup of coffee, it was as if they had survived cancer or some other serious illness together.

In August 2001, Davis wrote about Alfred Wilhelmi for *Atlanta* magazine. Researching for that article, he uncovered what he considered clear violations of medical ethics in the use of pituitary growth hormone. He thought that, however well-meaning their intentions, doctors had practiced just what the title of the article declared: "bad medicine." Davis was a sportswriter at this point, but he kept being drawn back to the story that was so central to his life. This time he described how convinced he'd been at twenty-two that knowing his risk would not affect his life. But, he said, "I've wrestled with the specter of CJD—that at any moment I might succumb to a gruesome disease—ever since. There were times when I ignored it and chose to party myself into oblivion. I've stared deeply into it and scared myself into bouts of depression. I've been so angry I could scarcely find my voice." He'd found his voice.

Gradually, as the cases started to taper off, Davis felt some relief about his own health, and the anger subsided. The victims he knew about were all among those who began treatment earlier than he had. Still, he wondered how many more were out there whose deaths had been misdiagnosed, or who might have died in an accident or some other way before their CJD manifested itself. An apology, David Davis thought, would at least give him some satisfaction—that someone had owned up, taken responsibility, implicitly admitted that mistakes had been made.

IN BRITAIN: "NEGLIGENTLY LETHARGIC"

Former patients, and the families of those who died because of the pituitary programs that spread from the United States around the world, found their collective voices in other countries. In Britain, they found it in court. In Australia, there was a massive government inquiry. In France, a criminal investigation. As health officials elsewhere were forced to face their mistakes, clues did emerge about how a therapy meant to cure had also killed.

Unlike the Americans, the British had immediate records of the children treated there with growth hormone. But the Department of Health decided not to inform them after the first CJD death in February 1985. There was nothing families could do anyway, no diagnosis or cure. They were kept in the dark about the disease hanging over them until four years later, when a second recipient died. Families of CJD victims in England blamed their government for not recognizing the possibility that pituitary hGH could transmit Creutzfeldt-Jakob disease. They sued the British Medical Research Council (the British equivalent to the National Institutes of Health) and the Department of Health for negligence. Other former patients wanted compensation for what their attorneys called the "psychiatric injury" of living daily with the fear that they'd been infected, that a time bomb might be in their brains.

The trial, in April and May 1997, revolved around how much was known about how spongiform encephalopathies like scrapie, *kuru*, and CJD were transmitted. In what year should health officials have recognized the danger? At first, attorneys for the victims thought that the program should have adopted the Roos gel filtration method of processing frozen glands from the very beginning, around 1963. But the Medical Research Council, which launched the program, had received advice that storing glands in acetone actually was safer, because acetone killed viruses.

The Americans had used acetone to store glands rather than freezing them, too. A British court document noted that, in 1973, the UK program sought advice from "suitable experts in the United States, Dr. Wilhelmi and Dr. Raiti, who stated that they considered the risk of viral contamination of hGH small and that no patients of theirs had been adversely affected despite the large numbers treated by them with hGH prepared from pituitaries stored in acetone." Hepatitis would have been the potentially deadly virus that most concerned doctors in the early seventies.

Even as Raiti and Wilhelmi reassured their British colleagues that pituitary hGH was not making people sick, some of the children in both countries already harbored the incubating CJD infection given to them unknowingly by pediatric endocrinologists. Even more tragically, a different set of U.S. experts—those in Carleton Gajdusek's laboratory—were already learning how spongiform encephalopathies spread and how difficult the infectious agent was to kill. Scientists in Gajdusek's lab had published studies and warnings in various journals in the late sixties and early seventies, including Gajdusek's experiment transmitting CJD from a human victim into a chimpanzee. The victims' lawyers argued that the key year in Britain had been 1974, because as the Medical Research Council looked into switching to processing frozen glands, it should have reviewed the safety of the entire program. At that point, the attorneys insisted "the literature trail would have led to the identification of the risk of contamination." They argued that these pieces of the puzzle could have been put together:

That CJD was transmissible by injection of brain tissue;

That there was a close similarity between the human spongiform encephalopathies and the animal varieties, particularly scrapie;

That the only safe working premise was that research data in relation to scrapie was directly relevant to CJD;

That scrapie was highly resistant to conventional forms of viricidal agent;

That acetone could not be relied upon to eradiate slow viruses (the prion);

That scrapie infected the pituitary;

That it was suspected then that other neurological diseases could be transmitted the same way.

In 1974, too, *The New England Journal of Medicine* published the letter describing transmission of CJD by corneal transplant; and Gajdusek warned in the *Journal of Neurosurgery* that extraordinary precautions should be taken when performing biopsies or autopsies on CJD patients.

Carleton Gajdusek was not available to testify in the London trial. He had pleaded guilty to sexually molesting a Fore boy he had brought back from New Guinea to live with him, and had gone to prison. But a virologist from Gajdusek's lab did support the British health agencies' argument, testifying that those involved with the growth hormone program could not have been expected to make a connection between transmissible dementias and pituitary hGH, in spite of the literature trail: "Awareness of the risk would have required a highly unlikely sharing of knowledge of veterinarians, neurologists, virologists and endocrinologists." The judge agreed—the disease had been too rare, the experts too specialized, the danger too remote. He did not find that the program officials had been negligent in 1974. Among other reasons, he noted that no government or research agency or pharmaceutical company anywhere in the world had exhibited concern that human growth hormone might transmit slow viruses. No one had put together the puzzle pieces by then, as far as the judge understood.

The year they should have known and acted, he ruled, was 1977. They should have responded urgently to Alan Dickinson, the scrapie expert who had spent a sleepless night thinking about how human growth hormone was processed and who contacted the Medical Research Council with his concerns. The year 1977 also was when Gajdusek's Nobel Prize lecture, warning about the risk of transmitting CJD in tissue, appeared in the widely read and multidisciplinary journal *Science*. The judge ruled that the British health agencies had been negligent when they did not immediately follow up on Dickinson's fears. They did ask Dickinson's advice; he thought the acetone preservation method might be better than the frozen method, which turned out to be wrong. But he had also insisted that both methods should be tested with scrapie-infected mouse brain. He had told them that the growth hormone program should exclude pituitaries from patients with dementia.

An unhurried year after Dickinson's warning, British health officials asked the advice of two academic virologists, who confirmed that there was a risk that pit-hGH could transmit CJD, though they thought it was remote. Even so, one virologist had stressed that the pediatric endocrinologists who were treating the children should be made aware of the "gruesome possibilities and their imponderable probabilities" and take ultimate responsibility when deciding whether or not to continue the injections. But the virologist's letter did not go to either the steering committee that ran the treatment program or to the doctor's committee responsible for patients. British pediatric endocrinologists remained uninformed that they might be lethally infecting kids they were trying to help.

Finally, in 1980, a sluggish three and a half years after Dickinson's initial alarm, the British changed their collection criteria to exclude glands from patients with dementia or CJD. That occurred, not in response to Dickinson, but only after a report by a Department of Health Slow Virus Group that had been established to consider Gajdusek's 1977 warning that tissue from CJD patients could remain infectious. Incredibly, the Americans did not do the same. In 1975—in spite of Wilhelmi's and Raiti's earlier assurances to their British counterparts that pituitary hGH appeared safe from viruses— the U.S. National Hormone and Pituitary Program had changed its instructions to pathologists, excluding glands from people who died of infectious or serum hepatitis, or from drug addicts who were at high risk for it. Those new instructions, however, made no mention of slow viruses, presenile dementia, or other names used at the time to describe CJD. According to the NIH, although Gajdusek worked at NIH and his papers were published in American journals, the pituitary program that operated in the United States under NIH auspices *never* excluded pituitary glands from patients known to have died of Creutzfeldt-Jakob disease.

The British judge ruled that there had been a "negligent failure" in the United Kingdom to take necessary steps. They had waited more than a year to seek expert neurological advice; they delayed eighteen months before instructing Dickinson to proceed with his tests of their extraction methods; they did not notify the endocrinologists who went on treating children; and they failed to investigate how glands were excluded or processed.

The "medical and scientific staff of the Department...who were fully alive to the potential risk of slow virus contamination of the human growth hormone, wanted the problem kept under wraps in the hope or belief that the risk would never eventuate into an awful reality," the judge wrote. "In my judgment an unwise philosophy pervaded both within the Department of Health and the Medical Research Council that the risk of slow virus contamination of human growth hormone was too awful to contemplate, or at least should not be the subject of public knowledge and the discussion even among clinicians, who owed a duty of care to their child patients." Both agencies had recognized the risk between 1976 and 1980, but did not protect the patients. The judge ordered compensation on behalf of all those who began treatment in Britain after July 1, 1977, with hormone prepared by the Wilhelmi method. The court later expanded the number of recipients who could be compensated, including some of the so-called worried well who suffered recognized psychiatric illnesses as a result of living with the threat of CJD.

Some noted afterward that the Medical Research Council had stockpiled pituitary hGH at great expense, and had weighed what appeared to be a theoretical risk on the one hand versus the risks of stopping treatment. They knew recombinant human growth hormone was almost ready for use. A medical risk is always theoretical, of course, until the worst happens. There was a lesson here for medical science, the attorney representing British victims suggested: "The saga perhaps demonstrates that we never know as much as we think we do."

He also described how the trial served as a public inquiry, especially for the parents who listened through weeks of testimony with "the dreadful burden of guilt.... It was they who made the decision to give [their children] this treatment, simply because they were short. The parents without exception—and most were there for most of the trial—ended the trial with a profound sense of relief at knowing exactly what happened, what had been decided and when. There is no doubt that it was a cathartic experience for them."

AUSTRALIAN CONCERNS
THAT AUSTRALIANS IGNORED

In Australia, someone had put together the puzzle pieces even earlier. Perhaps because the medical community there avidly followed Gajdusek's descriptions of *kuru* in New Guinea, which was an Australian territory, some of those advising the pituitary program realized by 1971 that hormones could possibly carry transmissible dementias. Nevertheless, Australia also failed to protect its patients.

In June 1994, the eight-hundred-page *Report of the Inquiry into the*

Use of Pituitary Derived Hormones in Australia and Creutzfeldt-Jakob Disease analyzed the findings of a government-ordered investigation conducted by University of Sydney law professor Margaret Allars. There had been only one CJD death in that country related to growth hormone, but more among women treated for infertility with a different pituitary hormone. The Allars report found that in 1971, Vincent McGovern, a representative of the College of Pathologists who sat on the Human Pituitary Advisory Committee, "raised the issue of the danger of unconventional slow viral infection of collected pituitary glands," and that the committee then wrote to Australia's College of Pathologists seeking advice. Two pathologists knowledgeable about slow viruses replied, sharing McGovern's concern:

"We both agree with the opinion given by Dr. McGovern. There is good evidence that Kuru and certain diseases of sheep rarely transmissible to man [are] caused by their small virus-like agents which are unusually resistant to heat, formalin and ultraviolet light. It is also possible that all commonly demyelinating diseases such as multiple sclerosis come into the same category. It is our opinion that pituitary glands should not be collected from patients who have died from demyelinating or chronic neurological diseases of the central nervous system." The Australian criteria were revised to exclude not just hepatitis and pituitary diseases but also neurological diseases of the central nervous system possibly due to viral infection. McGovern arranged for these new criteria to be published in the Newsletter of the College of Pathologists of Australia, years before anyone else appeared to take note of the risk.

But then, in July 1977, worried about increasing the yield of hormone, for some reason the Australian laboratory processing the glands redrafted the instructions and left out neurological diseases. The Allars committee didn't get an explanation. The inquiry found no record of any discussion of unconventional slow viruses among pituitary program advisors between McGovern's 1971 warning and 1980. That's when the Australians talked with the director of the British Medical Research Council, which was revising its collection criteria to exclude glands from CJD patients. A subcommittee of Australia's hormone program discussed doing the same at a May 1980 meeting, but decided that there was no evidence that Creutzfeldt-Jakob disease was present in the Australian population. Yet cases of CJD had been reported in Melbourne as early as 1963. The doctors and scientists on the subcommittee sought no outside expert advice. Allars found subcommittee members were "not to be blamed for their lack of expertise or lack of familiarity with the developments in knowledge of CJD. They were not neuropathologists or virologists. They are to be blamed for their failure to recognize the limits of their expertise and the need to seek advice."

Just as the British court found that the UK Department of Health should have acted on CJD contamination warnings by July 1977, Allars declared Australia should have acted at least by 1980, when the advisory committee instead "pushed aside the issue of risk of slow viruses, as evidenced in its minutes. I did not have sufficient evidence to be able to pinpoint precisely a time in the period between 1977 and 1980 when Australians... gained knowledge of the risk through their attendance at international scientific meetings with their English counterparts."

Another government scientist testified to the Allars committee that "from 1973 onwards, Health Department files expressed concerns about the possibility of transferring CJD by medical goods and instruments" and relayed them to the pituitary program advisory committee, "which the files show ignored the warnings." Two other prominent Australian medical experts agreed, telling the Allars committee: "We believe that it should have been apparent by the mid-1970s to biological scientists with a familiarity with the general scientific literature that CJD and related conditions were likely to be transmissible."

One of these experts, Wesley Whitten, had warned in 1966 that pituitary processing might not remove all viruses when he served as assistant of the National Biological Standards Laboratory (Australia's FDA). In 1978, the standards laboratory raised concerns about slow viruses when it evaluated an application from a company that sought to sell human growth hormone to Australians. Commercial pituitary hGH, which was allowed onto the U.S. market, was denied approval in Australia.

Yet the Australian government program continued, and a Health Department official argued that the perspective was different if one placed oneself back in 1977 or 1980. He was sure people were familiar with the scientific articles "but making the leap from saying that corneal grafts, that neurosurgical instruments transmit the CJD agent, to saying that this is a possibility through pituitary hormones, and then going further and saying it is such a possibility that the program should be re-examined and stopped is a substantial leap that was not made in this country and was not made in any other country."

In fact, in the United States, where the National Pituitary Agency had been cosponsored by the College of Pathologists and pathologists were listed on its letterhead, no one seems to have made even the first step, unlike pathologists in Australia.

Perhaps the most important conclusion drawn by the Allars inquiry was that when doctors ignore boundaries between treating patients and experimenting on them, the stage is set for tragedy. It is "a dangerous situation if no attempt is made to draw the lines between ordinary exercise of clinical judgment, research, experiment and clinical trial, even if those lines be blurred lines. The absence of lines is most dangerous when new advances in medicine are being explored." The committee added the lesson of lack of proper control, which it likened to "Dracula in charge of the blood bank.... It was a very narrow, a very self-interested group, who were running the Australian human pituitary program."

The Australians set up counseling services and support groups, established a trust fund to cover medical and other care costs for victims, and designated money for research. But some hormone recipients remained dissatisfied with the outcome of the inquiry. Australia's Senate Community Affairs Committee looked into their objections and issued yet another report in 1998; it quoted one former patient who complained that "no one will ever be made accountable for their improper actions." Instead, wrote another, the members of the Human Pituitary Hormone Program committee "sought kudos and career advancement ahead of prudent medical practice and patient safety."

In 1998, the Australian government issued a formal apology.

THE UNITED STATES KEEPS THE LID ON

Most pediatric endocrinologists in the United States insisted they never heard of CJD until 1985, and that they had no reason to know about a rare group of diseases linked to cannibals in the remote New Guinea jungle. Raymond Hintz remembered being aware in 1982, at an FDA conference on various tissue processing, that prion diseases might contaminate pituitary hormones. John Crawford, the Boston doctor who treated the tall girls, recalled knowing that there was a "theoretical possibility" pituitary hGH could carry CJD after the 1974 death of a Boston neurosurgeon who had operated on the brain of an infected patient. That recollection might have been hindsight, however. Robert Blizzard, in the grand tradition of the early endocrinologists who would experiment on themselves, was still giving himself cadaveric hGH injections as part of his small study on aging in 1985.

Al Parlow said he remained unaware that CJD could lurk in pituitaries as well as the central nervous system until Alan Dickinson's unpublished work, which he learned of in April 1985, in the office of the director of the National Institute of Diabetes and Digestive and Kidney Diseases. That was the meeting that sealed the fate of human-pituitary-derived hGH. One of Dickinson's colleagues attended the meeting to describe results of their experiment, which were published shortly after. In Parlow's mind it didn't really matter, though, because when he took over, he said, "I know how we did things—rigidly, compulsively, carefully, consistently, and at the highest level of operational standards....There were twenty-eight batches and each one of them a perfect batch. Never compromised." Almost as if they came from God.

While Parlow waited for his vindication, former National Hormone and Pituitary Program director Salvatore Raiti complained he was the sacrificial victim, the forgotten man. A defeated-looking man with an Australian accent, stooped shoulders, and thinning hair, Raiti was working in Baltimore emergency rooms just to make a living. "They took the program from us....I had to find another job." He complained that "I'm a forgotten soul. I did so much for so many people." He'd expanded the pituitary collection from 10,000 to 80,000 glands in just a couple of years of achievement, initiated the switch from acetone-stored to frozen glands. "I in a sense sacrificed an academic career. I expected some recognition....I waited twenty-five years. Nothing came."

Raiti said he, too, heard of CJD only in 1985, when Raymond Hintz notified him of the first death, and that there was no reason he should have recognized the danger earlier. "The NIH is not the NIH, it is not a single institute. It's ten or fifteen institutions. They each operated independently of each other, some rivalry between them. The people working with these viruses had their own little world." Even so, he said, if recombinant hGH hadn't been on the horizon when Hintz reported the first CJD case among hormone recipients, "I think people would have taken the risk" and continued the pituitary program. It was, Raiti pointed out, "only twenty something cases" out of perhaps 10,000 treated.

The decision makers at NIH, those higher up the chain, died without facing the public questions that their counterparts endured in other countries. Did they read any of Gajdusek's advice to pathologists? Hear about the concerns expressed in *kuru*-savvy Australia? Were they contacted in 1980 by the prominent French scientist Luc Montagnier, who said he warned doctors running the pituitary program in France, and reportedly warned program directors in other countries? Did they notice that the British excluded glands from CJD patients in 1980?

The questions of who knew or should have known in 1977 or 1980 at the least seemed less pressing, as no cases turned up among those who began their hormone therapy after Parlow took over the processing. Those who began receiving Wilhelmi's pituitary preparations after 1970, like David Davis and Tony Grossenburg, remained at risk. But they had not spent nine years taking pre-1970 preparations, and that was the average duration of treatment for known CJD cases in the United States. Father Tony Grossenburg rarely thought about the possibility that he'd been infected. When entering the priesthood, he had revealed to the Church his history with human growth hormone and the remote threat that hung over his health. After that, CJD only occasionally crossed his mind—say, if he stumbled a little as he paced while delivering a sermon.

Judith Fradkin believed they'd found all the CJD deaths from the past, and hoped there would be no more in the future. They had a few good years in 2000, 2001, and 2002 and thought at last the epidemic was over; then another case. And another. "You get your hopes up—it's always devastating when you hear of these." They no longer sent out letters. They just kept their website updated.

No one knew when those treated for height as children could finally release their breath. In 2002, the *Journal of Neurology, Neurosurgery, and Psychiatry* published a report of a forty-seven-year-old man in the Netherlands who had received just one dose of human-derived growth hormone, as part of a diagnostic procedure when he was a child. Thirty-eight years later, he developed CJD. This was the longest incubation period yet.

In the journal *Neurology* in 2003, epidemiologists concluded that preparations using Wilhelmi's methods carried the highest risk of infecting children in the United Kingdom, where thirty-eight had developed CJD, and most had been infected when they were eight to ten years old. In Britain, "the peak risk of CJD was estimated to occur twenty years after first exposure, and the estimated lifetime cumulative risk of CJD in Wilhelmi-treated patients was 4.5 percent." About one in twenty. Not great odds. On the other hand, the study concluded that "size-exclusion chromatography, used in non-Wilhelmi preparation methods, may prevent CJD infection." It was looking pretty good for Parlow's product, anyway.

PART 5

$35,000 an inch— and growing

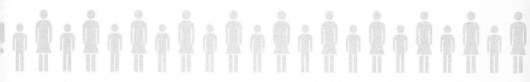

CHAPTER 12

a disease is born

BALLROOM IN
BASKETBALL COUNTRY: DAY ONE

The Human Growth Foundation 2003 annual meeting in Kansas City, Missouri, looked nothing like the parent organization Fred and Gwen Mahler remembered. The Mahlers were invited to a luncheon, along with Bob Blizzard, to honor their pioneering roles on behalf of the National Pituitary Agency—when Fred flew with jars of collected glands in his cockpit, and Gwen persuaded the Clipped Wings to champion the cause of dwarfed children. Fred had retired, and the two Mahler children whom Blizzard treated for height were grown: the Mahlers' son, about 5'8", had children of his own. Their daughter, though just five feet, resolutely pursued her dream to become a pilot like her dad. She'd recently ferried American troops into Iraq, and her parents couldn't have been prouder. She would be flying in to see them honored.

Gwen Mahler came thinking that she might pitch in again on behalf of the nonprofit group, just like the old days. Maybe a bake sale? Something to help raise money for kids with growth disorders? She was energetic as ever and ready to roll up her sleeves. But she'd been told by the director, Patricia Costa, that these days the Human Growth Foundation existed mostly on the Internet. It kept a website, published the informational booklets that doctors liked to distribute in their offices, and held this annual event. Gwen seemed a little puzzled. Where were all the families?

It was a blustery day in Kansas City, which was hosting a basketball tourney downtown. The purple banners of Kansas State's Wildcats fluttered on some buildings, a reminder of how sports reign in the Midwest. Basketball talk bounced through the hallways.

Many of the 120 or so people signing into the meeting at the Hyatt Hotel were area doctors and nurses seeking Continuing Medical Education credit. Required in most states to keep licenses current, the hundreds of courses, conferences, lectures, and informational luncheons that physicians must attend each year have spurred the creation of a whole medical education industry, one closely entwined with the pharmaceutical companies. At the Human Growth Foundation event, attendees entered a ballroom ringed by sales representatives who manned tables for each of the growth hormone manufacturers. The tables offered bowls of candy, stacks of brochures, piles of colorful giveaways bearing product logos: backpacks, pens shaped like teddy bears and lions, stuffed animals, and tape measures with their implied promise of growth. Cartoon characters and close-ups of grinning kids overlooked the displays from posters on the walls.

Since they all sell essentially the same product, the companies try to distinguish themselves in other ways. Genentech's sales rep touted their long-acting, or depot, delivery system. It didn't work as well for growth as daily injections, he acknowledged, but for teenagers who were the "least compliant group," as he put it, this was better than nothing. Pfizer/Pharmacia talked up a companion program that employed four nurses who did nothing but work on insurance appeals all day long. Novo Nordisk showed off its premeasured dose in a device that looks more like a pen than a syringe, aimed at enabling even young children to inject themselves. No one had achieved what one sales rep confided was the "holy grail"—a method to deliver growth hormone in a pill. He didn't think they ever would, though he'd heard that a rival company was at work on an inhaler. With people strolling from table to table and scooping up goodies, the scene in some ways suggested a bazaar, but none of the eager-to-chat sales staffers offered any bargains. Manufacturers hadn't been forced to lower prices significantly on growth hormone to compete. "It's pretty pricey," one company rep sympathized with two parents, but he assured them that "no one pays out of pocket" and that his company could start the therapy going while they switched to an insurer that would cover treatment.

Some had come to the meeting for both personal and professional reasons. One nurse also had a son taking growth hormone for height. She became concerned when he wore the same size T-shirt for six years, and worried that his asthma medication might have stunted his growth. Now he was a junior in high school and 5'10", not only normal but just above average for an American male. Still, the pediatric endocrinologist hoped to eke out at least another inch, and her son aspired to his full "genetic potential of six feet," and a chance to compete at basketball. He was a talented athlete relegated to the B teams by coaches because of his size. Her in-laws disapproved, and so she hid the medicine from them whenever they visited, but as soon as they left she took it out again. Another nurse admitted a bit self-consciously that she'd attended partly to investigate the therapy for her child, a middle school wrestler who weighed only sixty-four pounds. Though she knew that her son had probably inherited his slow road to puberty from his father, and that he didn't seem unhappy, she was anxious for him to be able to continue his sport through high school.

Though there weren't many families to hear it, the first night featured a panel on "Living with Short Stature." A pediatric resident with Turner syndrome shared her experiences, as did three adolescent boys accompanied by their mothers. The pediatrician-in-training had been given pituitary hGH briefly, until CJD swept it off the shelves; biosynthetic growth hormone arrived on the market too late for her. She ended up 4'8½" tall. Yet she talked about how she had never let her short stature stop her: from campaigning for student council in junior high school, from playing tennis, from graduating from college and medical school, or even from driving a car. In fact, she cheerfully offered to share the name of a great local garage where she got pedal extenders.

The mothers, on the other hand, talked more about living with growth hormone therapy than living with short stature. They were grateful that hGH seemed to be working for their sons. These parents had overcome the objections of relatives who thought they should just let nature take its course, and also of insurance companies that excluded growth hormone from coverage. None of their children had been diagnosed with GHD. One mother described how a pediatrician said her boy was the smallest eighteen-month-old the doctor had ever seen. Yet physicians kept advising her to wait and see if he would sprout. At age five, her son took an overnight stimulation test. The test had been "very traumatic," and his hormone level registered normal. Doctors pointed out that both she and her husband were short. But she knew they had to take action; when they plotted her son's growth, it looked as if he might end up around 4'10". At six, the boy went on growth hormone–releasing hormone as part of an experimental protocol, then on to hGH. Both her sons had also taken Lupron and, more recently, an aromatase inhibitor. Some doctors in the audience murmured their surprise.

Pediatric endocrinologists have experimented with Lupron for more than a decade to delay puberty, and possibly increase final height. Aromatase inhibitors, on the other hand, are newer and are used to treat breast cancer by making the body unresponsive to estrogen. In the 1970s, a man with a rare resistance to estrogen was described in the medical literature when he grew an additional ten inches after puberty. At twenty-eight, he had reached 6'8", and his growth plates still had not fused. From that case doctors learned how important estrogen is for growth plate closure, not only in girls but also in boys, in whom some testosterone naturally converts to estrogen. It occurred to more than one pediatric endocrinologist that if you could hold the growth plates open indefinitely by restricting estrogen, a patient could be made to grow well beyond puberty. In fact, possibly beyond any limits imposed by genetic potential. And unlike Lupron, aromatase inhibitors do not prevent the development of secondary sex characteristics; a boy's voice deepens and his beard starts to grow right on schedule with his classmates. However, the use of these two very potent medicines combined with hGH to treat height is not only unapproved and experimental but also controversial, especially outside a controlled study. They add to the already considerable expense. They carry risks, not all of them known yet. Among other things, estrogen is key to bone density and preventing fractures.

The mother speaking didn't notice the murmur of interest as she finished her account of her son's growth. At fifteen, he was 5'5" and as tall as his father. The doctors now predicted that he would reach 5'7". "We're keeping our fingers crossed," she said, and told the story of the time he was "demoted" to the B team in basketball and the coach phoned to explain that her son was "really gifted" but had to be cut from the top squad solely because of his height. They would keep hGH therapy going as long as there seemed to be a potential for more growth.

Her son, looking and sounding like a normal teenager, recalled being teased when he was very young—"Kids can be mean sometimes"—and he didn't think there was a good comeback. But he told the audience he played soccer, a sport in which he found that height doesn't matter a whole lot, and he was running track. He announced with pride that he'd just clocked the best time on his junior varsity squad, concluding: "If you don't let height control your life, you really can get past it."

Later, standing in the buffet line, the adolescent answered a more personal question without embarrassment: Had he minded delaying puberty? He replied that it had been all right. His mother was more adamant. She refused to let her son end up at a height unacceptable for a man. She'd been relieved and grateful to discover a pediatric endocrinologist who would ignore the growth hormone deficiency test results, who would treat her boys, and who would keep going until they got as tall as they could.

DAY TWO: EDUCATING DOCTORS
TO "OPTIMIZE HEIGHT"

The next day's schedule of talks, unlike the teddy bear pens or the panel of mothers, was not aimed at families. The events were called educational sessions. The assembled medical professionals learned that pediatricians, general practitioners, and nurses should not just dismiss kids with one normal test, or assume youngsters who came from short families had nothing wrong with them; and that endocrinologists shouldn't necessarily stop prescribing hGH when an adolescent reached normal height, or even stopped growing. Basically, growth hormone should be prescribed earlier, more often, and longer. Several speakers suggested patients with GHD should continue treatment during adulthood, when levels naturally decline, because of growth hormone's impact on energy and muscle mass, cardiovascular function and bone density.

In 1996, the FDA approved hGH for adults with growth hormone deficiency, though not for obesity or aging or bodybuilding or improved athletic performance or any of the other uses that make it a flourishing black-market drug. Among the goals of adult GHD treatment is the vaguely defined one of enhancing a patient's perception of well-being.

It's an area rife with abuse, acknowledged Wayne Moore, a pediatric endocrinologist at the University of Kansas who addressed the Human Growth Foundation meeting on the topic. The question of whether everyone with childhood GHD should receive lifelong treatment remained controversial, he acknowledged. Still, doctors should counsel young patients and their parents that the shots might need to continue even after the growing was done. He flashed a photo of a seventeen-year-old girl in a bikini onto the screen, taken eight months after she had reached full height. She still weighed the same 120 pounds, but complained that she didn't feel energetic enough to exercise the way she used to on growth hormone therapy, and that she'd gained some abdominal fat. Moore paused over the photograph of the adolescent after she resumed taking hGH, allowing the audience to fully appreciate her lean look in a bikini. She and her family, he commented, were satisfied with the results.

In another educational session, Sandra Blethen, a pediatric endocrinologist and Ph.D. working for the pharmaceutical manufacturer Serono, lectured that a doctor's goal should be to make kids as tall as possible, not just as tall as normal. She described how the aim in the pituitary era had been to give children just enough hormone to get them to a specified cutoff. By contrast, the recombinant era aimed at giving patients as much as they needed to "optimize height": "Our goal is to get a child to a height that reflects his genetic potential, not a minimally socially acceptable height."

Blethen predicted that, given the explosion of knowledge gained from the deciphering of the human genome, eventually there would be no such diagnosis as idiopathic short stature or even familial short stature or, possibly, constitutional growth delay. It probably would turn out that extremely short kids had gene defects, she said. Blethen thought late bloomers probably did exist, but the burden was on doctors like those she was addressing to be very sure that's what they were seeing. Early diagnosis was key. "It's often very sad to have a youngster come in...at fourteen or sixteen or eighteen asking you can't you please do something about their growth."

Raymond Hintz had been flown in to handle the most important topic of the day: "Is growth hormone therapy safe?" Hintz, the Stanford pediatric endocrinologist long associated with Genentech, had emerged as the hero of the CJD tragedy, and biosynthetic hormone contained absolutely no danger of Creutzfeldt-Jakob disease. Yet even decades and more than 100,000 worldwide pediatric patients later, the long-term safety of growth hormone treatment worried some scientists.

In 2000, A. J. Swerdlow, an epidemiologist at the Institute of

Cancer Research in England, wrote that there was still insufficient data to rule out the cancer concerns raised by the reported association of both acromegaly and IGF-1 with malignancies. He argued for a large study of cancer incidence in people treated with hGH as children more than ten years before.

Just a few months before Hintz stood up in Kansas City to address the safety issue, Swerdlow and his colleagues published the troubling results of a study in *The Lancet*. Looking at 1,848 young people who received pituitary growth hormone for GHD in the United Kingdom from 1959 to 1985, they found a "greatly raised" incidence of colorectal cancer. They also found "significantly raised risks of mortality from cancer overall," as well as deaths from two specific malignancies: colorectal and Hodgkin's disease. Admitting that the conclusions were based on small numbers—two colon cancer deaths—and "cannot necessarily be generalized" to patients receiving biosynthetic hGH in modern daily dosing regimens, the authors called the need for further data urgent: "Our data do not show conclusively whether cancer incidence is increased by growth hormone treatment, but they do suggest the need for increased awareness of the possibility of cancer risks, and for surveillance of growth hormone-treated patients."

A commentary in the same issue, coauthored by an American and a Canadian doctor, calmed nerves somewhat: the findings were "not definitive," although they were "somewhat worrisome"; they should be weighed against the established benefits of treating GHD. On the other hand, the commentary continued, the British findings were troubling enough that doctors should reassess the risks and benefits for controversial uses of growth hormone, especially when concentrations of IGF-1 that occur through puberty and then naturally decline now might be maintained for decades artificially.

The Swerdlow study received widespread publicity, including an article in *The New York Times*, and set off what one pediatric endocrinologist described as a "tizzy" among her colleagues. Was this going to be another tragedy, more friendly fire? Online advice doctors fielded worried queries from parents. The Lawrence Wilkins Pediatric Endocrine Society issued a special editorial in *The Journal of Clinical Endocrinology and Metabolism* stating that available pediatric data did not support "any concern for excess malignancy at this time." The editorial warned that failure to treat GHD could lead to premature mortality from heart problems. It questioned whether the malignancies Swerdlow found might be coincidence. It stated that careful monitoring had begun in the pituitary era and that after the introduction of recombinant hGH, the "monitoring of potential adverse effects was meticulously continued, facilitated by scrupulously maintained, and continually enlarging, databases involving both government and pharmaceutical companies in concert with pediatric investigators." Raymond Hintz served on the committee that wrote the editorial.

Hintz was again reassuring, in his avuncular style. He told the Kansas City audience that while every biological substance has side effects, the pharmaceutical company databases had been "gathered assiduously" and formed the "first line of defense." In Genentech's National Collaborative Growth Study from 1985 to 1999, there had been reports of adverse events in 7.2 percent of the 33,161 patients, and only 799 "serious adverse events," representing just 2.4 percent. There had been 156 deaths. The most common cause of death had been recurring brain tumors in children whose GHD had been caused by either a pituitary tumor or tumor treatment. There had also been twenty cases of leukemia. Four of those occurred in children without previous risk factors. There had been sixty-eight cases of carbohydrate intolerance, which includes several types of diabetes.

The other major database, Pfizer/Pharmacia's KIGS (originally named the Kabi International Growth Study), also reported minor side effects among its 27,952 young patients, and some cases of sodium and water retention. If ignored, this can cause symptoms that range from swelling to intracranial hypertension to cardiac failure. KIGS also listed instances of slipped epiphyses in the hip joint, scoliosis, and acromegalic changes such as growth of the nose or jaw. The question, as it always is in epidemiology, was how many of these adverse events would have occurred anyway in the same age group. His conclusion from the KIGS database was that there was no evidence of increased risk for developing new tumors during growth hormone treatment. But of course, longer follow-up on more patients was called for to "strengthen these reassuring conclusions."

Hintz worked to defuse Swerdlow's research; he flashed a slide quoting the caution published in the study itself that no one should "over interpret risks based on such small numbers." He had spoken to the authors, and if they had decided to write their paper just six months earlier, before the second colon cancer case turned up, "they would have had no paper." Unfortunately, it was impossible to do this kind of research in the United States, where there is no cancer registry with which to compare hGH patients, and where privacy laws would prevent scientists from viewing the records even if they had them. Tracking patients for years after they discontinued their shots and no longer saw their pediatric endocrinologists would be "ideal." But, Hintz said, "I think the best we can do is convince our pharmaceutical colleagues to continue these follow-ups on into adulthood."

Overall, he concluded, "there's a very low incidence of adverse effects" in what "has been a very well-studied group." The majority of serious problems arose in kids with risk factors, including Down syndrome with its known leukemia risk and Turner syndrome with its propensity for carboydrate intolerance and fluid retention. Hintz imparted the encouraging message that hGH therapy was "mostly" safe. "It's very strong mostly.... In most cases this is as safe as any biologically active agent that we give," he said, leaving the impression that only a scientist's instinct for caution kept him from being unequivocal.

Indeed, in the question-and-answer session, he and Sandra Blethen from Serono joked together that many of the potential side effects listed on the consent forms were there only to CYA, or "cover your ass." More seriously, Hintz added that doctors would continue reviewing the cancer data carefully, because he had personally witnessed the effect of IGF-1 in a test tube on cells: "There is a theoretical concern because growth factors are growth factors and they make tumor cells grow, too, but in the clinical setting we do not see anything that looks ominous at this point." Then he knocked deliberately on the lectern, quipping that he hoped it was made of wood.

As Hintz confided in the hallway, after CJD he would "never say never" again.

LILLY ASKS THE FDA
TO ADD SHORT STATURE TO THE LABEL

A few months later in 2003, Raymond Hintz traveled to Bethesda, Maryland, on behalf of Eli Lilly to argue that the FDA should approve growth hormone for use in short healthy kids. Lilly sought permission to sell Humatrope to treat what it termed non–growth-hormone-deficient short stature, which it simply defined as any child shorter than 98.8 percent of others the same age and gender, the shortest subgroup of children with idiopathic short stature.

If Lilly won approval, the company could legally market to the same group that Genentech had been criminally prosecuted for targeting, and insurance companies could no longer automatically deny reimbursement when stimulation test results came back normal. About 400,000 children in the United States between the ages of seven and fifteen met Lilly's definition. Even if doctors treated them all, there would still always be a bottom percentile. And many doubted the line would hold at only the very shortest. This struck some as the top of the slippery slope. Billions of dollars rode on Lilly's presentation to the Endocrinologic and Metabolic Drugs Advisory Committee, which would vote on a recommendation to the FDA's Center for Drug Evaluation and Research—especially since the FDA almost always accepts the recommendations of its advisory panels.

The FDA invited a Canadian researcher to present opposing arguments. He was Harvey Guyda, a professor of pediatrics at McGill University in Montreal, who'd been reluctant to come until he was told the FDA couldn't get anyone else. For thirty-seven years, he'd considered himself a member of the "pediatric endocrinology fraternity," as he liked to put it, a group that included old friends as well as colleagues.

Steeped in the values of the Canadian national health system, Guyda believed that doctors in the United States had been "brainwashed" into overprescribing hGH, starting with the influence of the pharmaceutical companies that pay for their training as young pediatric endocrinologists. In an interview the night before the FDA advisory meeting, while he ate dinner in the hotel where it would be held, Guyda bragged that 95 percent of Canadian patients treated through childhood for growth hormone deficiency still met the diagnosis when retested as young adults, unlike UK and U.S. patients. This was evidence that very few children without true GHD received growth hormone in Canada. Guyda believed in caution, and couldn't resist mentioning that Canada had suffered no cases of CJD from the pituitary hormone it processed. But he also objected to the treatment of idiopathic short stature with hGH as a matter of social justice. Why should such an expensive medicine go to possibly make someone who is healthy a little bit taller, when there were plenty of children within a few miles of Bethesda—and he nodded in the direction of the poor neighborhoods of Washington, D.C.—who might be severely growth hormone deficient yet didn't get medical care?

Still, Guyda wasn't looking forward to taking his public stand the next morning.

Before Lilly's application, the FDA had approved five pediatric indications for recombinant growth hormone. Besides GHD, chronic renal failure before kidney transplantation, and Turner syndrome, it added a rare genetic disorder called Prader-Willi syndrome in 2000. Prader-Willi children are born with slack muscles and missing the switch in the brain that signals they've had enough to eat, so that it's a constant struggle to restrain them from gorging. Families are forced to chain their refrigerators and lock their cupboards. Doctors thought hGH could improve muscle development in these children, reduce their fat, and boost their energy as well as their height. The following year, the FDA approved Pharmacia's application to add Small for

Gestational Age (SGA) to the label, but only for the 10 percent or so of tiny newborns who do not catch up with their peers on the growth charts within the first two years. Even after approval, some pediatric endocrinologists remained uncomfortable with giving toddlers such high doses of hGH.

Now Lilly asked for a sixth pediatric indication to bear the government stamp of approval: non–growth-hormone-deficient short stature.

In their written review of Lilly's evidence supporting the application, FDA staff noted that, if approved, non–growth-hormone-deficient short stature would break new ground. In contrast to the other indications, all of which "represent clinical conditions identifiable on the basis of defined clinical and pathological criteria," here was a group of potential patients who had nothing in common except size. Their short stature had no single known cause, and not all the various possible causes were even pathological. The children might have hormone deficiencies or dysfunctions that current testing did not detect; they might harbor genetic mutations or defects; or they might have inherited normal variations in growth patterns. That is, they could just come from extremely short families or families that produced late bloomers.

Also, the other approved conditions affected so few patients that they qualified as orphan indications. But using the traditional statistical definition of short stature, which was below the third percentile, an additional 1 million to 1.7 million children in the United States potentially could receive growth hormone therapy. On this basis, FDA staff estimated an annual cost of $18–$22 billion, compared with the $182 million annual cost for U.S. patients with GHD. In order to ease approval, Lilly had proposed a more restrictive cutoff: −2.25 SD (2.25 standard deviations below the mean, or average), which translated to the shortest 1.2 percent. Even so, the federal staff review noted, "the potential number of candidates for GH therapy is many multiples of the number of patients currently treated" and the cost would be "significant."

FDA staff also summarized the ethical concerns: there was the point that only the well-off would benefit; the question of whether this would shift resources from unmet medical needs; the difficulty of weighing the cost and discomfort of daily shots for years against any potential gain. How to balance the "potential stigmatization of normal children" against "the unhappiness, loss of quality of life, and educational/social disadvantages of short children"? How to differentiate between normal and abnormal when this was not strictly a medical definition but one that included social judgments? Last, there was the consideration of "avoiding unnecessary GH augmentation therapy." This decision might open the floodgates to parents who simply wanted to enhance their child's height at any cost.

Guyda interpreted the staff report as saying: Don't go there.

But FDA staff also statistically reviewed the research Lilly submitted and issued the judgment that pediatric endocrinologists had been anticipating—with either hope or dread—for decades. The NIH experiment, cosponsored by Lilly, and the only trial ever likely to be done comparing short normal kids who got GH with those who received years of placebo shots, *did* demonstrate that biosynthetic hGH increased their final height. The mean gain, or "treatment effect," was 3.7 centimeters (1.44 inches) by the company's calculation methods, a little less at 3.2 centimeters by the FDA's. On the basis of the NIH study, growth hormone therapy also appeared to be as safe for short normal patients as for any other group.

When the meeting opened, at eight-thirty a.m. on June 10, 2003, in a hall at the Holiday Inn Select, it was apparent that this was to be no head-to-head academic debate between Harvey Guyda's philosophy of medicine versus Raymond Hintz's. Lilly had flown in some of the country's most prominent pediatric endocrinologists as external consultants, there to answer any of the committee members' questions. Their experts sat in a row, a phalanx at Hintz's left hand. The company had prepared a briefing book three volumes thick, outfitted a pressroom with a free buffet lunch, and hired a public relations firm whose representatives circulated to answer reporters' questions.

David Orloff, director of the FDA's Division of Metabolic and Endocrine Drug Products, immediately set the stage by stating that, contrary to its usual practice, the agency would not make an oral presentation, because there was no disagreement on the facts in this case. He called on Lilly.

Hintz presented Lilly's basic argument, which was one of fairness. Why should a child the same height as those treated for GHD or Turner syndrome be denied the chance to be taller just because doctors didn't know the cause? All these children suffered from the same problem, short stature. He described this as height below the "normal range," noting that various medical societies define short stature as the shortest 2.3 percent for age and sex. In the United States, that means an adult man shorter than 5'3" or an adult woman under 4'11".

"So why should one treat short stature? Children and adults with short stature, irrespective of cause, may well have disadvantages compared to their peers," Hintz said. His second reason was simply that, in many cases, hGH therapy "corrects short stature."

In contrast to the FDA staff report, Hintz argued this decision would not break new ground, because every indication the FDA approved after 1985 had been for a condition that was non–growth hormone deficient. Essentially, the FDA had already gone there.

Gordon Cutler, the pediatric endocrinologist who'd initiated the controversial experiment at the National Institutes of Health in 1988, explained its significance. Cutler was no longer at the NIH; he now worked for Lilly as medical director for the Humatrope product team. Going back years, he noted, doctors had been concerned that growth hormone treatment in nondeficient children might accelerate their bone age along with their growth rate; that it would shorten their growing time, and therefore not add height in the end. But in this pivotal study bone age did not unduly advance and final height improved. "This is what we set out to learn sixteen years ago." Humatrope had boosted the patients as a group to a mean height just above the third percentile. Cutler suggested that the pivotal study actually underestimated the effect of hGH therapy; the children had been older

than was typical when they started, and received a lower and less frequent dose than currently prescribed.

Indeed, Lilly submitted a second, different study done in Europe
that compared short normal patients receiving low and high doses of
hGH, concluding that the larger dose stimulated more growth. There
had been no placebo group, but when each child's final height was
compared with the height doctors had predicted without treatment,
most of the children ended up taller by about two inches. Almost a
third beat the prediction by more than four inches. Cutler proudly
pointed out a single dot representing a child who grew more than six
inches taller than predicted. He acknowledged that height prediction
remained imprecise. Perhaps more significant, 94 percent of those
who got the high dose ended up in the normal range, "thus conferring
on these patients the lifelong benefit of normal adult stature." What
that benefit might be was unique to each person, according to Cutler:

"For one patient it may be a lifelong dream of becoming a pilot, or
pursuing any of the careers which encompass millions of jobs in the
United States for which there is a minimum height requirement. For
another child, it may simply be the desire to catch up to one's peers,
to reduce the likelihood of being repeatedly mistaken for a child three
or four or five years younger; or being teased, bullied, or excluded,
simply because of one's size."

In terms of risk, the Lilly team reported that no new safety concerns had emerged. There had been a cancer case in the pivotal study:
an eleven-year-old diagnosed with advanced Hodgkin's disease only
nine weeks into the experiment. They believed the boy must have had
the disease before starting on hGH. In the European study, a twelve-
year-old boy who'd received the lower dose of hGH for six and a half
years developed an unusual abdominal tumor and later died. This
was not a type of tumor associated with any other growth-hormone-
treated patient in Lilly's database or the literature. They thought this
also was unrelated to his GH exposure.

The other adverse events expected from previous experience with
growth hormone occurred no more frequently in kids treated for idio-

pathic short stature than in kids treated for other conditions, and the number of these "relatively mild and typically transient" events hadn't risen in the high-dose study.

Because Lilly knew the government had concerns about inappropriate use, the company proposed ways to maintain control. They'd chosen a height criterion that excluded all children in the normal range and almost half of those who met the medical definition of short stature. But Lilly argued against adding any other restrictions to the label. It should be left up to pediatric endocrinologists to decide whether to consider growth rate, bone age, chronological age, target height, predicted height, or psychosocial factors before prescribing. Lilly's proposed label only required that a patient be extremely short.

Instead of a more restrictive label, Lilly would make sure pediatric endocrinologists understood how to make an accurate diagnosis and were aware of the risks versus benefits of treatment. The company would include this information in its physician-to-physician educational sessions and Continuing Medical Education programs. There would be no direct consumer advertising. Humatrope would continue to ship only through closed specialty pharmacies rather than retailers. "So a patient cannot simply turn up at the GP's office, get a prescription for Humatrope and go to the corner drugstore and get it filled," promised Charmian Quigley, senior clinical research physician for Lilly.

The company would continue to monitor prescribing, and to screen for adverse events through its postmarketing database. The real defense against abuse, Quigley assured the panel, lay with the pediatric endocrinology community itself, which didn't support using hGH to make children with normal heights taller: "Pediatric endocrinologists are relatively conservative and view themselves, in fact, as the gatekeepers of growth hormone therapy." Besides that, insurance companies limit access in order to control costs. Assuming many pediatricians wouldn't make referrals and some families would decide against treatment, she estimated that only about 10 percent of eligible short youngsters would be taking hGH by five years after approval. About

30,000 to 40,000 new patients spread among the various pharmaceutical manufacturers. Which was closer to one in a thousand U.S. children rather than the one in a hundred who qualified according to the proposed label.

Members of the FDA advisory panel seemed willing to accept that Humatrope had made some non–growth-hormone-deficient short kids taller. But looking at the inch and a half or so average gain in the pivotal study, they asked about the benefit. Lilly had presented no evidence that extremely short kids had psychosocial problems or that Humatrope reversed them. The psychological data, the company acknowledged, had turned out to be "inconclusive." All the extremely short children had measured normal in terms of self-perception and behavior before they were assigned to either the placebo or the hormone group. At the end, self-perception remained equivalent in both groups. Parents, typically mothers, described some improved behavior in their adolescents who got Humatrope. But the numbers had been just too small to be statistically significant. The NIH managed to enroll seventy-one subjects; only sixteen who got Humatrope and nine who received the placebo stuck it out to the end of the experiment. The lack of scientific evidence that a few additional inches changed these youngsters' lives should not be held against their application, Lilly argued, since no other approved growth hormone use had demonstrated a clear psychosocial benefit, either.

Surprisingly, even the children who received placebo shots in the pivotal study ended up growing a little closer to average height than when they started. Called on by the committee to explain why kids on dummy shots also got taller, Gordon Cutler replied that most of the patients had significant bone age delay, which meant more time left to grow. Essentially, someone 4'9" might reach 4'10" with no therapy, but could get to 4'11½" with a low dose of hGH, and might make it to 5'1" with a higher dose, he said. Cutler threw in his opinion that there was "no such a thing" as a child who wouldn't respond to hGH treatment. Still, he acknowledged, the study revealed no way to predict in advance who would respond a little or a lot. Even growth velocity during the first six months of Humatrope showed a "very, very weak" correlation to the final outcome.

But then, committee members wanted to know, why not just wait a few years and see who would spontaneously catch up? And why not put an age restriction on the label so that doctors didn't launch into needless and expensive therapy for a child who might reach the normal range anyway? A committee member noted that at younger ages, height prediction is even less reliable. Another commented that Lilly's proposal seemed to swing open the door for Humatrope's use in cases of constitutional growth delay. Cutler assured them that "pediatric endocrinologists do not want to treat children who are going to end up at a normal height without treatment. And it's one of the things that they spend, you know, three years of intensive training trying to learn how to do." But a minimum age on the label "would become very complicated."

One of Lilly's consultants, Ron Rosenfeld of Stanford University, added that while some late bloomers did catch up, when it came to the extremely short group they were referring to, "very few" would achieve normal adult height: "Given the inability to predict effectively, and given the fact that these children are so dramatically short when they present to pediatric endocrinologists, it was our feeling that we could not discriminate between the group that would catch up and those that wouldn't, and our recommendation would be that all at least have access to growth hormone therapy."

"I beg to differ," Harvey Guyda shot back when it was finally his turn to speak, after hours of Lilly's presentation. "Short kids do catch up." He started his brief presentation by describing a study of almost five hundred very short children who ended up significantly closer to average by the time they finished growing, even though doctors had done nothing but measure them. Another researcher had followed 226 extremely short children and found two-thirds spontaneously achieved normal adult height, and that only 10 percent didn't reach a height about midway between their mother's and father's, the target some pediatric endocrinologists liked to refer to as a child's "genetic potential."

Guyda disparaged Lilly's research. He noted how many patients in the Humatrope trials had delayed bone age, signifying they were probably late bloomers, and that others also had conditions that did not fit the definition of idiopathic short stature. Mostly, Guyda challenged the "quite modest" results. Even moving a boy from the first to the third percentile, which the Lilly team had celebrated as a potentially life-altering crossing into normal stature, meant he would still be almost five inches below average. "So then it becomes a moot question: What's normal? Are you normal when you're at the mean? Are you normal at the fifth or tenth percentile, or are you still normal when you're at the third percentile?"

Both of Lilly's studies produced a high dropout rate. "And what we're arguing...is this benefit up here for these four or five patients." Guyda pointed to some dots on Lilly's charts. Then he pointed to dots representing the youngsters who got placebo injections but still spontaneously grew. Some of them had done as well as some of the European children on Humatrope. Half of those remaining at the end of the European study had been enrolled in a single Dutch center, Guyda noted. Perhaps their impressive final heights mostly reflected the fact they were Dutch, an exceptionally tall population. If the Humatrope had been so beneficial, why had almost half of the high-dose group stopped treatment?

Overall, Guyda remained unimpressed—except by the expense. While GHD kids achieved relatively good adult heights for about $10,000 per centimeter, people who begin with normal growth hormone secretion require higher doses to respond, therefore more biosynthetic hGH. He quoted an analysis that put the cost of treating idiopathic short stature as high as $40,000 per centimeter, or roughly $120,000 for three centimeters, which is just a little over an inch. "So these are very expensive centimeters."

And all to solve a problem that seemed social rather than medical.

When FDA committee members began to ask him questions, Guyda couldn't filter out a note of scorn; he derided the description of pediatric endocrinologists as effective "gatekeepers." He noted that

the last published statement of the Lawson Wilkins Pediatric Endocrine Society still advocated against using growth hormone for idiopathic short stature. Still, more than 10,000 U.S. children received
hGH for just that reason, including almost 25 percent of those in
Genentech's National Cooperative Growth Study database.

How did so many kids get prescriptions off-label, one committee
member wondered out loud, given all the controls that Lilly representatives had just described?

Guyda laughed and suggested someone from the other side should
field that question. So a Lilly consultant, pediatric endocrinologist
Margaret MacGillivray, from the University of Buffalo, helpfully
described for the committee exactly how it was done: "When you
apply to the insurance companies, you will get rejected. And then the
next thing is, you make an application for some of the foundations run
by certain pharmaceutical companies to assist you with a six-month
trial." Even without evidence of growth hormone deficiency, some
insurers would pay when a child showed a significant improvement in
growth rate during the first six months, as most did.

Then Guyda finished up, raising some final concerns about safety.
He mentioned a recent report of seven deaths of Prader-Willi children, deaths which might or might not turn out to be related to the
growth hormone therapy they'd been receiving. His point: "There
are surprises out there." Specifically, he worried about the long-term
impact on organs of prolonged elevated insulin levels, since growth
hormone can increase insulin resistance, an underlying cause of diabetes. He also wondered whether the recommended dose would
raise IGF-1 levels above normal. How might that affect tissues that
are especially sensitive during pubertal growth spurts? Would it ultimately cause cancers? "And I think that remains a big concern for me.
Even though there's no data to support the fact that's going to happen,
we can anticipate there may be something along that line."

When the questions ended, Guyda didn't stick around for the rest
of the meeting; he headed back to Montreal feeling, as he put it later,
as if he'd been a lamb led to slaughter.

The public comment section followed lunch, including dramatic pleas from two former hGH patients. The first was Nicole Costa. Blond, poised, and seventeen, she'd come with her mother, Patricia, who was executive director of the Human Growth Foundation. Her mother liked to brag that Nicole had been a poster child for growth hormone therapy almost her whole life, which had begun seven and a half weeks early by Cesarean section, and off the bottom of the growth charts.

Patricia Costa told the committee that the Human Growth Foundation received pharmaceutical industry money, including from Eli Lilly, but that she'd paid her own way and her daughter's to plead on behalf of short children.

Nicole Costa immediately grabbed the committee's attention as she took the microphone and said she felt lucky to be able to make her presentation without having to stand on a box. It was only because, even though she'd tested normal for growth hormone, her endocrinologist had had "the wisdom" to prescribe hGH. When she was six and a half years old, doctors predicted she would grow to only 4'8". Now she stood 5'2" even without high heels. In kindergarten, she hadn't been able to reach the water fountain. She sat alone on the benches at the amusement park waiting for friends to finish rides that she'd been too small to board. Her mother had to order her first communion dress made, since none off the rack were her size. In second grade, a teacher forced her to sit in a kindergarten chair because of the rule that every student's feet must touch the floor while the child was seated. Nicole Costa loved sports, but being tiny restricted her choice of what she could play. If growth hormone hadn't improved her stature, she was sure, she would never have been able to buy ready-made clothes in a department store, or reach the upper shelves in a supermarket, or drive a normal car. She begged the committee to give other children the chance she'd had: "the opportunity to reach...full growth potential."

Deno Andrews followed her, appearing even more dramatically at the microphone, on his knees. This, he said, before standing up, was two inches taller than the first endocrinologist predicted he'd reach as an adult. He was diagnosed with growth hormone deficiency, which made him lucky, because it meant he could receive hGH. That might never have happened if Andrews's mother had listened to the pediatrician who assured her Deno had nothing wrong with him, but was just a late bloomer and would eventually catch up. His mother, Mary Andrews, headed a parent support group called the Magic Foundation that, like the Human Growth Foundation, is devoted to growth disorders. It, too, received pharmaceutical industry funding, including from Lilly; and Deno Andrews, now in his thirties, added that he'd spent nearly three years as a growth hormone salesman for Serono. But Andrews declared that he'd paid his own way to tell the committee it was unfair that those not diagnosed with GHD didn't have the same medical opportunity that he had.

He described a miserable childhood, during which he was laughed at on the basketball courts, passed over when it came time to pick teams, called "midget, shrimp, small-fry, shorty, and a number of other derogatory terms" every day. No wonder he became a poor student. He didn't believe the studies that concluded short kids didn't suffer psychologically. Short kids developed tough exteriors just to attend school each day. So they lied to the researchers, telling them they were normal and things were all right. "I lied," Andrews said.

Giving short kids medicine was right: "It is as right as getting corrective lenses for eyesight that is abnormal. It is as right as an insurance company paying to repair a dent in a car. It is as right as getting a tutor or extra help at school for a child who isn't performing well." What would committee members do if they had a child who learned at a rate that was 2.25 deviations below average, Andrews asked. "Would you wait to see if they'd catch up? Or would you do something about it?"

QUALMS, AND A VOTE

When committee members began to discuss the decision, many revealed unease. The most critical questions came from Deborah

Grady, a professor of epidemiology and biostatistics at UCSF. An expert on menopause, Grady had been among those researchers who discovered that the FDA-approved hormone replacement therapy did more harm than good—after it had been prescribed for decades to millions of American women. Perhaps that made her more cautious. She said she doubted that a five-year-old could make an informed decision to commit to years of daily injections in hopes of growing an extra couple of inches, and thought there should at least be some minimum age for treatment.

Immediately, her suggestion was countered by George Goldstein, the industry representative on the panel. Though not allowed to vote, Goldstein sat at the table and could participate in the discussion. He warned that as a former pediatrician he would hate to wait until it was too late to make a child taller and then regret his decision. "The psychosocial consequences of this to the child, to the family, and to their respective communities are often only visible or, indeed, palpable years later." Unsurprisingly, he recommended approval.

But Grady persisted. "I was just going to point out that if you double [the] duration of treatment, you double the amount of time for potential adverse effects, and you at least double the cost." She'd done the rough calculation that injecting a child from age five to sixteen could add up to half a million bucks for the drug alone, not counting doctor visits and fees.

Cost also bothered panel member David Schade, chief of endocrinology at the University of New Mexico School of Medicine. He'd found Nicole Costa's and Deno Andrews's testimonies about the psychological burden of short stature "compelling." Yet Schade remained troubled by Lilly's failure to present data that such an expensive treatment produced a real benefit beyond height. He was having difficulty understanding "why we should actually spend $20,000 a centimeter...when Lilly has not even indicated that we are reducing by 10 percent the psychological trauma of being short."

Returning to the microphone on Lilly's behalf, Gordon Cutler agreed psychological studies remained "ambiguous," and that "psy-

chological benefit has not been shown conclusively for any indication." Still, pediatric endocrinologists saw children all the time who
felt handicapped by short stature. Cutler insisted that the real issue
remained that these children felt "disadvantaged" when they knew a
treatment could increase height, but the FDA denied it to them.

After more questions, the FDA's David Orloff told advisors what
to consider when voting, like a judge instructing a jury. He did not
want them to worry whether growth hormone to treat non–growth-
hormone-deficient short stature was merely cosmetic, or that their
decision might set a precedent for approving other drugs for what
some called cosmetic reasons—"usually those unaffected by the target
condition." They shouldn't be concerned that approval would put the
FDA on a slippery slope. As long as a therapy had been shown to be
safe and effective, the choice of whether to treat shortness—or bald-
ness or mild acne or fatness for that matter—belonged to patients,
their families, and their doctors.

Orloff gave advisors their charge: to decide whether they were
satisfied that Humatrope worked and was safe for non–growth-
hormone-deficient short stature, and whether its effect was "clinically
meaningful." He also wanted their suggestions about any more criteria
the FDA should add to the label. Last, he asked them what additional
information should be gathered even after approval, since to him it
was "quite clear that not all the questions about the safe and effective
use of this intervention in this population have been answered by the
studies to date."

Committee members immediately and unanimously agreed that
growth hormone treatment worked in short healthy kids; it was statistically effective; it had added height. None expressed doubt that
being at the extreme short end of the stick hurt. But most wrestled
with whether or not a few extra inches were "clinically meaningful."
One mused that it might be worthwhile to go from 5' to 5'2". Some
two inches might mean more than others. Several stated there just
wasn't enough data about quality of life to judge. One predicted widespread disappointment because such modest height improvements

didn't address the enormous pain of being extremely short. Another argued that only patients and their parents could decide the significance, which required fully informed consent: children needed to be told clearly that after all the shots, they might not get any taller. Or that they might possibly grow one to three inches.

The committee also struggled with safety. Grady emphasized that safety was "a very important issue here, because what we're talking about is treating otherwise perfectly normal kids who are short, for five to maybe ten years, at a time when they're young children up until they're pubertal—potentially a critical time for later events." Though they had data from GHD patients that she found "fairly reassuring," the one placebo-controlled comparison for non-GHD short stature had enrolled only seventy-one children and followed up fewer than half of them. Even so, she found the data "a little bothersome."

One death was reported in the treated group, she said, "versus none in the placebo group. There were five serious adverse events versus two. There was this report of a...tumor and Hodgkin's disease. And if you look at the adverse events, there was a report of more flulike syndromes, more infections, more pain syndromes, more bone disorders, lymphadenopathy (swollen lymph glands), reproductive abnormalities, fungal and parasitic infections and surgical procedures." Not statistically significant, Grady acknowledged, but "fairly different"—"more than a twofold increase in those things in the treated group." And that was in a trial so small that it hadn't turned up any cases of intercranial hypertension, a known potential side effect of growth hormone therapy, and a condition that she didn't consider trivial. "So I don't think we have really good data on safety." Grady advised the FDA to demand a mandatory registry for patients receiving growth hormone for idiopathic short stature, and a routine follow-up, at the least.

But her caution sparked another rebuke, this time from one of the few pediatric endocrinologists on the panel, Yale University's William Tamborlane. He argued that safety had been established by experience. A mandatory registry was unnecessary, Tamborlane continued, because practicing pediatric endocrinologists already collected data with the financial support of the manufacturers. He ridiculed Grady for downplaying the problems of growth-impaired kids the way her mother, ten or fifteen years earlier, might have dismissed weight reduction medication for overweight children by saying "You know these are perfectly healthy children—except they're fat."

Others on the panel defended Grady's safety concerns, however. "We're all a product of our experiences," David Schade noted. As an endocrinologist who treated adults, his experience included prescribing the diabetes drug Rezulin, which the FDA approved and then recalled from the market after patient deaths. Some problems didn't show up until you began treating many thousands of individuals, Schade pointed out. And with the approval of growth hormone for short nondeficient kids, doctors would suddenly be treating a huge population that would remain huge, because there would always be a lowest percentile. He knew that some adult patients who took growth hormone suffered serious side effects, and he could imagine potential problems when "we're adding a hormone that's already there, rather than a hormone to growth hormone deficient individuals."

Schade didn't understand why, out of 400,000 or more potential patients, the NIH and Lilly had managed to recruit so few to their clinical study. "So I'm concerned that we haven't looked at enough individuals in order to define the hazards of this drug." Therefore, he, too, thought the FDA should require close monitoring of nondeficient kids getting Humatrope.

Paul Woolf, chairman of medicine at Crozer Chester Medical Center, wanted the patients followed up for decades after treatment because "we really don't know, down the road, what will happen to these kids. I doubt whether growth hormone will initiate new tumors, but kids who already have tumors—could their spread be worse?" Had the advanced Hodgkin's disease found in one child in the pivotal study been accelerated by hGH treatment? "I mean, I have no idea. I don't know if anybody else has."

Another advisor pointed out that Lilly evaluated safety by comparing the children in the study with those taking growth hormone for other indications like Turner syndrome or GHD. Lilly had not compared the adverse events among children in their experiment with those among healthy kids the same age who did not take hGH. Also, Lilly sought approval for the high dose, though only thirteen children in the high-dose study had been followed to final height. A larger trial could not only illuminate safety but also establish which patients might respond to a lower dose.

The industry's representative jumped in to quell this rising call for more data. "If we were to wait to approve this until 'adequate' . . . safety data were obtained," George Goldstein said caustically, the cost of studying thousands of patients "prior to approval would make it, in a word, impractical." Lilly's postmarketing surveillance and the company's "renowned" vigilance would be enough, he assured them.

Committee members then took turns suggesting a variety of additional qualifications they would like to see on the Humatrope label before doctors prescribed it for healthy short kids. Perhaps the label should restrict use based on a child's age or growth velocity or bone age or serum IGF-1 level. There might be an indication of when to stop, some standard by which a physician could judge whether to continue treating: At final height? If the growth rate didn't improve by at least 50 percent? Or when velocity decreased so much that additional therapy would be unreasonable?

They wanted more information on who should not get it. For example, Schade said he'd seen no data on whether it was safe to prescribe growth hormone to a diabetic child, or about whether hGH significantly hiked insulin resistance in an obese child: "And that's of great concern because, at least in my state, and probably throughout the U.S., childhood obesity has become an epidemic." He also thought the FDA should look harder to find markers along the way of who would grow significantly. "If we don't have some handle on who's going to respond, we are going to be not only wasting a lot of resources, but basically causing a lot of children to take a lot of injections for no reason." Essentially, Schade worried how a physician could prescribe growth hormone intelligently. "I have problems with the concept of—quote—letting the private physician or family make the ultimate decisions. They can do that, but they need data, and they need the information on which to make those decisions and I just don't believe we have them."

Endocrinologist Nelson Watts, from the University of Cincinnati, agreed he didn't have the information to decide which children he should treat, what dose he should prescribe, or what he should monitor. He'd been thinking about the comment that Deborah Grady's mother might have pooh-poohed the need for drugs to treat childhood obesity. "An agent that reduced weight in obese children by 2 to 4 percent, that had limited safety data, might not be something to embrace," Watts said in Grady's defense. Since the reason to treat short stature seemed to be psychosocial, he suggested use be limited to those kids who had psychosocial issues.

When Grady's turn to speak came again, she argued against relying on physicians and insurance companies to control the widespread use of growth hormone on short kids. She wanted more criteria to justify prescribing than simply being measured in the shortest 1.2 percent. Lilly acknowledged that its definition of abnormal height was somewhat arbitrary; as a Lilly representative had put it, "normal changes." But in any other medical circumstance, Grady objected, a cutoff correlated with *something*. For example, a bone density score was used to initiate treatment because it correlated with increased risk of fracture. "And here we have no similar data on the correlation of this cutoff with any real outcome." Grady thought the earliest treatment age should be seven and that late bloomers should not get growth hormone, because they usually caught up sufficiently on their own. She also called for standards to stop ineffective therapy after a year or two. Otherwise a doctor might continue prescribing hGH to a child for a decade, with no way to judge whether the response was worth six or seven injections a week and a "whole lot of money."

Then they voted for approval, eight to two. Joining Deborah Grady against Lilly's application was Nancy Worcester, the consumer representative on the panel, a women's studies professor at the University of Wisconsin, Madison. An expert in some women's health topics, Worcester was the only advisor without a medical degree, and the only one to voice skepticism about Lilly's promise to curb abuse by educating pediatric endocrinologists as gatekeepers. She hoped there would be non-industry-sponsored education of doctors about such a controversial product. This was her first meeting, and she'd been trying to figure out when to discuss the broader social rather than only scientific issues. As she voted, Worcester explained that, besides safety, "I'm worried about the medicalization of shortness, and that it would actually increase the problem of stigma."

The advisors' approval made more news than their concerns. Summarizing the tally he'd taken during the voting, committee chairman Glenn Braunstein, chairman of medicine at Cedars-Sinai Medical Center, reported that half the panel had "a very large question mark" about whether the modest additional height represented a clinically meaningful response; three members thought Lilly had not sufficiently characterized safety in this group of patients. Two felt the data had not been sufficient to guide safe and effective use. All but one had called for a mandatory registry and follow-up of these new patients.

The next morning, in the hotel lobby, one of the committee members caught sight of Nicole Costa and congratulated her: "Your testimony—you made the whole thing go! You should be very proud of yourself."

THE NEWS REACHES FAMILIES
AT THE MAGIC FOUNDATION

The FDA made its decision just one month later, approving the use of hGH in children with non–growth-hormone-deficient short stature. The government accepted Lilly's definition and its proposed higher dose. The agency required one new criterion: a growth rate "unlikely to permit attainment of adult height in the normal range." The label now also precluded use in patients whose short stature "should be observed or treated by other means." The insertion of "observed" represented a nod toward those who argued that not all extremely short children require medical intervention.

But nothing specifically excluded treating constitutional growth delay, because there was no reference to bone age. The label contained no minimum age to begin therapy or minimum response to continue it; no reference to IGF-1 levels before or during treatment; no mention of psychological evaluation; no other additional criteria that the panel had discussed or that individuals on it had recommended. As for the nearly unanimous call for a mandatory registry, or for close monitoring and long-term follow-up, the letter of approval, signed by David Orloff on July 25, 2003, instead made some polite requests of Eli Lilly: "We encourage the continuation of your ongoing global post-marketing observational research program"—which included subsidiary studies on new tumors and on growth-predictors. The letter also requested that Lilly inform the FDA of any changes in the risk management plan.

The language about growth rate was, as one of Lilly's consultants, Ron Rosenfeld, acknowledged, "a *very* loose wording. It basically puts no restrictions on endocrinologists. . . . If they had wanted to be stricter they could have said, 'Limit its use to patients whose predicted adult height on the basis of bone age is below such-and-such.' But they don't tell you how one should predict what the adult height should be, so it really gives the endocrinologist a lot of discretion in terms of usage." And though Rosenfeld said he personally did not like to treat a boy with a predicted height above 5'4" or a girl predicted to grow over 4'11", if a family insisted, he would refer them to other doctors who might have different cutoff points. Other physicians' cutoffs were not necessarily wrong, but given that growth hormone treatment was neither a hundred percent effective nor a hundred percent safe, and cost the health care system so much, Rosenfeld did hope the medical community could police itself and practice responsibly. "But I don't have a hundred percent confidence in that. I believe that there will undoubtedly be physicians who will be much more liberal in the use of growth hormone either than I would or than I think they should."

The news of approval arrived just as the Magic Foundation held its ninth annual meeting in Chicago. Deno Andrews proudly strolled the lobby of the O'Hare Marriott with his wife, who had been his high school sweetheart, and a new baby snuggled on his shoulder. He also had embarked on a new business venture: CEO of a growth clinic that his mother, Mary Andrews, was opening on the bottom floor of the building where the Magic Foundation offices occupied the top. New Heights Medical Clinic in Oak Park, Illinois, anticipated serving families from throughout the Midwest, a commercial enterprise he hadn't mentioned to the advisory committee when he begged them to approve hGH for hundreds of thousands of new patients. New Heights was being outfitted with gay colors and pint-size furniture, and Deno Andrews pledged it would be a place where doctors and nurses talked to short kids in a way that was appropriate to a child's age, not size. But the clinic had not yet been able to hire a full-time pediatric endocrinologist. Long gone were the days when Robert Blizzard initiated a parent organization by promising his colleagues that the doctors could keep control; even so, the idea of literally working under a parent group made many pediatric endocrinologists uneasy.

The Magic Foundation is very much Mary Andrews's organization. She's everywhere during the annual event. She started this group in Deno's bedroom when he was a child because she felt frustrated by the role of parents in the Human Growth Foundation, what she described as the "You're only a mother" attitude. She had no problem challenging doctors, and she'd been a tiger while advocating for her son. Deno not only received pituitary hGH for his growth hormone deficiency; when she heard that Robert Blizzard was beginning an experimental program to investigate whether delaying puberty would improve final height, she took Deno to Virginia and talked Blizzard into trying the new treatment. When her son reached 5'3" at age seventeen, Blizzard asked him if he wanted to continue. Mary Andrews answered yes. Blizzard scolded her that if she couldn't keep quiet, he would expel her from the room. He asked the boy again, pointing out that 5'3" was normal. This time it was Deno who said he would like to be taller. Delaying puberty for three years resulted in some snide locker-room comments, but he knew it had been worth it to reach a final height of 5'7". Mary Andrews devoted the same fierce energy to building an organization, and the Magic Foundation had eclipsed the Human Growth Foundation as a place for families.

An annual meeting of the Magic Foundation is an event crowded with parents and children, because pharmaceutical industry subsidies help the organization keep hotel rates affordable. A vacation, as Mary Andrews likes to call it, that is a gift from the Magic Foundation to families of children with growth disorders.

On this summer day in 2003, toddlers who looked like infants and adults the size of children mingled with bridal parties in the hotel lobby. Most of those with growth disorders had visible syndromes that caused their short stature, like Russell-Silver syndrome, which is marked by distinctive features including a triangular-shaped face. The convention provided a place where kids with Russell-Silver syndrome could play together in the pool while their parents questioned the doctors. Placards on tripods outside each seminar announced not just the medical condition under discussion but the company sponsoring each presentation. Turner syndrome, brought to them by Eli Lilly; growth hormone deficiency, by Novo Nordisk.

In the growth-hormone-deficiency room, Barry Bercu, a pediatric endocrinologist at the University of South Florida College of Medicine in Tampa, flashed a shot from The Wizard of Oz onto the screen: Dorothy surrounded by Munchkins, most of whom were hypopituitary dwarfs. It was a "remarkable development," Bercu commented, that many of the Munchkins filmed in the 1930s wouldn't end up this short if born today, reminding the audience that growth hormone therapy really is a miracle.

On the other hand, Bercu went on, "different families have different attitudes about short stature." If short parents accepted their kids were small because of biology, that was okay. Most children he saw didn't have a pathology but were below average because of either familial short stature or constitutional growth delay. "You need to discriminate physiology from pathology," Bercu said. "The pathology you're gonna do something about. The physiology you *may* do something about." Sorting out the two could be difficult.

This was not a short-is-just-physiology kind of crowd, though, as the questions revealed. A family from Hawaii complained to Bercu that local doctors had found nothing abnormal in their son, whose small size wasn't remarkable in a classroom full of Japanese-American and Filipino-American children. They had to take him to Seattle to find a doctor willing to try him on a trial dose of growth hormone. He bulked up, could play club sports, became engaged in school, and improved developmentally. Bercu smiled. This was an argument "against the naysayers who are for not giving growth hormone to non–growth-hormone-deficient kids." Another mother radiated even more fervor, describing how her small-for-gestational-age son, a twin, not only grew on hGH but also began to see better and hear better, and was no longer startled at loud noises. Bercu responded indulgently that he hadn't heard about all those effects, but her testimonial might be worth following up with a study. He advised a Michigan couple whose doctor resisted increasing their child's hormone dosage because of concern about rising IGF-1 levels that he should go ahead and "push the dose." When they asked about delaying puberty with an aromatase inhibitor, however, he grew more cautious. On the other hand, he told the story of a 6'6" child psychiatrist with a very tall wife, who insisted that his child of normal height be tested for deficiency. No matter the height, "if your child is growing poorly, I think there's an indication to treat." Bercu listened sympathetically to their complaints about pediatricians who accepted limits for their children that they as parents found unacceptable. He made himself popular by describing his role as a physician as serving as a "consultant" to parents.

At times he even sounded more like an advocate for medical intervention than the parents. When a mother described her eighteen-year-old daughter's recovery from a tumor that resulted in some neurological problems and a final height around 4'7", Bercu suggested she investigate the possibility of limb lengthening. The procedure involves chiseling the bones apart, caging the legs in a metal device, and stretching them incrementally over many months as new bone fills in the gaps. "Four feet, seven inches is a disadvantage," Bercu insisted, endorsing the surgery idea with more and more enthusiasm as he went on, though the mother looked dubious. "Driving a car...to me it makes a lot of sense. It's not a minor cosmetic issue."

The next day, the news that the FDA had approved growth hormone therapy for short kids hit television, newspapers, and the Magic Foundation convention simultaneously. Mary Andrews reserved comment, though there was little doubt this decision would be good for both the foundation and the clinic. Deno Andrews was glad the FDA had listened. He believed that every child should be enabled to reach his or her genetic potential; even children who would be 5'5" without treatment deserved help if they had the capacity to grow more.

But even at the Magic Foundation convention, not everyone shared this opinion. British pediatric endocrinologist Richard Stanhope, there for his worldwide expertise on Russell-Silver syndrome, bluntly announced to the other invited speakers at lunch that he viewed giving growth hormone to short normal children as a form of "child abuse." Like Harvey Guyda, he remained unconvinced that the NIH/Lilly study did, in fact, treat normal children. The European studies Stanhope trusted found such children gained not one or two inches from years of shots but one or two centimeters.

The news also traveled fast to the children during their organized activities. Saturday night, the Smith family rushed through dinner in the hotel restaurant before a scheduled bingo game. Chip was an anesthesiologist, with silver hair and a square jaw, tanned and fit from mountain biking; Linda, pretty and blond and thin. They made a handsome couple, about equal in height, around 5'6". Linda joked that they never expected to produce basketball players. But they came to Chicago with their three boys and a girl because their second-oldest son, Scott, thirteen, had growth hormone deficiency. In spite of being treated for a year, he had not responded with the expected burst of height. Insurance covered the $3,000-a-month cost, minus a thirty-dollar monthly co-payment. He was happy, had friends, played tenor saxophone, wrote poetry, enjoyed debate. But they hadn't summoned the nerve to tell him he might need shots for GHD his entire life, let alone that if treatment failed he was expected to end up 4'8".

They worried about Scott's impending transition from middle school to high school. Mostly, they worried that the clock was ticking and the injections had not helped. Every month seemed like a lost opportunity. He had a significantly delayed bone age, but he was also entering puberty. Chip Smith was visibly frustrated that their local pediatric endocrinologist continued to refuse to augment Scott's dosage. The doctor didn't want to boost the boy's IGF-1 levels too high, fearing a possible prostate cancer link. From a Magic Foundation advisor, they'd learned about a more aggressive doctor in Chicago. They'd already made an appointment; he would see them in two and half weeks. They decided to take not only Scott, but also their youngest son, whose growth pattern also seemed unusual, for testing.

But at dinner, the oldest of their four children, fourteen-year-old Jeff, floored them by suddenly announcing he would like to get shots as well. Jeff hated needles. Not only that, he was closing in on his parents' height and showed no abnormal growth pattern; his bone age was right on target. Well built, with sandy, bushy hair, he was a good-looking teenager around the tenth percentile for his age. But Jeff had heard people talking all day about how the FDA now would allow doctors to treat normal children with hGH, and he'd heard the children gained an average of two inches. He decided he wanted those two inches.

Chip Smith told his oldest son that what counted was in his heart, not his height. He mentioned watching a panel of Russell-Silver dwarfs at the conference, who spoke about how they led normal lives. They were short, Chip said carefully, "but attractive." He and Linda mentioned Jeff's college fund: Would he choose to spend it on an extra two inches if it meant not being able to afford his dream school and he had to attend an in-state college instead? They tried to get Jeff to think about this, advising him that life is made of trade-offs. Then the children headed off to play bingo.

With the kids gone, Chip acknowledged he would find it difficult to say no. Although at age fifty he knew that two inches were not that important ("I still found him attractive," Linda chimed in, smiling at her husband), he couldn't argue with Jeff's feeling that it would mean a lot in high school. "Growth hormone's like aspirin," he repeated several times. The leukemia scare had been debunked, he said. He was not thinking of Jeff now, but Scott, fifteen months younger and still in the third percentile, getting pudgy, loosing muscle mass and, Chip thought, energy—all symptoms of growth hormone deficiency—because their doctor insisted on playing things safe. Chip Smith was a physician and said he could write the prescription himself. But he didn't want to play endocrinologist. He wanted the endocrinologist to do more. "Don't tell me about IGF levels, look at the child!" He banged his fist on the table. "There's no downside! He's not gonna get sick from it."

The next morning over breakfast in the same restaurant, while their children slept in, Chip and Linda Smith debated about rescheduling their appointment and bringing all four kids to see the new pediatric endocrinologist in Chicago. "Obviously our fourteen-year-old has been thinking about this," Linda said. They believed he worried he would end up 5'6". Both his grandfather and his father were 5'6". Jeff, however, thought that was short. The doctor had actually predicted he would reach 5'8". But from everything he'd heard this weekend, Jeff was afraid he wouldn't get to that height without medical help. If the new pediatric endocrinologist would be willing to treat their oldest son as well as Scott, the Smiths thought they'd be willing to let Jeff make that decision for himself. "He wants to maximize his growth potential," Linda explained.

CHAPTER 13

now what?

"WELCOME TO GROWTH CITY"

Now that the FDA had declared human growth hormone a safe and effective way to make short kids taller, many families would feel encouraged to seek treatment. More urgently than ever, each pediatric endocrinologist needed to figure out a personal standard.

A few months after the FDA action, a committee of the Lawson Wilkins Pediatric Endocrine Society published new guidelines for practitioners. The paragraph on idiopathic short stature noted that the government had approved growth hormone to treat extremely short children unlikely to catch up in height, but also that the decision relied on only two studies, neither of which had appeared in peer-reviewed journals. The paragraph ended: "The long-term consequences of treating otherwise healthy children with GH remain uncertain." This cautious tone differed sharply from the impression created by the phalanx of prominent pediatric endocrinologists who had lined up for Lilly. The next annual meeting of the Lawson Wilkins Pediatric Endocrine Society promised to be lively.

It seemed fitting that the society invited Stanley Prusiner to kick off the meeting, which took place in May 2004. Prusiner had won the Nobel Prize for describing the prions that cause Creutzfeldt-Jakob disease. Many of those pediatric endocrinologists who gathered to hear him at San Francisco's Moscone Conference Center vividly remembered when Carleton Gajdusek addressed an earlier convention; Gajdusek had warned that every one of their pituitary hGH patients might turn out to be infected with CJD. Fortunately, that terrifying worst-case scenario never materialized. Still, as Prusiner described the ongoing search for ways to detect and cure CJD, he served as a reminder that some of the doctors in this hall had unknowingly broken the first rule of medicine: Above all, do no harm.

The conference didn't devote much time to dwelling on the past, however. Immediately, it turned to the current dilemma: Which short children should be entitled to growth hormone? The keynote speaker, a prominent German researcher and pediatric endocrinologist, Michael Ranke, chided his profession. They needed better ways to find the kids most likely to benefit from hGH. They should develop more standard measurement methods and better growth prediction models. Once they ordered therapy, they should keep weighing how well a child responded against the enormous price tag, and against how much more improvement seemed likely. "Too often we are opting to continue treatment for a few centimeters of gain."

But during the question-and-answer session, American pediatric endocrinologists protested that families wouldn't let them stop. One physician for a prepaid health plan described two boys with pituitary tumors who had reached six feet thanks to hGH but insisted on getting two inches taller. "My patients feel a sense of entitlement," she complained. At the cost of another $20,000 each, "should we be terminating growth hormone if a patient has reached an adequate height?"

Yes, Ranke answered. "Adding another inch is actually a waste to society."

Ranke didn't operate in America's consumer-driven health care system, however. Not only did U.S. families feel entitled to decide how tall is tall enough, but hGH doses are based on body weight, making teenagers the most profitable pediatric patients for hormone manufacturers.

Downstairs, on the first floor of the conference center, a vast exhibition attracted doctors between sessions. They crammed the exhibition hall, collecting free items and carrying their freebies from booth to booth in gift tote bags emblazoned with drug company logos. Genentech's sales staff wore denim shirts that proclaimed: "Welcome to Growth City."

The FDA has warned both Genentech and Lilly about the lack of balance in their growth hormone promotional material. In 1997, a letter from the Division of Drug Marketing, Advertising and Communications informed Lilly that some of its panels about hGH for Turner syndrome violated the Federal Food, Drug, and Cosmetic Act by burying the risks in a small block of text at the bottom. In 2000, regulators told Genentech to immediately desist describing its Nutropin Depot, a long-acting form of hGH delivery that requires dosing only once or twice a month, in a way that misled patients into believing it was as effective for growth as daily injections, when studies showed it was not.

More recently, just a month after the agency approved Lilly's application for short stature, the FDA's regulatory arm warned Genentech to immediately cease using promotional material that omitted all information about the risks of growth hormone therapy. Specifically, regulators complained that Genentech's panels at a Turner Syndrome Society meeting the previous year violated the law by suggesting the company's products were safer than had been demonstrated.

At the Moscone Center, Lilly's booth attracted special interest. The company's new booklets about Humatrope for idiopathic short stature were not on display but in a cabinet, available to anyone who asked. A sales representative explained that Lilly had promised the FDA not to market Humatrope directly to anyone but pediatric endocrinologists. But a Lilly representative in a particular region might "facilitate" getting information to other types of physicians interested in learning about growth hormone for idiopathic short stature, he

In one, half of a group of short children would be randomly assigned
o receive hGH, while the other half received $100,000 to $150,000
vorth of excellent psychological counseling, to see which group ended
p happier. A second study would just hand "short children $100,000
equal out life's opportunities." The audience laughed.

An endocrine researcher also challenged the panelists, objecting
their assumptions that hGH didn't have a significant potential to
rm kids with idiopathic short stature. The NIH/Lilly study hadn't
n large enough to prove there was no additional danger for these
s, he argued. "And it didn't continue decades into adulthood.
ess a child is extremely short and really distressed, I wouldn't
t to expose him to risk." When Lilly's Quigley responded that
stry databases didn't demonstrate that patients receiving growth
one for idiopathic short stature faced any higher risk than those
g it for other reasons, the researcher shot back: "I don't think we
he data on elevated IGF-1s and cancer."

stly, those pediatric endocrinologists who spoke up searched
sonable ways to chart the ethical minefields in their practices.
tell somebody that I treat, 'I'm going to stop your growth hor-
ecause ten million children are uninsured'?" one asked. Any
saved would not necessarily find its way to underserved chil-
pointed out, or even go into health care.

her wondered what was wrong with the formula he already
ating a child who was not growing at a normal rate and con-
ntil the patient reached final height. "Children do have north rates and a right to their genetic potential," he said.

ssue of genetic potential is a very, very slippery slope," Ron
answered. What's the genetic potential of a child who has
ts with an inherited form of dwarfism, or with familial
re, or idiopathic short stature, for that matter? "I prefer the
... to help a child reach normal."

ther doctor wondered how they defined "normal." He
that people accept that it's normal for females to be shorter
So, how about considering what's normal among each of

explained. For example, a Lilly representative might pull together a
group of pediatricians who would be making referrals to the same
growth clinic and bring in a pediatric endocrinologist to speak to
them. Or a representative could provide a pediatric endocrinologist
to talk to a quarterly journal club, where doctors discussed the latest
medical literature. "Pediatric endocrinologists interacting with other
doctors ... giving peer-to-peer talks.... Here's the newest things going
on." He hesitated, then refused to say any more.

OPENING THE BLACK BOX

Later in the conference, hundreds packed an upstairs hall for the session called "Opening the Black Box of Idiopathic Short Stature." It was
sponsored by an unrestricted grant from Eli Lilly. "By happenstance,"
the moderator announced, the first speaker was also from Lilly.

Charmian Quigley, the senior clinical research physician who had
made Lilly's major scientific presentation to the FDA advisory committee, told her fellow pediatric endocrinologists that the NIH/Lilly
"gold-standard study" of short kids with normal hormone levels had
"demonstrated efficacy [while] raising no new safety concerns." Children with non–growth-hormone-deficient short stature were likely to
end up seven to eight inches shorter than average, she emphasized,
and doctors already gave hormone to equally short children who had
other conditions. It was the fairness argument, and didn't rest on
whether or not life improved for any patients. Quigley acknowledged
that the study produced "limited psychosocial data."

None of the panelists who followed her debated the FDA's wisdom, either.

Ron Rosenfeld argued that many apparently healthy but extremely
short children would turn out to have significant genetic pathologies,
perhaps a "molecular defect" involving IGF-1, which mediates the
effect of growth hormone after birth. He predicted that kids with
constitutional growth delay also "are going to turn out to have genetic
and molecular abnormalities."

The last two speakers, both from the University of Wisconsin in Madison, had been challenging their colleagues since the early nineties to reach a consensus on the ethics of growth hormone treatment, yet they also did not object to the idea of giving medicine to apparently healthy kids.

David Allen agreed with Lilly that the cause of short stature shouldn't matter. Most of the 40,000 to 50,000 U.S. children who already received hGH every year didn't suffer from classic growth hormone deficiency. He did think there should be evidence of disability to justify starting treatment and evidence of a good response to justify continuing it, given the enormous expense. He felt uneasy "simply reinforcing more advantages for the well-to-do." But without a profession-wide standard, doctors found it hard to deny parents who could pay out of pocket, especially when the FDA "sends out the message that it's reasonable to act on the desire to be taller."

Allen described a ten-year-old whose parents insisted their daughter needed growth hormone to be able to play a full-size violin. They could pay, and he pointed out that "in our country we have freedom to spend money the way we want." But if parents weren't footing the bill, perhaps pediatric endocrinologists should assume that kids below the first percentile had a disability and treat them only until they reached a height in the normal range, say the fifth percentile. Then doctors could defend prescribing on the basis that they'd achieved a therapeutic effect.

Norman Fost, who spoke last, congratulated his colleagues on having given up trying to distinguish between enhancement and disease, a distinction he found "morally irrelevant." Fost recalled a 1991 conference held in Wisconsin where pediatric endocrinologists had pretty much agreed that when Billy and Johnny had the same predicted height, only the one with growth hormone deficiency was entitled to therapy to boost him above 5'3". Fost thought either both Billy and Johnny were entitled or neither was, as long as the therapy was safe and effective. "The definition of disease is hopelessly vague," he explained. Therefore, Ron Rosenfeld's prediction that eventually

scientists would find a molecular basis for idiopathic sh[ort stature or] constitutional growth delay wouldn't resolve arguments [about whether] or not those conditions should be treated, or even whe[ther they were] diseases.

What bothered Fost was cost. Because of cost, "we [shouldn't do] this if it makes life better in some way," he argued. [...] been proven. So even if hGH effectively added inche[s ...] not feel entitled to it. He questioned whether it [...] spend $1 billion for a "marginal gain in height" whe[n ...] dren lived without health insurance and sometime[s ...] treatment for appendicitis. A smattering of appla[use ... the] room.

Fost then took a mild swipe at the drug c[ompany ...] sponsored continuing medical education can p[romote ...] low benefit therapies." Continuing education [...] the benefits seem dramatic in order to convi[nce ...] prescriptions. Fost concluded, like his colleag[ues ...] ing on pediatric endocrinologists to set mo[...] optimizing height, but reaching normal ran[ge ...]

As the panelists wound up, the first d[octor to the] microphone to ask a question appeared [...] Lantos, a University of Chicago professor [who criti]cized the ethics of growth hormone ther[apy ...] note that not only did Eli Lilly help fu[nd the Pedi]atric Endocrine Society annual meeting [, but one of the] panel—Norman Fost—had no report [... from Eli] Lilly. "I understand it might be hard to [find people] that don't have drug company involve[ment ...]

Why didn't pediatric endocrino[logists ... treat]ing children with idiopathic shor[t stature ...] demanded. If they truly believed th[at ... medi]cally justified because short kids su[ffered ...] they should want to conduct two [... that might] never be done:

the various ethnic groups in the United States? Besides, another questioner asked, why had the panelists assumed that taller people have an advantage. Shorter folks have the most basic advantage: longevity. People who are tall die at earlier ages on average than people who are short.

As the session ended, two men exiting the hall chuckled over John Lantos's proposal to give a child the choice between money and shots. "I'd take the extra inches," one said. But others grumbled that the panelists had basically agreed that it was all right to try to make your kid taller if you had the money to pay for it.

A few members of the audience crowded Allen and Fost for more guidance. A pediatric endocrinologist complained he felt pressured to continue prescribing hGH into puberty. He wanted to know if Allen thought it was all right to stop and see whether a child grew normally at some point. Allen assured him that, indeed, it was "criminal" to prolong treatment, given that two-thirds of the cost occurs when children require higher doses in puberty. A woman described for Allen how, as the only pediatric endocrinologist in her area, she dealt with parents who felt entitled to GH therapy for their short kids while her HMO overflowed with young patients who have life-threatening diabetes. Her supervisor regularly criticized her for ordering too many test strips for diabetic children to measure their blood sugar levels, yet she witnessed hundreds of thousands of dollars spent on augmenting the height of healthy children by an inch or two. She shook her head as if truly baffled. Why weren't her fellow specialists focused on treating the rising numbers of diabetic youngsters instead of height? she wondered out loud.

When Allen was free to stroll into the corridor, he said he sensed that pediatric endocrinologists felt swelling pressure to treat short children and that they "are starting to push back." Not only had the government expanded approval of growth hormone, but several companies stood poised to market recombinant IGF-1. Experiments were under way investigating whether adding drugs to delay puberty or drugs to prolong puberty could make kids significantly taller. Put them all together, he said, "and doctors are going, 'Whoa, I hope it doesn't work!'"

In the corridor, though, a different type of expert was also handing out advice, and he didn't sound nearly so sanguine that pediatric endocrinologists as a group would push back. He was David Sandberg, a psychologist who specializes in psychosocial issues of growth, and a critic of how much growth hormone doctors prescribe without scientific evidence that they're helping short kids live happier lives. As Sandberg explained his views, an endocrinologist stopped to ask about a patient. The boy wanted to try out for basketball in spite of his size; should he be encouraged? Sandberg replied that he wouldn't discourage a tryout, but he might suggest: If not basketball, how about swimming? It's the kind of strategy to help short kids cope that is a David Sandberg specialty.

DAVID AND GOLIATH

Back in Buffalo, New York, four months after the Lawson Wilkins Pediatric Endocrine Society convention in San Francisco, Sandberg made his way down the hallway of the endocrine clinic at the Women and Children's Hospital on a warm September morning. As he passed the familiar murals of polar bears and pandas that decorated the clinic walls, he spied two brothers as they headed to the waiting room. Both were patients he had seen for several years but not recently. The boys were happy to see him, and Sandberg extended his hand for a shake.

"You look like..." he began.

"Like I've grown?" shouted Robert,* a blond eleven-year-old and the more outgoing of the two boys.

"No, I was going to say, 'like you've matured.' Do you know what that means?"

Robert pursed his lips and bounced around for a moment before thrusting his hand in the air as if he were in a classroom.

* All patients' names and some identifying details have been changed.

"I know. It's like I'm acting my age."

"Right," said Sandberg. "That's exactly what I meant."

Sandberg chatted for another moment or two, then told the boys and their mother he would see them a little later in the examining room. Sandberg is a boyish, bespectacled, 5'9" thorn in the side of those within the medical establishment—certain pediatric endocrinologists and the pharmaceutical companies—who believe growth hormone is the obvious answer for kids who are normal but much shorter than average.

As a pediatric psychologist, his work at the hospital sets this pediatric endocrine clinic apart from others. The clinic's endocrinologists see between 220 and 250 new patients a year specifically to evaluate their growth, or lack of it. Some of these children turn out to have serious conditions, like kidney failure, thyroid disease, Turner syndrome, and Prader-Willi syndrome. Some are short because their bodies don't manufacture enough growth hormone. Some are short because their bodies can't utilize the growth hormone their bodies make. And some are short and nobody knows why. Most patients have been referred by pediatricians; others because parents are concerned their children seem smaller than normal.

In the clinic's crowded conference room several residents, fellows, and nurses gathered around a long table piled with folders, thick and thin, along with Styrofoam cups and a large thermos of coffee. On a shelf sat the new growth charts that Lilly representatives had furnished, complete with a bright red line marking the 2.25 standard deviations below average that defines non–growth-hormone-deficient short stature. Parents watching a doctor plot their child's growth curve couldn't possibly miss how far above or below that magic red line their child ranked, even from across a room.

Lilly's detailers had also dropped off a video touting the recently approved use of growth hormone for short stature. They were familiar visitors to the Buffalo clinic, where the company paid the salary of a nurse and where the former director, Margaret MacGillivray, also served as a Lilly consultant. MacGillivray had been among the phalanx of pediatric endocrinologists who appeared in Bethesda on Lilly's behalf to urge the FDA approval. Thanks to the addition of healthy, short kids to the label, sales of Humatrope had jumped 21 percent in the final months of 2003, compared with the same period a year earlier. MacGillivray believed short youngsters suffered, and therefore she supported using growth hormone for children with idiopathic short stature. The tension between her and David Sandberg was so obvious that he had arranged his schedule to avoid running into her at the clinic.

MacGillivray wasn't there on this particular day, but pediatric endocrinologist John Bouclis was. He's a solidly built Greek who grew up on the island of Crete and still talks with a thick accent made even less intelligible by his staccato delivery. He entered the conference room with a sigh. He'd just seen a fifteen-year-old boy and had to deliver bad news. The boy's X-rays showed that his growth plates had closed. The boy's father was 5'11", his mother 5'6", his sister 5'3"— and he was 5'2". There was no possibility for any more growth. Even growth hormone would do nothing.

"Everybody is crying in there," Bouclis said, throwing his hands in the air. "They don't know how this can be. But it's too late."

There was a pause in the busy room, but only briefly as doctors and nurses and social workers picked up whatever files they needed and hurried on to the next patients.

When Sandberg moved from the conference room to an examining room, his pace slowed down. He would slouch against a wall and begin to chat with his young patients as if he had all the time in the world. Through subtle questioning, his goal was to determine how well they were coping in the world. Were they bullied at school? Were they babied at home? How were they doing in school? Did they have close friends? Hobbies?

A boy entering middle school and only in the fifth percentile for height sat on the examining table glumly, clearly wishing he was somewhere else. He'd been diagnosed with idiopathic short stature, and because he had been adopted, it was not certain if he was short because his biological parents were short or because recent medical problems, including a tonsillectomy, might have slowed his growth. Sandberg eased into the visit by talking about sports. Had the youngster followed the World Cup game? What did he think of the two teams? The boy, who had started out saying he didn't care who won, became engaged in the conversation and admitted he rooted for Canada.

When talking to young patients, Sandberg frequently steers the conversation to school sports, a subject that almost always comes up when short boys are involved. Sometimes the kids themselves are worried they won't be chosen to play because of their size; more frequently parents fear that if their short sons play they will be hurt. Or they fear their sons won't have the same opportunities to participate as taller classmates. Sandberg believes far too much value is placed on athletics versus other school activities like band or chorus, but acknowledges that team sports have become a rite of passage for boys. He also knows that unless a child is truly growth hormone deficient, the injections probably will make almost no difference physically in a child's height and athletic performance. Nevertheless, he views sports as a "proxy for inclusion" and pays close attention to what his young patients say.

When the sixth-grader told Sandberg he'd been playing some hockey, Sandberg seized the opportunity to tell him about another patient who came to the clinic—a high school kid—who also played. "This boy keeps an eye out for whoever is coming at him, playing 'smart,'" Sandberg explained—without ever mentioning that this is what a small guy needs to do on the ice. Then he steered the conversation to household chores. Sandberg wants to make sure that these kids who look younger than their ages are treated, at least at home, according to chronological age and not height. Finally, he asked about the growth hormone injections. The boy complained that his dad slopped the alcohol all over. Sandberg suggested he might like it better if he did it himself, but the child demurred. He wasn't quite ready.

When Sandberg visited an older patient, a seventeen-year-old born with vision impairments and multiple hormone deficiencies,

Sandberg quickly realized that the high school junior had few friends. This especially concerned Sandberg because the teenager's eye problem would likely mean he would be unable to drive, another difference that would set him apart from others his age. But Sandberg remembered the young man's interest in drawing and writing from a previous visit, and suggested he might enjoy working on the school newspaper or yearbook, places where both talents would be useful. Before leaving the room, he handed the teenager his card—rather than giving it to the mother—and invited him to visit across the street, where Sandberg had an office in a faded gray Victorian with a pink door. "You're a bright guy," Sandberg said. "Let's talk about colleges." As he moved down the hallway to the next examining room, he worried aloud about the adolescent's lack of friends. "Friendships are essential to moving forward. They're one of the essentials of childhood."

As he made his rounds, Sandberg also asked about school— specifically about report cards. On this day, all were doing well but Jeffrey—one of the two brothers he'd spoken to briefly in the hallway. Both boys had gotten growth hormone injections for several years. But Robert, at eleven, and Jeffrey, at twelve, still looked far smaller— and younger—than their years. A stranger would peg them for eight or nine. They were growing, but very slowly.

Nevertheless, in the examining room with their mother, when Sandberg asked how they were doing, Robert said he was happy because he was growing, offering as proof his ability to go on two rides with height restrictions at an amusement park a few weeks earlier. Sandberg joked with the boys, then guided the conversation to school. The brothers looked at each other and then at their mother. There was an incident, the mother reported, adding that her sons would soon be switching from their small school to a much larger one.

Jeffrey had been diagnosed with attention deficit disorder, a learning disability, and was taking Ritalin, which he didn't like (and which some studies have linked to poor growth). He was the only child that morning who said he was picked on because of his height. Other kids, he complained, set him up to ask the teacher questions that got him into trouble. Because of his misery, his mother had arranged for her sons to switch to the larger school, but in the meantime Jeffrey had refused to return to the classroom. With some gentle probing from Sandberg, Jeffrey explained that the previous week during a ball game, another boy refused to let him have a turn and tossed the ball over Jeffrey's head, he thought on purpose. In response, Jeffrey had called the boy a name. Now he was afraid to go back to school.

Sandberg asked him if anyone spoke up for him when he got picked on. "I do," Robert responded brightly, patting his older brother on the back. "But you're not always there," Jeffrey said in a low voice. Sandberg asked about the new school they would be attending and suggested they discuss some ideas for dealing with the teasing that they would inevitably encounter. Would Jeffrey be willing to come and talk to him for some tips? Jeffrey looked skeptical. "You mean, like a shrink?" Sandberg smiled and shook his head. "No, I don't shrink. Like a coach. There are some moves you can make to avoid situations like the one that just happened." He asked what lines Jeffrey used when other kids commented on how young he looks. When Jeffrey shrugged, Sandberg supplied some possibilities: "Can you tell them, 'I'm growing slower than other kids but I'll catch up'?"

In fact, Sandberg knew Jeffrey might never catch up in height. But he doesn't think that matters. "It's all about the story you tell yourself," Sandberg explained later. Jeffrey had told himself the story that his problems with the other boys in his school were because of his height, yet he had many other problems, including learning difficulties and an absent father. He had focused all the blame on his size. His younger brother, Robert, who was even smaller for his age than his brother, had no problem making friends, and with his exuberant personality it was easy to see why. Unlike Jeffrey, Robert seemed very much at home in the world; he had somehow mastered the moves.

Robert admitted that his problem at school was the opposite of his introverted brother's: sometimes he talked with his friends when he should be listening to the teacher. He had an impish charm, and although he was eleven years old and at least five inches below average on the charts, he participated in track, baseball, and basketball. When someone told him he looked ten, he didn't say that he was taking growth hormone. Instead, he told Sandberg, he had a stock answer. "I say I may look ten, but I act twelve."

Robert's positive outlook extended to the growth hormone treatment as well. He was sure it was making him grow even though, in fact, his growth was not impressive and there was no evidence the shots were having any effect. "Everyone's a happy customer," is how Sandberg later described this phenomenon that families using growth hormone tend to attribute any growth they experience to the shots. "That's what makes it such a great product." Kids who grow five inches tend to credit all five to the treatment—not realizing that it's more likely responsible for an inch or maybe two at best. When the drug fails to significantly boost growth rate, according to Sandberg, doctors often blame the patient, assuming the child is noncompliant and skipping doses.

CHALLENGING ASSUMPTIONS

The pediatric endocrine clinic in Buffalo is unique in several ways, not least because it offers the services of psychologists. The clinic receives funding through the Buffalo Children's Growth Foundation, and raises additional money through the United Way and local organizations not only to pay the psychologists but to provide an array of social programs for patients and their families.

When Sandberg first arrived at the clinic in 1990 he'd had little experience working with short children; his area of expertise was intersexuality—children born with disorders of sexual differentiation. Based on the medical literature and what he'd heard from doctors treating short kids, he fully expected this patient group to be burdened with psychological problems. "So I was surprised when I wasn't seeing psychopathology," he recalled. "According to the literature, these kids were depressed, they were socially withdrawn, they were performing poorly in school. If you look at these older papers, that is what they were saying. But I was not seeing it. What I *did* see was that these kids were reporting teasing and juvenilization. But they didn't seem to be dysfunctional."

Given the discrepancy between the patients he was seeing and the literature he was reading, he began to question the findings of the older studies. "There were very few psychologists working on this topic, and the largest group was acting as consultants for Genentech."

Within a few years he was not only questioning the long-held notion that short children suffered psychologically and socially because of their height, but also challenging those who supported that view. In a 1994 article in *Pediatrics*, he concluded: "Short stature does not appear to be associated with clinically significant psychosocial morbidity. Severity of the height deficit does not correlate with the level of behavioral adaptation. These observations challenge the justification of providing growth hormone therapy for all short children to improve their psychosocial functioning."

But his was a lone voice in the wilderness at a time when enthusiasm for the drug was growing. Four years later, a Genentech-sponsored psychologist, Brian Stabler, presented results of a study suggesting growth hormone could improve the behavior of short children—just as tall girls reportedly behaved better once they began treatment. Sandberg remained unconvinced. In an article in the *Journal of Clinical Endocrinology and Metabolism*, Sandberg concluded: "Adult height and degree of growth over the course of GH therapy were unrelated to Quality of Life outcomes." Four years later, in a paper he coauthored with British researcher Linda Voss, he wrote: " 'Short stature' as an isolated physical characteristic appears to hold little value as a predictor of the individual's psychological adaptation or quality of life. In order to avoid the unwarranted medicalizing of healthy short stature, clinicians would be well advised to incorporate factors" besides size.

Sandberg *does* believe teasing can make a boy's life miserable. The most common problem parents of small boys bring into the examining room is bullying, and Sandberg does not make light of it. Study after study has shown that children who are tormented by bullies perform more poorly in school because they do not want to be there, and suffer higher rates of loneliness, depression, anxiety, and even suicidal thoughts than their peers. Short boys are, in fact, bullied more than twice as often as their taller peers, and parents' fears about the short- and long-term psychological damage it causes when they are tossed into trash cans, harassed in school hallways and at bus stops, or ostracized in lunchrooms are well founded. Yet despite the prevalence of bullying (more than 20 percent of teens and preteens in U.S. schools suffer from bullying), and variety of young victims (short kids, obese kids, kids who get insulin shots, any child who is different in any way), parents come to growth clinics and request growth hormone injections with the belief that it will stop bullies from picking on their short sons. Sandberg tells parents it won't. "First, if growth hormone works at all for your child, it won't work for a while," he explained. "But you have to deal with the teasing now. Let's talk about how."

THE ROAD TO THE GROWTH CLINIC

Children arrive at the Buffalo growth clinic because their parents or pediatricians feel something's not right. A parent may notice a child still fits last year's clothing; a pediatrician may detect that a child is slipping from his expected trajectory on a growth chart, the pediatrician's most important tool for spotting growth problems in children. Ideally, pediatricians weigh and measure a child at each visit and carefully plot the results.

But little about figuring out a child's growth is ideal. It's hard to get an accurate height measurement, and mistakes are common. Kids slouch and fidget from one minute to the next, don't look straight ahead, don't keep their heels to the wall. People are elastic, taller in the morning than later in the day. "The ideal child to measure would be rigid," one study put it. "A living subject, however, is of no fixed height." Babies and toddlers present even more of a problem, since they are measured lying down with someone (preferably two people) to stretch them out; this can differ from standing height by as much as an inch.

Determining how a child is growing over time multiplies any inaccuracies. Measurements frequently differ when taken by different people, and especially when the same equipment is not used each time. Experts also disagree about how many months apart the measurements should be taken to have value. Even the season of year matters: children grow less in autumn and winter.

John Bouclis said that he can find an additional four to five centimeters "ninety-nine percent of the time" simply by stretching an infant to his full length. "When you are figuring the growth rate, that can mean a difference of sixteen centimeters [just over six inches]," he added.

Not only does he see children who've been mismeasured, but he sees children whose real problem is not height but weight. Bouclis thinks the pediatricians "punt," as he put it, sending the family to a growth clinic because they have a hard time telling the parents their sons should diet. Obesity, which is dramatically increasing in children, complicates efforts to figure out a child's growth pattern. It typically lowers growth hormone levels, but doesn't seem to prevent kids from growing taller at a normal or even faster rate. However, it also may prompt earlier puberty, leaving less time to grow.

Other common errors pediatricians make, said Bouclis, include forgetting to record the date, transposing height and weight data, failing to plot at the closest month of the child's age, or using an inappropriate growth chart to compare that boy or girl with others. For decades doctors used charts based on old data: the heights of 10,000 infants and children living in Ohio between 1929 and 1975. Most were white, middle-class, and fed with formula, which meant they tended to gain weight faster than breast-fed infants. Significantly, the charts did not account for children of other races and ethnicities who might be smaller. In addition, these all-important charts that are used to determine how far above or below average a child is ended at age ten for girls and eleven for boys, making it difficult to track and compare the growth of adolescents. It was not until 2002 that new growth charts, developed by the National Institutes of Health, the National Center for Health Statistics, and the Centers for Disease Control and Prevention, finally became available to pediatricians.

Determining a youngster's accurate height, growth rate, and where he or she stands compared with peers comes before the trickiest part of all: making a prediction. But height prediction since Wettenhall and Roche used it nearly fifty years ago as a crystal ball for their patients has not improved greatly. Predictions are fairly accurate when assessing large populations of children, but are far less precise when it comes to forecasting the height of an individual child, particularly one who is at the far end of the range—either very tall or very short. In fact, different height prediction methods produce different results for the same child. A recent study followed sixty-nine boys with constitutional delay of growth and puberty until they reached age twenty-two. The researchers discovered that *none* of the methods currently used accurately predicted which of the boys ended up 5'3" or less.

Yet doctors decide whether to give years of therapy to children without growth hormone deficiency on the basis of what those predictions tell them is a child's fate without treatment. And they judge how well the growth hormone works based on those same faulty predictions. They also still use those predictions to stunt tall girls; Bouclis acknowledged that he will occasionally prescribe estrogens if parents and the girl are insistent enough.

When children walk through the clinic's door, either through a pediatrician's referral or because of a parent's concern, they undergo a rigorous workup that usually includes blood tests and X-rays to rule out any of the number of diseases implicated in short stature. During this initial workup, the psychologists ask parents, as well as the child, to fill out questionnaires aimed at revealing any psychosocial problems the child may be experiencing.

When the test results are back the medical doctors call the parents with their diagnosis. Sandberg calls later to sum up his findings based on the psychosocial questionnaires. But ideally he wishes that he and the doctors could sit down together first and determine what additional assessments need to be done, either medical or psychological, and then, "in a single voice," outline treatment options to families based on various services available at the clinic. Too often, he said, the decision to give a child growth hormone is made because a boy's height is in the lowest percentiles—or the parent says he gets teased, or the child starts crying. The response, he said, is, "Treat him." A better response, Sandberg believes, would be to tell parents, "Let's get some more information. I think we can help, but I'm not sure yet what will be helpful." Sandberg says he isn't "expecting the endocrinologists to do it, but I am expecting them to say some of the treatments we provide cannot clearly differentiate between the medical and the psychological."

Even at Children's Hospital, however, that doesn't happen. Time, Sandberg acknowledged, is part of the problem. "Collaboration is very complex. You have to make time." And the dynamics of interacting with the families and running a clinical practice make it difficult. Finally, attitudes are hard to change. Medical doctors tend to see the role of psychologists as subordinate: to soothe kids and help families understand what's going on while they, the pediatric endocrinologists, figure out how to treat the patients.

THE TICKING BIOLOGICAL CLOCK

Time presents a different type of problem for the pediatric endocrinologists. For children whose short stature is not the result of any apparent disorder, the decision to pursue growth hormone can be a tough call. Teresa Quattrin, a pediatric endocrinologist and director of the clinic, agreed in large part with Sandberg's complaints about the overuse of growth hormone. She is sympathetic to the notion that an additional one or two inches may not make a great deal of difference in the quality of adult life for the child who receives years of growth hormone shots. She also knows firsthand that helping a boy achieve his genetic potential is not clear-cut, either: She grew up in Venice, in a large family with brothers who range from five-five to above six feet.

Quattrin attended medical school in Italy before continuing her training in pediatric endocrinology in the United States in time to experience the CJD tragedy and see it as a cautionary tale. "In 1985, I was in the room with Margaret MacGillivray when she got the call about CJD," she said. "I will never forget that. I will never say a medicine is safe. We physicians have to be humble. We're not." She tells parents, "We don't know what growth hormone will do thirty years from now."

Answering questions over lunch in the hospital's cafeteria, Quattrin worried aloud about the long-term side effects of growth hormone therapy. She wondered what hGH might be doing at the tissue level to the children who are treated with it for years, and if the dosage levels are really what they should be for her young patients.

Multiple large case-control studies in the past five years have reported positive associations between high circulating levels of the insulinlike growth factor (IGF-1) and breast, prostate, colon, and lung cancer. She's also concerned that the drug could in some cases be curtailing a child's growth by advancing his bone age: "The databases don't show it, but we see it all the time."

Short stature, she emphasized, is not like other childhood diseases such as cystic fibrosis, diabetes, or leukemia, where the chance of long-term drug side effects are outweighed by the immediate seriousness of the illness. Beyond that, she wondered, "What right do you have to be 5'8" when people aren't getting vaccinations?"

On the other hand, when confronted with pleading, anxious parents and children who have often picked up on their parents' anxiety, she admitted she "wimps out." No doctor enjoys confronting a weeping family like the one Bouclis encountered in the examining room a few hours earlier.

Nature applies pressure, too. Unless a child's growth has been monitored regularly and carefully throughout childhood, and a growth problem caught early, the chance of intervening before the end of puberty closes the door to growth is poor. Often, however, a child is nine or ten by the time parents become aware that he is substantially shorter than his classmates and not catching up. Conservative doctors may prefer to watch and wait—and to measure regularly for a period of six months, just to be sure that a child's growth is not progressing as it should. But not only can parents be insistent that something needs to be done immediately, doctors know that puberty is looming. And as Quattrin put it: "Puberty can stab you in the back."

Puberty is a double-edged sword. The accompanying growth spurt is generally double that of the prepubertal growth rate and contributes more than 15 percent to the child's total adult height. It is more rapid than any other in a child's life except for the nine months he or she spends in the womb. But the estrogen that fuels the pubertal growth spurt also causes the epiphyses to close.

Nobody can honestly predict with great accuracy how much time is left before the growth plates fuse. Puberty, it seems, is like a fingerprint or snowflake: no two experiences are alike. Some growth spurts are breathtaking; others sputter out and end without the startling increase in height parents may have witnessed in another child or remembered from their own youth. A father may recall that he added another inch or two after finishing high school, while his son didn't grow at all after eighth grade. Within the same family, one daughter may begin menstruating at eleven and grow no more than an inch, while her sister will take another four years—time that allows her bones to continue lengthening—before her first menstrual period. And for most children, when puberty ends, so does growth. But not always. Some continue to add inches through their teens; some adults report they were still growing during their college years. Even after the epiphyses close, the spine continues to grow.

As a result of puberty's unpredictability and height prediction's unreliability, Quattrin said she's becoming more aggressive about treating children early, then stopping to see what happens. "I'm trying to catch up little kids to the fifth or tenth percentile," long before they hit puberty. She takes it case by case. But if she doesn't see growth failure, if she just sees shorter-than-average parents with a shorter-than-average child, Quattrin will tell them: "This stature of 5'4" or 5'5" didn't affect you. You have a beautiful wife, a beautiful child, a good job. Would you like to be taller? Yeah. Would you have liked green eyes like your father?"

HALTING PUBERTY WITH DRUGS

In recent years parents have begun asking doctors at the clinic to delay their child's puberty with a cocktail of drugs in order to buy time for additional growth. David Sandberg cautions, however, that delaying puberty in normal children can be more psychologically traumatic than being shorter than peers.

"It's the most counterproductive thing you can do. At our clinic, three-quarters of kids feel they are treated younger than their chronological age prior to puberty. And it's more insulting to be seen as *younger* than their age than *shorter*," he warned. "The implication is that the onset of puberty is less important than adult height. And there's no data to support that. Ironically, it used to be common before growth hormone came along to give boys a bit of testosterone to kick-start puberty in a low enough dose that it wouldn't prematurely advance bone age. There is some data that it provides some comfort. But it's cheap. There's no money to be made in it."

In fact, a recent study disputed the importance of adult height in the marketplace, the oft-quoted axiom that taller men make more money just because they're taller. The researchers concluded that there *is* a wage disparity between taller and shorter white males, but that it's not the result of adult height; it's related to how tall a boy was at age sixteen. The wage gap was between those who were late and early maturers, a reflection perhaps of a late-blooming boy's lower participation in sports, clubs, dating, and other activities where he could build self-esteem and social skills. Social exclusion and a feeling of not fitting in has long-term economic consequences for shorter teens, whether or not they end up as short, average, or tall adults. The economists who wrote the study concluded that if hGH made kids taller teens, it might boost their future earnings.

But Sandberg finds psychological well-being more complex. "The schema they [drug companies] are selling is that to be short is to be unhappy. That flies in the face of common sense. Think about it. If our happiness depended upon a single characteristic, we'd be very vulnerable. And you should look to the physician to correct that—not be part of it."

Many of the short children he sees have multiple problems: broken homes, absent fathers, learning disabilities, poorly functioning families. Yet pediatricians refer them to the clinic for short stature and growth hormone treatment. He understands the time limitations on doctors, and attributes some of their referrals to their training. "Doctors are not trained to be critical, they're trained to help. But just because somebody comes in and says, 'I need an antibiotic,' you don't prescribe one." Likewise, "when a parent is saying, 'My kid's not doing well—he's unhappy,' it's usually many things together," not simply short stature. "I'm saying we need to evaluate, determine what the problem is."

But that kind of thorough, thoughtful evaluation doesn't fit into a fifteen-minute office visit. And while insurance will usually cover a child's visit to a pediatric endocrinologist, it is less likely to pay for sessions with a psychologist. Moreover, a referral to a psychologist with its implication of mental illness is less palatable to some parents than a recommendation for a drug: it's easier to tell people you're going to the doctor for some pills than to a psychiatrist to learn how to cope.

Sandberg wishes more families were given the option: "If more time were taken to talk to kids, to find out what they're really worried about, and what they expect, some kids may be willing to take another route." It takes skill and time to determine what the child himself wants versus what his parents want. Sandberg also believes it's ethically important for the sake of informed consent. "Do doctors explain fully that we really only know the short-term side effects because we only follow these patients until they stop the treatments? Don't we have an obligation to talk about the plausibility, the theoretical plausibility, of problems in the long term?"

When Sandberg is particularly frustrated with what he considers the lack of thoughtfulness on the subject of growth hormone, he is less charitable to the medical profession. "You know, I think medicine risks being complicit with the social prejudices."

But he acknowledges that doctors who are reluctant to prescribe growth hormone may find themselves overruled by parents who shop for another pediatric endocrinologist who will. In some instances, parents unhappy with a child's growth rate under the treatment of one doctor will switch to another who offers to try a larger dose.

Sometimes parents don't agree and the child is caught in the middle. In March 2004, a judge ruled in favor of a Louisiana mother who insisted her eleven-year-old son receive growth hormone, over the objections of the boy's father. Sometimes parents' motivations cause Sandberg to despair. "There are some parents always pushing their kids," he explained. "They're always looking for that edge—the right neighborhood, the right school. Growth hormone is one more way to give what they believe is an advantage. And the kids who will get this so-called advantage are the ones with good insurance, the middle- and upper-middle-class kids. Height will become one other feature that leaves some people in the underclass."

Meanwhile, short kids from poorer families with no health insurance often don't see a pediatrician, much less a pediatric endocrinologist, relying instead on emergency room care, which rarely entails measurement. Their growth patterns remain uncharted. For these kids, growth problems that could indicate real illness or disorders are discovered too late or not at all.

THROUGH THE EYES OF CHILDREN

Each summer for the past few years Sandberg has met with a variety of parents at the Magic Foundation's two-day conference. The first year Sandberg was invited, he wasn't quite sure why; his views were widely known and out of the mainstream. Nevertheless, he gamely went, hoping to get his point of view across while offering advice on how parents could help their short children cope. He spoke at the convention in the summer of 2003 to a group of parents of girls with Turner syndrome.

First, he held up a photograph of former presidents Clinton and Bush, as well as presidential candidate Ross Perot in campaign mode. Making a reference to the often cited fact that taller presidential candidates generally win elections, he deadpanned: "Poor Ross Perot. He's only made billions." Then he rattled off the facts, as he sees them, about short stature and psychological well-being. He told the group that short stature "is not associated with significant psychological dysfunction, but it can be a self-fulfilling prophecy." A child's height, he said, is associated with teasing and babying, but "that's not the only influence on that child. Look at her global adjustment, her intellectual capacity, her social support of peers, adults, and teachers. Look at her temperament—for some kids, it rolls off easily when they're called a name. Others will be devastated."

He warned parents who might be considering delaying their daughters' puberty in hopes of gaining more height with growth hormone that it is not clear that taller adult stature is better than on-time puberty. (Sandberg had tried to interest Genentech in a study on the impact of puberty at twelve versus fifteen. "No one is interested in finding data that on-time puberty in Turner syndrome is more important than additional height," he said. They didn't want that kind of data, he suspected, because girls weigh more at age fifteen than they do at twelve, and if they were to begin growth hormone at fifteen, according to weight, doctors would prescribe much more.)

Later that afternoon Sandberg attended another workshop where a group of young adults born with Russell-Silver syndrome were offering advice to parents of children with the same disorder. If short children grow up to be unhappy adults, the five women and one man who took turns on the podium that afternoon should have been miserable. All but one were well under five feet, some barely four feet tall, yet they assured the audience they were content, even happy, with their lives. Their message to the worried parents in the audience was to lighten up about their children's height.

"Your children are going to be okay," said one. "They'll learn to drive a car. They'll get married. Don't worry." What was more important, they all agreed, was that parents not lower their expectations just because their children were shorter. "Expectation is very important," said another. "Demand they give you their best."

Their comments reminded Sandberg of the verses he kept on the wall of his office in Buffalo. Written by the English poet and dramatist Edward Young, they expressed a similar sentiment, couched in the language of the eighteenth century. The first lines read:

> Pygmies are pygmies still, though perched on Alps.
> And pyramids are pyramids in vales.
> Each man makes his own stature, builds himself.

The remarks of those very short Russell-Silver adults who emerged self-confident from a childhood of teasing inspires Sandberg to continue battling his Goliath—the pharmaceutical companies and doctors who, he thinks, too easily succumb to their message. In 2004, he published an unusual study in *Pediatrics* showing how adolescents in sixth through twelfth grades view one another. More than nine hundred children in public middle school and high school in Buffalo were measured in the fall when school started. The students were not told they were participating in a height study. Although there were several parts to the experiment, perhaps the most interesting—and revealing—was the "play." Each student was asked to pretend he or she was directing a play and needed to cast various parts based on twenty-eight different descriptions, which the researchers provided. The descriptions included such phrases as "Is very shy and doesn't join in," "Gets picked on," "Is too bossy," "Everyone likes to be with," and "Is not good at sports." The study was designed to assess how children characterized their peers, whether height played a role in a child's popularity. If short children truly are as unpopular as growth hormone enthusiasts claim, they would have been disproportionately labeled with the negative characteristics. What Sandberg's researchers found, however, was that a child's stature had little impact on his or her social standing. Very short children, as well as very tall kids, had friends and were just as well liked by their peers as their average-size schoolmates.

Sandberg concluded that extremes of stature have "minimal detectable impact on peer perceptions of social behavior, friendship, or acceptance." Furthermore, he warned in the journal article, "if problems with peer relationships are identified among short or tall youths, then factors other than stature should be considered as etiologically important." In other words, if a child claims he's bullied by other kids because he's short, the problem probably lies elsewhere and should be explored, and the sooner the better.

In spite of the publicity his peer-reviewed study had received, and praise for its methodology, the pediatric endocrinologists Sandberg worked with didn't seem to believe its results. Some referred to Sandberg's research findings simply as his opinions, which infuriated him. Especially since he thought they were the ones making medical decisions based on opinion, not science.

If people are sincerely concerned about the psychological well-being of children, Sandberg pointed out, medical centers could take the tens of thousands of dollars a year that it costs to possibly make one child a little taller later, and use it for psychological services to help many short children with their problems now. Also, Sandberg argued, drug companies should spend some of their time telling people not to give short kids a hard time. They could spend money on education and public service announcements. "Even Philip Morris tells people not to smoke."

In the end, however, Sandberg said he was happy to see the kids, for whatever reason they come in the door. If parents think it's height that is causing all the problems, fine. As long as he can spend sometime with the kids. And maybe help them tell a different, better story about themselves.

a new normal?

IF FIFTY YEARS of treating height tells us anything, it's that temptations to improve on heredity are powerful, especially when parents believe it will make their children's lives better. Mothers and fathers of tall girls hoped massive doses of estrogen would give their daughters an adolescence without misery, and a better chance to find husbands and happiness.

The history of growth hormone reveals powerful financial incentives for drug companies, and some doctors, to stoke these temptations. Growth hormone therapy spread to short healthy children long before there was scientific evidence it boosted their height, and although it cost some families hundreds of thousands of dollars. Its use continues to expand despite uncertainty about the long-term risks of adding more hormone to children whose bodies already produce normal amounts, and despite the lack of proof that treatment for height improves quality of life.

At the pace that medical science is uncovering what genes do and how to tweak them, it's not difficult to imagine a future in which treating healthy, normal children to reach or surpass their predicted genetic potential becomes commonplace. So many characteristics might multiply a child's odds for success and happiness: from calmer temperament to better muscle coordination, from photographic memory to the kind of intelligence that measures high on standardized tests. Whatever the technology—swapping genes, inserting synthetic genes, using drugs to turn bits of DNA on and off—temptations to improve inheritance will multiply as well.

The history of treating children for height suggests that these future therapies will not necessarily be sold to doctors or to the public as cosmetic or even acknowledged as enhancements. They may begin as long-sought cures for recognized and devastating diseases. But once such cures exist, they will find new uses.

As with height, some parents will pursue every chance to improve on a child's heredity; others will hear their son or daughter diagnosed with a condition that can be changed, and feel pressured to take what the doctor offers. But when does a disadvantage become a disease? Who will be considered too moody? Too uncoordinated? Too forgetful or unintelligent? Both culture and drug marketing departments will redefine normal.

When biosynthetic growth hormone was first approved, Genentech immediately doubled the number of its potential customers simply by changing the definition that most endocrine clinics used to diagnose growth hormone deficiency. Children who had previously tested normal suddenly were not normal. Ron Rosenfeld was at Stanford University with Raymond Hintz at the time: "And Ray and I well remember calling up families and saying, 'Remember we told you your child wasn't growth hormone deficient? Well, we've changed our mind, your child *is* growth hormone deficient! Come on in and get this new growth hormone!'

"All of these levels are arbitrary, and it was as good an arbitrary point as any," Rosenfeld said with a shrug. "And no endocrinologist contested that, because we were all anxious to open up the opportunity of growth hormone therapy to as many children as possible."

Similarly, the pharmaceutical giant Eli Lilly redefined how short is too short. The traditional cutoff point that doctors used to define short stature was the third percentile: any boy or girl whose height fell below 97 percent of others the same age and sex. But Lilly knew the FDA would be reluctant to approve growth hormone use for 1.7 million U.S. kids. Besides, the traditional definition of short stature was also arbitrary. Being among the shortest 3 percent doesn't correspond with any particular disease, or even any particular height, since percentiles differ depending on whether a child is being measured against schoolmates in the Netherlands or schoolmates in Japan. So the company adopted the strategy that only a fraction of extremely short kids should qualify, the shortest 1.2 percent. It invented a new diagnosis for them: non–growth-hormone-deficient short stature. And it argued they are not normal, though their hormone levels are.

The company's strategy succeeded in adding at least three-quarters of a million potential new customers with the imprimatur of the FDA, whose mission is to regulate treatment for disease rather than to authorize drugs for enhancement. A social problem became an official medical disorder. No longer "short normal," as they'd been termed in the medical literature for decades, the very same kids are frequently now described in the very same journals as "short but otherwise healthy." And many pediatric endocrinologists argue they cannot justify refusing growth hormone for kids taller than the arbitrary cutoff. Now that short stature has been labeled a disease, parents won't be denied a cure.

There will always be a shortest 1.2 percent, of course, so the FDA's action means there will always be children with non–growth-hormone-deficient short stature. As more than one doctor has pointed out, if all those who qualify get a prescription and grow taller, then every girl or boy who stands just above them on the growth chart will take their place among the lowest 1.2 percent and by definition cross the line from healthy to unhealthy. By this logic, and perhaps for the first time, medicine will be making some kids sick simply by making others better. When asked why the company chose that particular cutoff, Lilly scientist Charmian Quigley explained that normal is not a fixed concept. "Normal," she said, "changes."

WE WROTE THIS BOOK anticipating tough decisions ahead for parents as normal continues to change. Parents who are already given genetic choices express a strong cultural preference for height. Sperm banks report that women want the fathers of their babies to be tall. Ads in Ivy League newspapers for egg donors specify height, not to mention coloring and SAT scores. Now that some couples at fertility clinics use preimplantation technology not just to screen an embryo for chromosomal defects, but to select their baby's sex, certainly some will want to screen an embryo for its potential to grow six feet tall. As genetic technologies develop, perhaps pediatric endocrinologists will no longer be able to say Scottie dogs have Scottie dog puppies, and Great Danes have Great Danes. And perhaps it will no longer be socially acceptable for Scottie dogs to have mere Scottie dogs.

Will there be even more stigma attached to someone who is different, when that difference can be prevented? Will society lose something of value by eliminating conditions at the extremes? Such abstract-sounding questions are already real and personal when it comes to stature. When researchers found the gene for achondroplasia, then quickly identified genes for some other inherited forms of dwarfism, the Little People of America faced what it would mean to eliminate embryos that carry the genes that make them who they are—people who do not think of themselves as defective.

In 1995, the group unexpectedly found itself at the center of the debate over the potential use of genetic testing for eugenics, and issued a thoughtful but anguished statement. Couples could be told if an embryo carried a rare form of dwarfism fatal in infancy. But expectant mothers could be urged to test routinely for genes that cause short stature, then pressured not to give birth to a baby who was less than perfect. Insurance companies might refuse to cover such pregnancies to term and families might find themselves condemned for knowingly bringing such babies into the world. "What will be the impact of the identification of the genes causing dwarfism, not only on our personal lives and our needs, but on how society views us as individuals?" the statement asked. Especially given "the traditional desire of parents to create perfect, healthy children."

That's why some people with dwarfism greeted the discoveries with excitement while "others reacted with fear that knowledge from genetic tests such as these will be used to terminate affected pregnancies and therefore take the opportunity for life away from children such as ourselves and our children." Mostly, Little People wanted it recognized that they are people of worth. "We as short-statured individuals are productive members of society who must inform the world that, though we face challenges, most of them are environmental... and we value the opportunity to contribute a unique perspective to the diversity of our society." They were arguing for their right to exist.

Scenarios in which twenty-first-century families pursue the genetically perfect child not only ignore the value of diversity but also overstate the role of genes. Very few single genes predetermine destiny. Mostly, we inherit propensities that are influenced by environment. Even height, with its strong genetic basis, is also powerfully affected by nutrition and, as cases of psychosocial dwarfism reveal, nurturing. One of the ironies is that, as growth hormone use spreads, the United States has stopped getting taller. Children in the Netherlands continue to gain stature in each generation, while the U.S. population does not. Some have theorized that Dutch society does a better job of seeing that all its children eat well, exercise, and get access to good health care in the womb and while growing up.

When medical science begins to reach for the microscope as often as the stethoscope, DNA testing will identify some defects and abnormalities in every person. There are questions, though: Which ones will match up with disability or disease? Which differences will we choose to fix? Which will we accept and live with, as we always have? How much variation will we accept? Once there's an ability to choose or alter more inherited characteristics, what will be considered normal? The gene therapy that makes life livable for a patient with muscular dystrophy might boost the muscle power of a kid struggling to keep up, or race ahead, in gym class. A drug that interferes with the ravages of Alzheimer's disease might improve memory and grade point averages for healthy children. How will parents respond when a son or daughter wants the chance to be made not just taller but also smarter, like the kid next door?

A HALF-CENTURY of attempts to alter height offers some cautions:

Because a treatment gives someone more of what the body produces naturally, like a hormone, that does not make it safe. Because it has minor side effects in the short run when given to a few people doesn't mean it won't cause major illness years later, or when given to a lot of people. Children are developmentally vulnerable, and the effects of medication on them are less studied, partly because ethical concerns protect them from experimentation. Yet off-label use is a form of experimentation that's widespread when it comes to children. From a medical point of view, a risk remains theoretical until something bad happens.

Doctors make decisions on the basis of their personal and cultural as well as medical beliefs. Once a treatment exists, its existence becomes a reason to use it. So the rationale for giving medicine to healthy short children keeps changing: to alleviate suffering, to treat growth failure, or to fulfill genetic potential. Because short stature is a lifelong disadvantage, because it's probably a genetic defect, or because we're able to optimize height and that's what families want. The reasons keep changing as the prescriptions keep mounting.

Experiments become treatments not only before all the risks are fully known but also in the absence of clear benefits. Even the growth hormone manufacturers, largely thanks to the efforts of David Sandberg, admit there is no proof that short kids have significant psychosocial problems and no conclusive evidence that growth hormone

therapy makes them happier. Weighing unknown risks versus undoc-
umented benefits is one thing for an adult, and another when making a decision on behalf of a child. For that matter, how much risk *is*
acceptable when considering children who have no health problems
but are extremely short?

Virtually every relationship in medicine has changed since the days
when Maurice Raben first tried hGH from the laboratory on a boy
with hypopituitary dwarfism and then the federal government distributed it free and only to those who needed it most. The consequence
is that there's more information available for medical consumers than
ever before, but much of it's connected to commercial interests with
huge financial incentives to promote medical treatment, tout benefits,
underplay potential dangers, expand uses, and play up stigma if that's
what it takes to sell their products. There's been no incentive to conduct an expensive follow-up and see how things turn out for patients
like Laura and the other Tall Girls decades down the road.

Although there are pediatric endocrinologists critical of their specialty's ties to industry, many argue that their individual judgments
aren't clouded by a few free growth charts or pens, or even by who
supports their research, pays them to speak to other physicians, funds
a nurse or a student for their clinic, or finances their journals, societies, and continuing medical education. Patient groups argue that the
substantial corporate funding their organizations receive doesn't bias
the information they distribute or the public stands their leadership
takes. A parent making a decision about the rest of a child's life, however, has no way to know.

"Of course we're influenced," acknowledged Ron Rosenfeld, who
besides prestigious academic affiliations has financial ties to the
growth hormone manufacturers Genentech and Lilly, and the recombinant IGF-1 manufacturer Tercica. "That's why advertising budgets
are so high, that's why marketing VPs make so much money. But having said that, I do have confidence in the ability of the majority to
balance these things and come up with an informed opinion to give
patients. And I think that some responsibility must lie on the part of

patients to accept the fact that doctors aren't gods and they can be influenced and they don't always know what's best and there has to be some degree of *caveat emptor* in the consumer."

In other words, medicine has graduated from the era of "Doctor knows best" to an era of "Buyer beware."

For their part, doctors complain they're pressured by parents who feel entitled to make their kids taller. Some physicians resist. Often, however, parents and doctors share the same wish to do something for a child. Except for insurance companies, which are the real gatekeepers, most of the forces described here are arrayed on the same side: that of doing more rather than less. The scientific curiosity of specialists, their personal and professional inclination to fix things, the building of academic careers and departments and medical practices, along with the profit incentives of drug manufacturers combine easily with the wishes of unhappy children and anxious parents.

IT'S HARD BEING a parent, and some of the most difficult decisions lie between accepting a child as he is and helping him become someone other people are more likely to accept and admire. Parents who say society should just be more accepting of difference don't get any help from a medical establishment that argues short kids should be treated because they can be treated. Parents, too, are under increasing pressure to give their children every possible advantage they can afford, and every opportunity to fulfill their potential.

One lesson for those who only want to make their children happy is the one every parent already knows but hates to acknowledge: the gratitude of a child is unpredictable. As novelist Margaret Atwood warned in an article in *The New York Review of Books*, parents who choose their children's features will inevitably have chosen wrong when the child reaches adolescence. " 'I didn't ask to be born' will be replaced by resentments such as 'I didn't ask to have blue eyes,' or 'I didn't ask to be a math whiz.' "

Undoubtedly, thousands of adults are pleased they're taller than they might have been because their families gave them injections. Yet some people have spent decades of adult life wondering whether pituitary hGH poisoned them with CJD, even resenting the feeling that they were part of some experiment. Some graduated from a childhood that focused on every inch—and which made them feel they could never quite measure up in the eyes of their parents—into an adulthood in which they blame every failure on height. Stature became their defining characteristic and an ongoing source of self-consciousness. Perhaps that's why the Tall Girls who took their pills ended up less satisfied with their final heights than the Tall Girls whose parents decided against treating them.

Other adults remain bitter their families never gave them the chance to try growth hormone. Otherwise, there wouldn't be websites devoted to those following the latest news on height, or people willing to undergo a procedure as risky and painful as limb lengthening. Men would rather be tall. That probably will not change. Neither will the fact that for most people, whatever their height, parts of childhood and adolescence are painful. Adolescence is a stage of life when happiness and self-confidence are so elusive that they might be considered abnormal; a time when feeling different can be both excruciating and completely normal.

Some things do change, however. The Tall Girls grew up into societies in which being a tall woman was no longer considered a pitiable fate. The practice of giving girls estrogens for height didn't wind down because doctors reversed course, but because fewer and fewer mothers brought their daughters in for treatment. John Crawford, who treated hundreds of girls, recalled that in the 1950s "too tall" was 5'6", then 5'8", then 5'10", then 6', and finally, by the 1990s, he had "no more customers." Culture and opportunity changed. Marriage was no longer the only agenda; girls were allowed to compete at sports without being considered unladylike, and to take on careers once reserved for men. Some women turned being tall into their biggest advantage, on the modeling runway, on the college basketball court. Parents of the Tall Girls in the 1950s and 1960s failed to imagine a future when many flight attendants and nurses would be male; pilots and doctors could be female; and girls who didn't make the grade as ballerinas could dream, instead, of becoming astronauts or running for president of the United States.

Society's changing for short people, too. Courts have repeatedly ruled that employers cannot discriminate on the basis of height unless they can show that it actually matters for the performance of a particular job. U.S. Army recruitment starts at 5' for a man, and 4'10" for a woman.

These court decisions came about because height restrictions excluded not just women, but rapidly expanding ethnic groups as well. The United States has never been a more demographically diverse society, with waves of immigrants coming from other parts of the world with shorter populations. They bring with them sports, such as soccer and martial arts, that offer athletic opportunities for kids who cannot all grow up to be point guards or linebackers. With the world more interconnected than ever before, the idea that a tall blond man of Germanic descent makes a more successful salesman, as described by the professor who conducted that well-cited study of hiring preferences in the 1970s, sounds as dated as life before personal computers. How many employers in the future will choose the taller job applicant over the one who speaks three languages?

Diversity is not just socially valuable, but also biologically advantageous. Scientists who decipher the human genome are finding that human beings exhibit much more genetic variation than anyone ever imagined. If a society can tolerate more variety, perhaps fewer adolescents might be made to feel abnormal, and fewer adults might feel the need to give them medical treatment in hopes of pushing everyone closer to average.

In 2000, and again in 2004, the shorter presidential candidate won. In 2006, a movie incarnation of British secret agent James Bond stood gun in hand, bristling with cool machismo, and under six feet for the first time in the series. The six-foot female costar of a long-running television show about life in the White House towered over her male costars, including the shorter-than-average actor who played the president. Cultures do change.

This book began with Laura. It should conclude with her as well. She recently had another breast cancer scare. After a routine mammogram she was told that because her breast tissue was dense and there appeared to be something suspicious, she should travel to Boston's Brigham and Women's Hospital for a more sophisticated mammographic examination. When she told the doctors there her history of hormone treatment, "they were aghast, just like all the other doctors I've seen," she said. After several needle biopsies, she underwent a lumpectomy, which showed severe hyperplasia, a condition that may turn cancerous. They suggested she was at high risk for cancer and should be closely followed.

But Laura also had good news to report. She and her husband had purchased an old rustic summer camp several years earlier on a lake in Maine, and moved permanently to a town nearby on the coast. Her parents, sisters, and brother and their children gather at the camp for weeks during the summer. Laura's two oldest nieces are taller than she is, hovering a little over six feet. The older one earned herself a four-year basketball college scholarship. The younger one hoped to do the same.

IN AUSTRALIA, Alison Venn's group published a third paper in 2005 based on the data collected on the Tall Girls. In this study they established that the psychological outcomes among both treated and untreated women were poor. The two groups suffered equally high rates of depression, leading the investigators to conclude that the intended psychosocial benefit of treatment was negligible.

Their findings, they wrote, "highlight the importance of attending to the mental health of adolescents presenting for management of conditions where self-concept and body image are a primary focus." On a more positive note, the researchers reported, in a fourth paper published in 2006, that among the women who had children in both groups there was no difference in ability to breast-feed.

Venn's researchers continue to mine their data for other information on the Tall Girls. They are preparing a paper on mammographic breast density, a marker for breast cancer. Although they have seen cancers in the group, it may never be possible, given the small size of the study population, to draw conclusions overall about the effects of the treatment on cancer risk. Investigators in Sweden, where cancer registries are maintained, hope to have better luck comparing their treated tall girls with those in the population who have developed the disease. They have obtained access to medical records from sixteen hundred women.

In Australia, where Venn's fertility research received a lot of media attention, she believes the treatment is still offered. She received inquiries from a couple of clinicians about the safety of lower doses of hormones, which they were giving or planning to give their patients. "Our response was that we are not in a position to be confident that any treatment will be safe," she replied.

MORE PRADER-WILLI DEATHS led to warnings that human growth hormone should not be used in those children with the syndrome who are severely obese or have serious respiratory impairment.

IN 2005, the FDA approved the first new drug in two decades to treat short stature: recombinant IGF-1 for severe primary insulin-like growth factor deficiency; the term was coined to describe children who produce enough of their own growth hormone but still grow poorly because of low IGF-1. "By being specifically targeted and having an FDA indication, it really codifies the disease," Tercica's president and CEO buoyantly told *BioWorld Today* after the federal government decided to allow the company's product, Increlex, onto the market and granted it orphan drug status.

Some pediatric endocrinologists believe there are just handfuls of documented cases of severe IGF deficiency in the world. Others believe that a significant number of children diagnosed with idiopathic short stature have some degree of IGF deficiency, especially those who do not respond well to human growth hormone therapy. Lacking IGF-1, they are unable to translate growth hormone into growth.

In a replay of Genentech's strategy with growth hormone decades earlier, Tercica received orphan drug status based on the rarity of the disorder, then immediately set out to expand the market. How many children have this form of growth hormone resistance, beyond those with the extremely rare condition called Laron dwarfism, is the billion-dollar question. Tercica, a California start-up that licensed recombinant IGF-1 from Genentech, is already clinically testing Increlex in slightly taller children with somewhat higher natural levels of IGF-1 than those for whom the FDA approved the drug.

As Tercica's president and CEO celebrated its approval, he described to the business press how sales reps and managers would be dispatched to talk to pediatric endocrinologists "who form the basis of this short stature market." Increlex was Tercica's first product, the first brick in what its CEO called "building a franchise in short stature and associated metabolic disease." Again, echoes of the recombinant growth hormone story.

Tercica explained its business strategy for attracting investors in a filing with the Security and Exchange Commission. It began with the approval to treat 6,000 or so youngsters in the United States and an equal number in Western Europe whose lack of natural IGF-1 made them unable to respond normally to growth hormone. This represents about a $200 million annual market. It would then "capitalize" on the broader opportunities of treating short stature. Tercica estimated some 60,000 children evenly split between the United States and Western Europe have short stature with some lesser degree of growth hormone insensitivity, representing a $1 billion annual market opportunity. The company would conduct continuing medical education programs, medical symposia, and regional speaker programs "aimed at establishing awareness of Increlex in the physician community."

Injections of IGF-1 can induce hypoglycemia, which can lead to convulsions, comas, and death. It was originally developed by Genentech for diabetes, then discontinued when it was linked to accelerating retinal damage in diabetics. As to the role IGF-1 might play in malignancy, scientists continue to investigate why so many studies find a relationship between elevated levels of IGF-1 and different types of cancers. It may not cause them, but may be involved indirectly, or facilitate an existing cancer's growth or spread.

There is increasing evidence from the laboratory that the IGF-1 genetic pathways play a key role in longevity, though it is a complicated one. Mice with a gene mutation that makes them growth hormone deficient have lived twice as long as normal. Rodents with growth hormone resistance, or IGF-1 deficiency, also live greatly expanded spans. The oldest living mouse on record was a Laron dwarf. These laboratory Methuselahs have prompted some gerontologists to express concern about giving children either extra hGH or IGF-1.

UCLA pediatric endocrinologist Pinchas Cohen, an IGF-1 researcher, calls these fears that are based on laboratory mice speculative. But recently, Cohen coauthored a study of Ashkenazi Jewish women who lived past ninety-five and their short daughters, finding many of them shared a gene mutation that made cells less responsive to IGF-1. The same genetic mutation that made them short seems to have helped them live long.

Who will determine what is considered a normal level of IGF-1?

IN SEPTEMBER 2006, David Sandberg left Buffalo to head up a psycho-endocrine unit at the University of Michigan in Ann Arbor, a unit that has focused on diabetes rather than height and has fewer research ties to growth hormone manufacturers. Sandberg is devising a program there that will help families decide whether growth hormone or psychotherapy is most appropriate for their child. He also works with families to define their goals for growth hormone therapy, which will help them decide when to start and stop treatment.

TWO PRINCETON ECONOMISTS confirmed in 2006 that taller people earn more in both the United States and Britain; each four-inch increase corresponds to 10 percent more earnings. A 6'2" American man was 3 percent likelier than a 5'10" man to become an executive and 2 percent likelier to be a professional. But the economists offered strong evidence that this so-called height premium has less to due with discrimination or social stigma than with intelligence. Taller people, on average, were smarter, and gravitated to higher-paying occupations.

These researchers also agreed that height at age sixteen predicts future earnings better than final height. They suggested that this was not because shorter kids don't pick up social skills. Instead, both teen height and cognitive ability could reflect prenatal health and childhood nutrition. Ending up tall doesn't make you smart. But a healthier start might make you both smarter and taller, and it's intelligence that might make you wealthier.

A COMPREHENSIVE REPORT on the National Hormone and Pituitary Program for those who had been treated with cadaveric hGH upped the CJD toll in the United States to twenty-six confirmed cases as of November 2006. The report added that "none of these people began treatment with hGH after 1977," when Dr. Albert Parlow's laboratory began processing. It was the first public credit Parlow had received by name.

As of 2006, thirty-four people treated with pituitary growth hormone made in the United States had died of CJD, including two in Brazil and six in New Zealand. In New Zealand, 15 percent of those who received Wilhelmi's product perished because the hormone they received did not go through the same filtering process as it did in the U.S. when it was put into vials.

The odds of getting CJD stood at 1 out of 300 in the United States, but for those who began treatment before 1977 they were about 1 in 104, less than 1 percent. Among those who started treatment before 1970, 1 in 52 people developed CJD, about 2 percent. The incubation period has not ended. The U.S. government could not identify confidently which preparations were high-risk or risk-free and so continued to decline to share with former patients information on which preparations they were given. Two patients, at most, the government said, received hormone from the batch that infected a chimpanzee with CJD.

Freedom of Information Act requests languished for years at the National Institutes of Health, and several former patients reached out-of-court settlements without receiving the documents to which they were legally entitled.

THE NUMBER of French CJD victims who had been treated with human growth hormone for height stood at 110 when, in February 2008, French courts brought to criminal trial seven doctors and former senior health officials who had administered its pituitary program. The now elderly men faced manslaughter charges for allegedly ignoring the CJD contamination that prompted the United States, Britain, and other countries to close down their pituitary growth hormone distribution in 1985, while France continued until 1988 and did not inform families of the risk. One of the defendants was also charged with accepting bribes and illegally selling pituitary by-products. All seven pleaded innocent, arguing that they had acted according to the medical knowledge of the time. More than two hundred family members of children who died of CJD after taking human growth hormone to grow taller crowded the courtroom, demanding justice from the French government beyond monetary payments they had already received.

Worldwide, around two hundred people are known to have died of Creutzfeldt-Jakob disease from infected pituitary human growth hormone. Confidence that those who took commercial hGH made from pituitaries had escaped CJD because the companies used Roos gel filtration methods was shaken by a letter to the *Journal of Neurology, Neurosurgery and Psychiatry* in 2008. Austrian doctors reported they had autopsied a thirty-nine-year-old man who died of the disease twenty-two years after taking KABI's product for growth.

THE FOLLOW-UP SURVEY of pituitary hGH recipients in the United States proved useful once again, in the wake of the British study that found higher cancer rates in those treated in the United Kingdom with growth hormone during the pituitary era. Like the British, the Americans found two former childhood patients who as adults had died of colon cancer. The small number made it impossible to say whether or not there is an increased risk of colon cancer for everyone receiving hGH. The National Institute of Diabetes and Digestive and Kidney Diseases has asked the FDA and the pharmaceutical companies to "watch for colon cancer" in people treated with biosynthetic human growth hormone.

IN THE FEW YEARS since the FDA approved growth hormone for approximately one out of every one hundred children in the United States, short stature has increasingly become big business. Sales of all brands of hGH increased during the first year that the shortest kids could legally be targeted. Lilly's Humatrope gained most, and in 2006 raked in $460 million worldwide, 40 percent more than it had four years previously. Genentech has also received permission to market its product for children with non–growth-hormone-deficient short stature. The latest cost estimates for treating height are more than $50,000 per inch.

Generic hGH went onto the market in Australia, where it brought down the price. Generics loomed in the United States despite the objections of the biotechnology industry and some of the major pharmaceutical companies. Other manufacturers continued to seek the holy grail, hGH in pill form or in an inhaler.

EVEN LESS PROVEN THERAPIES that manipulate puberty in the interests of adding inches continue to gain popularity, including the use of gonadotropin-releasing hormone agonists, such as Lupron, to delay the onset of puberty, or aromatase inhibitors, such as Tamoxifen, to hold the growth plates open.

IN 2007, Congress passed the most significant reform of the FDA in forty-five years, spurred by deaths from the use of the painkiller Vioxx, and a series of scandals involving the failure of various companies to inform the FDA of negative data, as well as the failure of the agency to monitor drug safety after approval. The pharmaceutical industry agreed to sponsor the reform, which will beef up the FDA's authority to require surveillance of drugs after they are on the market. It also attempts to limit conflicts of interest on the agency's advisory panels. Consumer groups hailed the legislation, while noting that it does not change the system that uses drug company funding to finance the regulatory process.

Also in 2007, the Justice Department scored another victory against off-label marketing of growth hormone. Pfizer subsidiaries agreed to pay civil and criminal fines totaling $34.7 million to settle Justice Department charges that stemmed from the promotion and distribution of the growth hormone Genotropin by Pharmacia before the company's acquisition by Pfizer. One of the subsidiaries pleaded guilty to offering a kickback to increase Genotropin sales.

Congress also turned its attention to pharmaceutical company marketing tactics and the influence of drug manufacturers on continuing medical education.

IN 2007, a group of researchers announced they had found the first of what are probably many gene sequences linked to normal variations in human height. The difference in just one letter in a person's genetic code made about half a centimeter's height difference among the study subjects. Those born with a gene containing two copies of the height-conferring letter were nearly a centimeter taller than those with different versions of the gene. It was hailed as the first convincing evidence of how DNA could affect normal variation in human stature. The researchers noted that mutations of genes such as these might lead to extreme short or tall stature and that one day such information could help diagnose children who are extremely tall or short for no known reason.

"By defining the genes that influence normal variation in stature, we might also someday be able to better reassure parents that their child's height is within the range predicted by DNA, rather than a consequence of disease," one of the scientists said. But the story of altering height so far shows that hearing a child is healthy is no longer enough.

And what about the someday when people can choose, or choose to change, DNA? Surely the same knowledge can be used to go beyond genetic potential rather than be restricted by it. Predicted range will not be reassuring, when there are the tools to do even better. The temptations are just beginning.

ACKNOWLEDGMENTS

We would like to thank the Fund for Investigative Journalism, whose generous award supported reporting for this book.

The people who gave us their time, especially those who shared the details of their lives, made this story possible. To name just some of them: Father Anthony Grossenburg, Patsy Grossenburg, Lucille Sluder, Laura Cooper and her mother, Shirley, Fred and Gwen Mahler, Chip and Linda Smith, and Janet Cregan-Wood. We wish them good health, and hope they obtain some satisfaction that telling their stories through us might help others. Not only did multiple conversations with David Davis inform the book, but his excellent and dogged reporting on the tragedy that overcame the National Pituitary Agency's program laid some of the groundwork.

Valerie Wheat, librarian at the Archives and Special Collections of the University of California San Francisco Library and Center for Knowledge Management, was especially helpful as we negotiated the archive's vast volume of Choh Hao Li's papers. The Regional Oral History office of The Bancroft Library at the University of California, Berkeley, provided excellent oral histories of Genentech founders and early employees. Journalist Jennifer Cooke managed to send us documents from Australia even while wildfires blazed there. Washington D.C., attorney Lewis Saul kindly dug into his memory and his files. Penny Jones graciously housed and fed Christine Cosgrove in Melbourne.

We also thank the many pediatric endocrinologists and other doctors and scientists who gave their time to be interviewed, some more than once.

Our agent, Candice Fuhrman, recognized the worth of the project, found it a publishing home, and kept the faith. Jessi Hempel and Chez Shadman ably aided us in our research. Sheila Himmel, Dr. Irene Solomon, Vince Cosgrove, and the founder of DES Action, Pat Cody, read versions of the manuscript and deserve special appreciation. Any mistakes are not theirs but ours. At Jeremy P. Tarcher, our editor, Sarah Litt, provided many valuable comments, and publisher Joel Fotinos exhibited remarkable patience.

We also thank our husbands and our children, who are all closer to perfect than we are. This book is dedicated to them.

GLOSSARY

ACETONE—A colorless liquid used as a household solvent, as the key ingredient in nail polish remover, and as a preservative for pituitary glands in some processing methods.

ACHONDROPLASIA—A condition caused by genetic mutation that leads to disproportionately short arms and legs, a large head, and short stature. This is the most common type of dwarfism.

ACROMEGALY—A disorder caused by excessive growth hormone resulting in abnormal growth of hands and feet and facial bones, including the brow and lower jaw. Lips, nose, and tongue can also enlarge, as can the heart and other organs. The late wrestler-turned-actor Andre the Giant had acromegaly, and was 224 cm tall.

AMINO ACIDS—The basic building blocks of proteins in the human body and elsewhere. They are small molecules that link into chains.

ANDROGENS—Hormones made by the testes and adrenal glands. They affect the growth of bone, muscle, fat, and other tissues, and are necessary for masculine characteristics. Testosterone is the primary androgen.

AROMATASE—A protein that helps convert androgen hormones to estrogens, which stimulate the growth of the long bones and eventual closing of the growth plates. If aromatase is inhibited, estrogen is blocked and the growth plates remain open.

AUXOLOGY—The science of human physical growth.

BIOSYNTHETIC HUMAN GROWTH HORMONE (also called recombinant human growth hormone, or r-hGH)—Growth hormone manufactured using biotechnology, or gene splicing. Genentech first introduced it to the U.S. market in 1985.

BONE AGE (skeletal age)—The measurement of biological maturity based on stages of bone formation, as distinguished from chronological age.

BOVINE SPONGIFORM ENCEPHALOPATHY (BSE)—Commonly called mad cow disease, a form of Creutzfeldt-Jakob disease that is found in cattle and transferred to people who eat infected beef. People with the infection are said to have a variant form of CJD, or v-CJD.

CENTILE (see also Percentile)—A measure of comparison with others in a population. The centiles on growth charts are based on groups of children the same sex and age. The centile number indicates what percent of girls or boys the same age are shorter than the child being measured.

CHROMOSOME—Long, threadlike pieces of DNA in the center of each cell. Every human cell normally contains twenty-three pairs of chromosomes; one set of each pair is inherited from the mother, one set from the father.

COLUMN CHROMATOGRAPHY—A method for purifying proteins by passing them through a tall glass column that traps some molecules and allows others through. In the version called gel filtration or size exclusion chromatography, the column is packed with fine porous beads that separate proteins on the basis of size.

CONSTITUTIONAL GROWTH DELAY—Delayed growth in height and sexual maturity that often runs in families. More boys than girls are late bloomers, as people commonly term those with this growth pattern.

CREUTZFELDT-JAKOB DISEASE (CJD)—A form of transmissible spongiform encephalopathy, a fatal neurological disease that leads to a recognizable spongy pattern of brain lesions, and that can be inherited, arise sporadically, or be transmitted. In the case of children who received human growth hormone from infected cadavers, it was transmitted by doctors who gave them injections. Such cases (induced inadvertently by medical personnel or procedure) are called iatrogenic CJD.

DEVELOPMENT—The body's progression to physical and sexual maturity.

DIETHYLSTILBESTROL (DES)—An orally active synthetic nonsteroidal estrogen first synthesized from coal tar in 1938 and later prescribed to pregnant women in a misguided attempt to prevent miscarriage.

DNA (deoxyribonucleic acid)—The substance found in the nucleus of cells that contains the genetic blueprints that direct a cell to produce the proteins it needs to carry out its function.

DOWN SYNDROME—A chromosomal abnormality that affects both mental and physical development, leading to short stature and a characteristic facial appearance.

DWARFISM—Extreme short stature that can be caused by a medical or a genetic condition, and that can describe those whose bodily proportions are the same as in average people or those whose head, trunk, and limbs are disproportionate. More than two hundred types have been diagnosed. Heights of adults with dwarfism range from about 2'8" to about 4'8".

ENDOCRINOLOGY—The study of the endocrine system, a system of glands that produce and control hormones.

EPIPHYSIS—The end of a long bone that is initially cartilage and is separate from the long shaft. It converts to bone in a process called ossification that occurs gradually as a child grows. Eventually, the epiphyseal center, commonly called the growth plate, hardens and fuses with the shaft of the bone. Completion of the process, the closing of the growth plates, is known as epiphyseal fusion.

EUGENICS—Originally, the science of bettering the human race, chiefly through selective breeding. The term, coined by Francis Galton in the nineteenth century, acquired especially sinister connotations in the Nazi era. More recently, it has been applied to efforts to improve hereditary characteristics through such new technologies as embryo screening and genetic engineering.

FOOD AND DRUG ADMINISTRATION (FDA)—The U.S. federal agency charged with overseeing safety in food and drugs.

GENE—A unit of heredity that parents pass to offspring, made up of DNA and usually containing the directions to make a protein.

GENETIC POTENTIAL—The idea that people have a potential limited by or determined by genes. While some genes do determine a single characteristic, most traits are the product of a combination of inheritance and environment. The most important factor influencing height besides genes, for example, is nutrition.

GIANTISM (gigantism)—Acromegaly when it occurs in childhood; abnormal growth caused by an excess of growth hormone.

GLACIAL ACETIC ACID—A corosive acid. (Acetic acid is what makes vinegar smell sour.)

GLAND—Organ or tissue that secretes a substance used by the body. Endocrine glands are those that release hormones into the bloodstream.

GONADOTROPIN-RELEASING HORMONE (GnRH)—A hormone secreted by the hypothalamus in the brain. During puberty it increases and is responsible for the adolescent growth spurt. Blocking it delays puberty.

GROWTH FACTORS—Chemicals produced by cells in a variety of body tissues that affect growth. They act alone or interact with one another and with hormones.

GROWTH HORMONE DEFICIENCY (GHD)—Lack of growth hormone. It has also been called hypopituitary dwarfism, meaning extreme short stature caused by the lack of a pituitary hormone. It can occur congenitally, or because of a tumor, or surgery or radiation for a tumor. Some cases are of unknown origin. It is rarely inherited.

GROWTH HORMONE–RELEASING HORMONE (GHrH)—Another hormone secreted in the hypothalamus of the brain that influences growth, by playing a role in the pulsatile secretion of growth hormone.

GROWTH HORMONE RESISTANCE (growth hormone insensitivity)—A rare condition that makes some people unable to use the growth hormone that their bodies secrete in normal amounts. Laron dwarfism is a form of extreme short stature caused by growth hormone resistance or insensitivity. There is evidence that Pygmies may as a group have growth hormone resistance, which would explain their short stature.

GROWTH PLATES—A common term for the area in the long bones where bone tissue is formed. It consists of cartilage, which is re-formed into bone over time. When this process is finished, it is said that the growth plates are closed, meaning that almost all growth is complete.

GROWTH VELOCITY—The rate of growth in height, weight, and so on.

HORMONE—A chemical substance secreted from a specific tissue, usually into the bloodstream, where it travels throughout the body and regulates many processes, including growth, development, and reproduction.

HUMAN GROWTH HORMONE (hGH)—A hormone secreted in the pituitary gland that, among other effects, promotes growth throughout the body.

HYPOPITUITARY DWARFISM (growth hormone deficiency)—A form of extreme short stature caused by lack of growth hormone. Hypopituitary dwarfs often are less than five feet tall, but are normally proportioned. It is not usually an inherited condition, and can be caused by pituitary tumors or radiation therapy.

HYPOTHALAMUS—A region of the brain that, among other functions, secretes hormones to signal the pituitary gland either to produce or to stop producing other hormones that regulate growth and development. Growth hormone–releasing hormone produced in the hypothalamus stimulates the pituitary to make growth hormone.

IDIOPATHIC SHORT STATURE (ISS)—Extreme short stature that is not inherited and has no known cause. The term traditionally applied to those in the bottom third percentile of height for gender and age.

INSULINLIKE GROWTH FACTOR (IGF-1)—A biochemical substance secreted by the liver that plays a key role in growth. Increasing growth hormone levels increases IGF-1. Recombinant IGF-1 is now being manufactured and marketed for severe short stature caused by IGF-1 deficiency.

INTRAUTERINE GROWTH RETARDATION (IUGR)—Growth retardation that occurs in the womb for a variety of reasons. About 90 percent of children born small for gestational age catch up by age one or two.

LUTEINIZING HORMONE—A hormone involved with the timing of puberty. Blocking it delays sexual maturation, and is used to treat precocious puberty as well as to treat height by giving children more time to grow.

MENARCHE—The first menstrual period.

MET-LESS hGH—Recombinant hGH that has the same number of amino acids as hGH found naturally in the human body. The first biosynthetic human growth hormone, manufactured by Genentech, had an extra amino acid, methionine.

MIDGET—A historic term for those with growth hormone deficiency, describing people with short stature whose bodies were proportioned like other people's. The term's associations with nineteenth- and twentieth-century freak shows makes it offensive.

MID-PARENTAL HEIGHT—The average of maternal and paternal height used in a formula to predict a child's final height.

MONOMERIC—Consisting of only one component.

NATIONAL HORMONE AND PITUITARY PROGRAM—The continuation of the National Pituitary Agency. It operates now as a laboratory that extracts hormones for use in research but not in humans.

NATIONAL INSTITUTE OF DIABETES AND DIGESTIVE AND KIDNEY DISEASES (NIDDK)—The current name for the institute within the National Institutes of Health that is involved with research of endocrine diseases. Its predecessors, the National Institute of Arthritis and Metabolic Diseases and the National Institute of Arthritis, Metabolic, and Digestive Diseases, oversaw the federal program to distribute pituitary human growth hormone.

NATIONAL PITUITARY AGENCY (NPA)—An agency launched in 1963 under the auspices of the National Institutes of Health to collect pituitary glands from cadavers, process human growth hormone, and distribute it free of charge to those with hypopituitary dwarfism. Its name was changed to National Hormone and Pituitary Program.

NON-GROWTH-HORMONE-DEFICIENT SHORT STATURE—A designation for the shortest 1.2 percent in the United States who have normal levels of growth hormone. Eli Lilly won approval from the FDA in 2003 to add this diagnosis to the label of their growth hormone product, making it legal to market to children who are short but otherwise healthy.

OFF-LABEL—A description for drugs for indications that have not been approved by the FDA and so do not appear on the label. While doctors may use their medical judgment to prescribe a drug for any purpose for which they believe it will be effective and safe, it is illegal for manufacturers to market drugs for off-label uses.

ORPHAN DRUG STATUS—The FDA designation given to drugs that are approved for diseases or conditions affecting fewer than 200,000 patients in the United States. This status assures them a monopoly for seven years. Congress designed this program in order to encourage manufacturers to develop treatments for rare diseases.

PERCENTILE (see also Centile)—A measure of comparison with others in a population. For example, when a child is in the third percentile of height, 97 percent of children the same age and gender in the population are taller.

PITUITARY GLAND—A pea-size gland that sits at the base of the brain, below the hypothalamus, and that releases multiple hormones, including growth hormone. The pituitary controls almost all the other endocrine glands, which is why it is sometimes termed the master gland.

PITUITARY HUMAN GROWTH HORMONE (cadaveric hGH, pituitary hGH, or pit-hGH)—Growth hormone extracted from human pituitary glands taken from cadavers. Its use was ended when cases of Creutzfeldt-Jakob disease emerged in individuals who had received injections of pituitary hGH.

PRADER-WILLI SYNDROME—A genetic disorder affecting about one in 12,000 to 15,000, typically causing short stature, as well as poor muscle tone, cognitive disabilities, and a chronic feeling of hunger.

PREMARIN—The commercial name for a drug derived from the urine of pregnant mares (thus the name). It became one of the most widely used drugs in the United States, and was the form of estrogen most commonly used for hormone replacement therapy.

PRION— A misfolded protein that causes neurodegenerative disease in humans and animals. Prion diseases include scrapie in sheep, and *kuru* and Creutzfeldt-Jakob disease in humans, among others. These diseases, also called transmissible spongiform encephalopathies (TSEs), were known as slow viruses before wide acceptance of the theory that they are caused by prions.

PROTEIN—A large molecule, made up of amino acids, that performs various activities in a cell.

PSYCHOSOCIAL SHORT STATURE—Short stature caused by physical and emotional deprivation that retards growth.

PUBERTAL GROWTH SPURT (adolescent growth spurt)—The increased rate of growth in weight and height that occurs during the five to eight years after the onset of puberty, when people reach peak height velocity.

PUBERTY—A dramatic increase in the secretion of sex hormones that marks the end of the juvenile stage of childhood and the start of sexual development.

RECOMBINANT HUMAN GROWTH HORMONE—See **Biosynthetic human growth hormone.**

SCRAPIE—A transmissible spongiform encephalopathy that kills sheep. It was a scrapie researcher who realized that, just as scrapie was impervious to normal methods for killing viruses and bacteria, CJD might survive the pituitary processing used to extract human growth hormone from cadavers and to treat children for height.

SECONDARY SEXUAL CHARACTERISTICS—Physical traits associated with the beginning of sexual maturation. In boys, these include facial hair and muscularity; in girls, the development of breasts and adult fat distribution.

SMALL FOR GESTATIONAL AGE (SGA)—Low birth weight, 2,500 grams or less for normal gestation length. The FDA has approved the use of biosynthetic hGH for children born with SGA who do not catch up to their peers. The vast majority of SGA babies do catch up within the first two years.

STIMULATION TESTS (provocative tests)—Tests using a variety of agents that stimulate growth hormone production in order to measure levels and to determine whether or not someone has growth hormone deficiency.

TESTOSTERONE—A hormone made in the testes that influences growth, as well as sexual maturation.

TRANSMISSIBLE SPONGIFORM ENCEPHALOPATHY (TSE)—See **Prion**.

TURNER SYNDROME—A disorder in which girls are missing all or part of an X chromosome, and consequently have little or no ovarian function. Lack of estrogen due to ovarian failure requires that they be given estrogen when they reach the age of puberty. They tend to be very short, although they produce adequate growth hormone.

NOTES

page INTRODUCTION

vii **"It is as right as"** Testimony of Deno Andrews, Endocrinologic and Metabolic Drugs Advisory Committee Meeting, Tuesday, June 10, 2003, Holiday Inn Select, Bethesda, Maryland, Department of Drug Evaluation and Research (CDER).

CHAPTER 1. "TALLNESS CAN BE A REAL HANDICAP FOR A GIRL"

3 **A week before** Information about Laura's experiences was gathered between 1999 and 2006 during lengthy interviews with Christine Cosgrove by telephone and e-mail, and in person in New Hampshire with Laura, her parents, and her sister, Cathy.

5 **"man must be"** Hugh Morris, *The Art of Kissing*, quoted in Ralph Keyes's *The Height of Your Life* (Boston and Toronto: Little, Brown, 1980), p. 135.

5 **"Tallness can be"** Georgiana P. Riegal, "Help for Tall Girls," *Parents*, November 1942, p. 98.

5 **"soft and low"** "The Low-Down for Tall Girls," *Los Angeles Times*, October 5, 1948.

5 **"If you are over five feet eight"** John Robert Powers, "Minimize Figure Faults by Improving Posture," *Los Angeles Times*, September 20, 1950.

6 **"A tall woman's problem"** John Robert Powers, "Tall Problem Solved by Right Foundations," *Los Angeles Times*, January 11, 1952.

6 **At the movies...Ingrid Bergman** Keyes, *The Height of Your Life*, p. 238.

6 **In 1948, Gimbels** "New Shop Is Opened for City's Tall Girls," *New York Times*, November 5, 1948.

6 **"lopped off a few"** "Fashion Caters to Tall Women," *New York Times*, April 25, 1949.

7 **Kay Sumner, a Disney animator** Lucille Leimert, "Confidentially," *Los Angeles Times*, June 23, 1947.

7 **It was not only the womanly** Joyce Lee, "Tall Girls: The Social Shaping of a Medical Therapy," *Archives of Pediatrics & Adolescent Medicine*, October 2006, p. 3.

7 **"I am sorry to say"** Walter C. Alvarez, "Dr. Alvarez Says: Tall Girl Can't Expect Drug to Halt Growth," *Los Angeles Times*, April 23, 1953.

8 **"may have found it"** E. Kost Shelton and Robert F. Skeels, *Endocrine Treatment in General Practice*, ed. Max A. Goldzieher and Joseph W. Goldzieher (New York: Springer, 1953).

8 **Theoretically, that left Shirley** John Gillis, *Too Tall, Too Small* (Champaign, IL: Institute for Personality and Ability Testing, 1982), p. 141.

9 **At 5'10", Jean Shrimpton... Veruschka** Heights for the models were reported at www.swinginchicks.com, consulted July 18, 2001. Reported heights of models, actors, and actresses are unreliable, however, according to Keyes.

10 **As for jobs** United Airlines, http://www.united.com/page/article/0,3361,00. html. Matthew C. Keegan, "The Original Eight: Genesis of the Modern Day Flight Attendant," http://www.thearticlewriter.com/OriginalEight.htm.

11 **"Girls who normally"** "New Treatment Helps Tall Girls," *The Boston Sunday Globe*, March 5, 1967.

12 **"According to the best"** Gertrud Reyersbach to Shirley Moore, November 7, 1968.

14 **"turning tortoises into hares"** H. N. B. Wettenhall, "The Tall Child," *Clinical Paediatric Endocrinology*, ed. Charles Brook (Oxford: Oxford University Press, 1981), p. 134.

16 **One hundred times the amount** Angie S. Graham, Drug Information Coordinator, Department of Pharmacy, Stanford Hospital and Clinics, e-mail to Christine Cosgrove, January 23, 2003.

CHAPTER 2. PLAYING GOD WITH HORMONES

18 **In 1938, Charles Edward Dodds developed** The history of the development of synthetic hormones and Dodds's role is taken from several books on the subject of DES. These include Robert Meyers, *D.E.S.: The Bitter Pill* (New York: Seaview/Putnam, 1983); Cynthia Laitman Orenberg, *DES: The Complete Story* (New York: St. Martin's Press, 1981); and Barbara Seaman, *The Greatest Experiment Ever Performed on Women: Exploding the Estrogen Myth* (New York: Hyperion, 2003).

18 **its molecular composition** Orenberg, *DES*, p. 11.

18 **"They had problems"** Meyers, *D.E.S.*, p. 41.

18 **When given to pregnant mice** Ibid., p. 54.

19 **the companies set the stage** Seaman, *The Greatest Experiment*, pp. 43–44.

19 **"no national catastrophe"** Meyers, *D.E.S.*, p. 64, citing the 24th edition of the *Dispensatory of the United States of America*.

19 **Dodds was knighted** Seaman, *The Greatest Experiment*, pp. 41–42.

20 **During the years that Dodds** John Crawford, telephone interview with Christine Cosgrove, December 15, 2000. The German and Austrian reference: "Thus I would guess that it was [the Austrian Jakob] Erdheim or one of his group rather than [Bernard] Zondek who should be credited with giving Albright the idea that estrogen could be employed to moderate exuberant statural growth in childhood." Crawford, e-mail to Christine Cosgrove, February 13, 2004.

20 **Reyersbach had been born** Prudence L. Steiner, "Recollections of Gertrud C. Reyersbach," *Jewish Women's Archive*, http://www.jwa.org/discover/recollections/reyersbach.html (consulted August 8, 2007); Reyersbach obituary, *The New York Times*, April 5, 1999.

21 **Crawford, the youngest** Crawford obituary, *The Boston Globe*, May 2, 2005.

21 **These doctors at Massachusetts General** Gertrud Reyersbach, "Effect of Diethylstilbestrol on Growth and Skeletal Maturation in Adolescent Girls with Tall Stature," *American Journal of Diseases of Childhood*, 94 (1957), pp. 453–454. Also John Crawford, telephone interview with Christine Cosgrove, December 15, 2000.

21 **From the start, this treatment** Heather Munro Prescott, "What Is 'Normal' Adolescent Growth?" Paper presented at the History of Childhood in America Conference, August 5–6, 2000, Washington, D.C.

21 **Even so, desperate parents** W. A. Marshall, "What Can We Do About Tall Girls?" *Archives of Disease in Childhood,* 50 (1975), pp. 671–673.

21 **For example, in 1965** Carol Walters, e-mail to Christine Cosgrove, November 13, 2002.

23 **Growing up in this privileged** "Child Healer Helped Preserve Native Birds," *Australian,* August 12, 2000; Wettenhall obituary, *Age,* September 12, 2000; Christine Rodda, "A Tribute: Dr. Norman Wettenhall," *Endocrine Society of Australia Newsletter,* April 2001.

23 **Yet, Wettenhall was a man** George Werther, conversation with Christine Cosgrove, May 2, 2004, San Francisco.

23 **Pediatrics, which had** Heather Munro Prescott, *A Doctor of Their Own* (Cambridge, MA: Harvard University Press, 1998), pp. 10–11.

24 **Some doctors complained** Sydney A. Halpern, *American Pediatrics: The Social Dynamics of Professionalism, 1880–1980* (Berkeley: University of California Press, 1988).

24 **A decade later** Leonard Engel, "Cortisone and Plenty of It," *Harper's,* 1958, pp. 57–62; "Mayo Clinic Celebrates the 50th Anniversary of the Discovery of Cortisone," Mayo Clinic press release, August 10, 2000.

25 **"too confident of their powers"** Michael Bliss, *The Discovery of Insulin,* (Chicago: University of Chicago Press, 1982).

25 **the New York endocrinologist...claimed success** M. A. Goldzieher, "Treatment of Excessive Growth in the Adolescent Female," *Journal of Clinical Endocrinological Metabolism,* 16 (1956), pp. 249–252.

25 **A year later, Laura's doctor** Gertrud Reyersbach, "Effect of Diethylstilbestrol on Growth and Skeletal Maturation in Adolescent Girls with Tall Stature," *American Journal of Diseases of Childhood,* 94 (1957), pp. 453–454.

26 **He noted in a later publication** H. N. B. Wettenhall, Christine Cahill, and Alex F. Roche, "Tall Girls: A Survey of 15 Years of Management and Treatment," *Journal of Pediatrics,* 36 (4) (1975), pp. 602–610.

26 **In the next few years** S. C. Freed, "Suppression of Growth in Excessively Tall Girls," *JAMA,* 166 (1958), pp. 1322–1323; M. J. Whitelaw and T. N. Foster, "Treatment of Excessive Height in Girls: A Long-term Study," *Journal of Pediatrics,* 61 (1962), pp. 566–570.

27 **Nurses at private girls' schools** Alison Venn and Jo Rayner, interviews with Christine Cosgrove, September 17–19, 2003, Melbourne, Australia.

27 **in 350 B.C., Aristotle** James Tanner, *A History of the Study of Human Growth* (Cambridge, England: Cambridge University Press, 1981), p. 8.

27 **In the centuries** Ibid., p. 65.

27 **That year, a Frenchman** J. M. Tanner, *Fetus into Man: Physical Growth from Conception to Maturity* (Cambridge, MA: Harvard University Press, 1990), p. 6.

28 **Typically between birth** Robert H. Shmerling, "Medical Myth: Can We Predict Height?" Aetna InteliHealth, February 11, 2003, http://www.intelihealth.com/IH/ihtIH/WSS/35320/35323/360788.html?d=dmtHMSContent, consulted March 4, 2008.

29 **Two scientific methods** For nearly half a century, growth experts have debated the relative merits of two methods for height prediction: one developed by American Nancy Bayley, known as the Bayley-Pinneau method, and the other developed by

James Tanner and colleagues in Britain. To use the Bayley-Pinneau method, radiologists first assign a child his or her bone age by referring to the Greulich and Pyle atlas. The child's X-rays of left hand and wrist are compared with those in the atlas. The reference standard for a particular age is based on the median of X-rays taken of many children at various ages. On the basis of a child's bone age, the Bayley-Pinneau tables enable pediatric endocrinologists to ascertain estimated adult height by considering the percentage of skeletal maturity a child has already attained and what percentage is left. These tables draw from records of the Harvard Growth Study in Massachusetts and the Institute of Child Welfare, in Berkeley, California, and cover ages from seven years to maturity for boys and six years to maturity for girls. In the Tanner-Whitehouse method, the radiologist assigns a numerical value to a dozen or so individual bones of the hand and wrist, the sum of which provides a maturity score. Reference scores are based on data obtained from several thousand X-rays of children. Tanner, "Growth at Adolescence" (Oxford: Blackwell, 1962); T. W. Todd, *Atlas of Skeletal Maturation (Hand)* (St. Louis: C. V. Mosby, 1937); W. Greulich and S. I. Pyle, *Radiographic Atlas of the Hand and Wrist* (Stanford, CA: Stanford University Press, 1959); Nancy Bayley and Samuel Pinneau, "Tables for Predicting Adult Height from Skeletal Age: Revised for Use with the Greulich-Pyle Hand Standards," *Journal of Pediatrics*, 40 (1952), pp. 423–441.

31 **A child in Denver** E. F. Harris, S. Weinstein, L. Weinstein, and A. E. Poole, "Predicting Adult Stature: A Comparison of Methodologies," *Annals of Human Biology*, 7 (3) (1980), pp. 225–234.

31 **"Although our predictions"** J. M. Tanner, R. H. Whitehouse, and W. A. Marshall, *Assessment of Skeletal Maturity and Prediction of Adult Height (TW2 Method)* (London: Academic Press, 1975).

31 **Similarly, Bayley pointed out** Nancy Bayley et al., "Attempt to Suppress Excessive Growth in Girls by Estrogen Treatment: Statistical Evaluation," *Journal of Clinical Endocrinology & Metabolism*, 22 (1962), pp. 1127–1129.

31 **One astute observer** Edgar J. Schoen et al., "Estrogen Treatment of Tall Girls," *American Journal of Diseases of Children*, 125 (1973), pp. 71–74.

31 **Roche developed a third method** A. F. Roche, H. Wainer, and D. Thissen, "Predicting Adult Stature for Individuals," *Monographs in Paediatrics* (Basel: S. Karger, 1975). Roche refused to be interviewed for this book.

32 **front-page story** John Yeomans, "Girl, 13, with Figure 35-24-35," *The Sydney Sun*, September 18, 1964.

32 **more sensational headline** "Drug Turns Young Amazons into Beauties," *Daily News* (Australia), September 18, 1964.

33 **"interfering with Nature"** "We Can Stop Girls Growing Tall," *The Sun*, September 18, 1964.

34 **Besides the side effects** The description of the office visits was provided by George Werther, interview with Christine Cosgrove, September 17, 2003, Melbourne.

34 **Werther believed Wettenhall** Ibid. Some girls felt these exams went beyond clinical and were abusive. One girl filed suit, but it was thrown out of court, according to Werther.

34 **One woman visiting** Jo Rayner, a nurse and researcher for the Tall Girls study, interview with Christine Cosgrove, September 19, 2003, Melbourne.

35 **"Various parts of my body"** The writer is a woman who was measured but ultimately not treated for tall stature. Her story, edited slightly for spelling and punctuation, was published anonymously in *Tall Girl Newsletter*, August 1999.

CHAPTER 3. TWO GIRLS, TWO CONTINENTS

38 One was Janet Cregan-Wood Information about Janet Cregan-Wood came from multiple interviews in person in September 2003, from e-mail exchanges, and from an unpublished manuscript about her experiences written by Cregan-Wood and her partner, Ed Wolf.

38 He took a detailed medical history George Werther, conversation with Christine Cosgrove, May 2, 2004, San Francisco.

39 Nevertheless, in the 1960s Pediatric endocrinologist Alan Rogol, telephone interview with Christine Cosgrove, November 4, 2002: "It started in Melbourne....Wettenhall's data is what we based what we did on. Norm was a friend of my boss, so we were aware of his data at that time." British pediatric endocrinologist Charles Brook, telephone interview, April 29, 2003: "The seminal name in treating tall girls in Europe is Norman Wettenhall....He really was the person who started the whole idea of treating tall girls, and it was taken up in this country principally by a chap called...W. A. Marshall, who worked in Tanner's clinic....When I went to work with Prader in Zurich in 1972, he was using—everybody was using Wettenhall's regimen for treating tall girls. That is, they were using large doses of estrogen."

39 "Perhaps the most common concern" H. N. B. Wettenhall and A. F. Roche, "Tall Girls Assessment & Management," *Australian Paediatric Journal*, 1, p. 210.

40 "A very tall person" H. N. B. Wettenhall, "The Tall Child," chapter 8 of *Clinical Paediatric Endocrinology*, ed. Charles S. D. Brook (London: Blackwell Science, 1981), pp. 134–140.

40 "This form of treatment" Editorial, *British Medical Journal*, April 20, 1963.

40 "I wonder what right" Dr. Stickler, "Abstracts," *The Journal of Pediatrics*, April 1967, p. 676.

40 "resist parents" Lawson Wilkins, quoted in Heather Munro Prescott, "What Is 'Normal' Adolescent Growth?" Paper presented at the History of Childhood in America Conference, August 5–6, 2000, Washington, D.C.

40 "They all belonged" Pediatric endocrinologist Irene Solomon, interview with authors, June 30, 2003, San Francisco.

41 He believed that by treating John Crawford, interview with authors, May 2, 2004, San Francisco.

41 "I was the radical" John Crawford, interview with Christine Cosgrove, December 15, 2000, Boston; and letter to Laura Cooper, October 26, 1998.

41 Gallagher urged restraint, and quotations following Gallagher, *Medical Care of the Adolescent* (New York: Appleton-Century-Crofts, 1960).

42 He also opposed Heather Munro Prescott, *A Doctor of Their Own* (Cambridge, MA: Harvard University Press, 1998), pp. 111–112.

44 Shirley remembered reading As it turned out, Shirley was probably correct. "Estrogen affects the way bile is metabolized, and thus it can lead to gallstones....Women on Premarin have two and a half times as many gallbladder operations as other women." Susan Love, *Dr. Susan Love's Hormone Book* (New York: Random House, 1998).

46 They had recently diagnosed A. L. Herbst, H. Ulfelder, and D. C. Poskanzer, "Adenocarcinoma of the Vagina: Association of Maternal Stilbestrol Therapy with Tumor Appearance in Young Women," *The New England Journal of Medicine*, 284 (1971), pp. 878–881.

46 Decades later, a doctor A. L. Herbst, e-mail to Christine Cosgrove, August 14, 2005.

46 **As early as 1953** W. J. Dieckmann et al., "Does the Administration of Diethylstilbestrol During Pregnancy Have Therapeutic Value?" *American Journal of Obstetrical Gynecology*, 66 (1953), pp. 1062–1081.

47 **11,000 prescriptions were written** *The Wall Street Journal*, quoted by Meyers, *D.E.S.*

47 **acquired a bad reputation** Crawford, telephone interview with Christine Cosgrove, December 15, 2000.

47 **"for girls worried about"** Wettenhall et al., "Tall Girls: A Survey of 15 Years of Management and Treatment," *Journal of Pediatrics*, 36, (4) (1975), pp. 602–610.

48 **"annoying hypertrophy"** Doug Frasier and Fred Smith, "Effect of Estrogens on Mature Height in Tall Girls: A Controlled Study," Letters to the Editor, *Journal of Clinical Endocrinology & Metabolism*, 1968.

48 **rise in cholesterol** J. A. Leuven et al., "The Effect of Large Doses of Ethinylestradiol on Apolipoprotein Levels in Excessively Tall Prepubertal Girls," *Metabolism*, 35 (10) (October 1986), pp. 978–980; M. Weninger et al., "Increase of Serum Lipids and Serum Lipoproteins in Girls Under Therapy with Estrogen and Norethisteron for Height Reduction," *Acta Paediatrica Scandinavica*, 76 (3) (May 1987), pp. 500–503.

48 **Wettenhall's chapter** H. N. B. Wettenhall, *Medical Care of the Adolescent*, 3rd ed. (New York: Appleton-Century-Crofts, 1976), p. 575.

48 **"Why is it"** A. F. Roche, H. Wainer, and D. Thissen, "Predicting Adult Stature for Individuals," monograph in *Paediatrics*, 3 (1975).

49 **tall girls were treated** Nadine Brozan, *The New York Times*, February 11, 1976.

49 **case of a girl** Angela Haines, *The New York Times Magazine*, April 4, 1976.

50 **"school corridors are filled"** Letter to the Editor, *The New York Times Magazine*, April 25, 1976.

51 **"was conceived at a time"** "Report of the Conference on Estrogen Treatment of the Young," *Pediatrics*, 62 (6) (1978), supplement.

51 **"The human experiment"** Ibid., p. 1217.

CHAPTER 4. "A GLAND LOST IS A GLAND WASTED"

57 **They invented imaginative** James Tanner, *A History of the Study of Human Growth* (Cambridge, England: Cambridge University Press, 1981).

57 **physicians began to realize** R. Tattersall, "A History of Growth Hormone," *Hormone Research*, 46 (1996), pp. 236–247.

58 **Cushing correctly theorized** Harvey Cushing, *The Pituitary Body and Its Disorders* (Philadelphia: Lippincott, 1912).

59 **They could cure** Tattersall, "A History."

59 **until 1921, when one of Cushing's** The colleague was Choh Hao Li. D. Perlman, "Scientist's Life a Feast of Learning," *San Francisco Chronicle*, January 11, 1971.

60 **Cushing charged that the companies, and quotations following** H. Cushing, "Disorders of the Pituitary Gland, Retrospective and Prophetic," *The Journal of the American Medical Association*, 76 (25) (June 18, 1921), pp. 1725–1726.

60 **A British physician wrote** Tattersall, "A History."

60 **And many did remain cautious** See Sheila M. Rothman and David J. Rothman, *The Pursuit of Perfection: The Promise and Perils of Medical Enhancement* (New York: Pantheon, 2003).

60 **That fact struck a blow** M. Grumbach, "Herbert McLean Evans, Revolutionary in Modern Endocrinology: A Tale of Great Expectations," *Journal of Clinical Endocrinology and Metabolism*, 55 (6) (1982), pp. 1240–1247.

61 **Evans continued to refine** See C. H. Li, *Current Biography*, April 1963, pp. 17–19.

61 **"A short time ago"** A. Wilhelmi, handwritten letter to Li, in Choh Hao Li Papers 1935–1984, MSS 88-9, Archives and Special Collections, Library and Center for Knowledge Management, University of California, San Francisco (UCSF). Referred to hereafter as the Li Papers.

62 **That explained why** M. S. Raben, "Treatment of a Pituitary Dwarf with Human Growth Hormone," *Journal of Clinical Endocrinology and Metabolism*, 18 (1958), pp. 901–903.

62 **In the early 1950s, doctors treated** Tattersall, "A History."

62 **They tried thyroid preparations** Rothman and Rothman, *The Pursuit of Perfection*.

62 **Big doses of thyroid** Robert Blizzard, interview with Susan Cohen, June 2003, University of Virginia.

63 **"Growth hormone, to date"** Tattersall, "A History."

63 **Raben experimented** C. T. Sawin, "Maurice S. Raben and the Treatment of Growth Hormone Deficiency," *The Endocrinologist*, 12 (2) (March/April 2002), pp. 73–76.

63 **Across the country** Li Papers.

63 **Because of these symptoms** Sawin, "Maurice S. Raben."

64 **Paper from Lawson Wilkings** Ibid.

64 **Raben's short letter** Ibid.

64 **Those who knew Raben** Ibid. The editorial opinion that Raben belonged to a generation of physicians who did not rush to patent is also Sawin's.

64 **He stored them in acetone** Ibid. Sawin offered this vivid description of Raben's lab during pituitary processing.

65 **A textbook in the 1950s** Max A. and Joseph W. Goldzieher, *Endocrine Treatment in General Practice* (New York: Springer, 1953).

65 **"The world's first Pituitary Bank"** Press release draft, UCSF, June 22, 1960. Li Papers.

66 **For example, an eleven-year-old girl** Ibid.

66 **Perhaps UCSF wanted** Roberto F. Escamilla, "Clinical Studies of Human Growth Hormone in Children with Growth Problems," in *Hormonal Proteins and Peptides*, ed. Choh Hao Li (New York: Academic Press, 1975), vol. 3, pp. 147–190.

66 **Li had already distinguished himself** Along with Harold Papkoff, he isolated monkey and human growth hormone. R. David Cole, "Choh Hao Li, April 21, 1913–November 28, 1987," *Biographical Memoirs*, National Academy of Sciences, www.nap.edu/readingroom/books/biomems/cli.html.

66 **Born in China** History.library.ucsf.edu.

67 **Slim, tall (5'11")** *Current Biography.*

67 **Li's wife later described** "Dr. C. H. Li Cover Story," manuscript, Li Papers.

67 **He even negotiated** Li Papers.

68 **FDA approval** October 17, 1967, In a letter to John B. Saunders, Roberto Escamilla wrote: "The long-term goal is to acquire ample knowledge as to the advantages and disadvantages of hormone therapy with HGH, including dosages, the optimum length of treatment and contraindications to therapy. To acquire all the information required by the Food and Drug Administration to produce this hormone commercially after its eventual synthesis." Li Papers.

68 **In 1958, the physician** A. Colegrove, "New 'Growth Drug' Means Hope for Girl Doomed to Lingering Death," *San Francisco News*. The clipping was included in a letter from Peter Forsham, director of the University of California Medical Center Metabolic Unit, October 6, 1958, denouncing its inaccuracies. Li Papers.

68 Those working for the Pituitary Bank Pituitary Bank Foundation Tenth Annual Meeting minutes, September 20, 1972; Pituitary Bank Foundation Eleventh Annual Meeting minutes, September 12, 1973. Li Papers.

68 They courted the public Pituitary Bank Third Annual Meeting minutes, September 8, 1965. Li Papers.

69 They successfully prompted "Gland Pledges to Be Sought," *Eugene Register-Guard*, June 5, 1964.

69 A television audience was told Li Papers.

69 they acknowledged that the primary purpose Letter from R. Escamilla to C. S. Cullen, Dean of the Medical School, June 6, 1967. Escamilla argued that the bank needed to exist in spite of competition from the National Pituitary Agency in order to continue the basic research that Evans and Li had started. He also noted that Li's hormone preparation method led to a hormone that was "superior" to others, an interesting point given the future tragedy with the NPA's product. Li Papers.

69 A radio broadcast "Substance of Stature," Broadcast 7029, *University Explorer*, CBS Radio Network, January 19, 1964. Li Papers.

69 The bank was more successful Pituitary Bank Foundation, Growth Hormone Committee Meeting minutes, February 27, 1974. Li Papers.

69 The Pituitary Bank began scrounging Pituitary Bank Foundation Fifth Annual Meeting minutes, September 13, 1967. Li Papers.

69 Requests from people Various such letters of request are found in the Li Papers.

69 The bank adopted the motto Report on the bank's 1964 collection and publicity efforts (unsigned). Li Papers.

69 A brochure for the public "The University of California Pituitary Bank." Li Papers.

69 Yet even with cadaveric hGH unavailable "The unanswered question, 'does growth hormone do anything to stature or metabolism in patients without growth hormone deficiency?' is the central theme of future Human Growth Hormone Committee endeavors." Minutes, Human Growth Hormone Committee Meeting, Pituitary Bank, March 15, 1966. Li Papers.

69 A group of clinicians Escamilla, "Clinical Studies."

70 One of these early subjects Ibid.

70 "When you have a new drug" Blizzard, interview.

70 Bob Blizzard biography Ibid.

71 there were about twenty pediatric endocrinologists F. Lifshitz, "Robert Blizzard—A Legacy," *Growth, Genetics and Hormones*, 19 (4) (2003).

71 pioneering branch An excellent description of the growth of this field can be found in Sydney A. Halpern, *American Pediatrics: The Social Dynamics of Professionalism, 1880–1980* (Berkeley: University of California Press, 1988).

73 "We were giving" Blizzard, interview.

73 "tooth and nail" "It would be a travesty if the tooth and nail competition of New York were to be transferred to California," William E. Latimer, Physician Coordinator of the NPA, to Li, May 17, 1963. Li Papers.

73 Her daughter Sandra Mrs. Bonnie Sharkey to Dr. Charles L. Blumstein, St. Rita's Hospital, Lima, Ohio, November 19, 1963. Li Papers.

73 "example of how doctors" Pathologist C. L. Blumstein, November 25, 1963. Li Papers.

73 Alfred Wilhelmi helped launch Minutes of the Ad Hoc Committee on Human Pituitary Collection, January 8, 1962. Wilhelmi was one of the original six

members of the committee because he had been producing hormone for the Endocrinology Study Section of the National Institutes of Health. Li Papers.

74 **Wilhelmi required pituitaries** The need to protect the vested interests of those already collecting pituitaries, while expanding the numbers of glands processed for scientists as well as patients, was set out in "A Proposal for the Support and Coordination of Collection of Human Patients," a draft document for what became the National Pituitary Agency. Li Papers.

74 **He is a man who makes** Liftshitz, "Robert Blizzard." This is an impression confirmed by talking with his colleagues and former patients.

75 **They saw the new agency** "I realize this is a well-intentioned type of bottleneck; but, nevertheless, there is considerable difficulty in the practical matter of working through the Agency." H. David Mosier to Li, March 9, 1967. In a letter to Li dated March 12, 1963, Mosier, a pediatrician on the faculty of the California College of Medicine at UCLA, described meeting with Blizzard and complained that he didn't seem to "make allowance for supporting local efforts." Li Papers.

75 **Some pediatric endocrinologists** Later, the government had trouble tracking down what became of all the NPA-issued hormone and determining whether or not it had ever been used in the studies for which it was requested. It is widely acknowledged by pediatric endocrinologists that they saw the NPA primarily as a treatment program, though the agency couldn't call it that.

75 **And Wilhelmi and Li were guaranteed** Notes of the Third Meeting of the Medical Advisory Board of the National Pituitary Agency, May 2, 1964. Li Papers.

76 **The first NPA newsletter** National Pituitary Agency newsletter, first edition. Li papers.

76 **there were only about 100,000 autopsies** This was as of 1958, and pituitaries were collected in only a small fraction of those brain examinations. In 1962, an estimated 15,000 pituitaries were collected for use in scientific investigations in the United States. T. Dull, J. Mahoney, and P. Henneman, "Human Growth Hormone—A Scientific Exhibit," prepared for the Annual Meeting of the American Medical Association, June 1963.

76 **"without allegiance to this"** National Pituitary Agency newsletter, first edition.

76 **To overcome the medical community's suspicion** Notes of the Fifth Meeting of the Medical Advisory Board of the National Pituitary Agency, March 27, 1965.

76 **Among other members in those early days** Fred Mahler and Gwen Mahler, interview with Susan Cohen, March 28, 2003, Hyatt Hotel, Kansas City, Missouri.

77 **Other parents also** Lucille Sluder, telephone interview with Susan Cohen, June 25, 2004.

79 **The FDA agreed** Notes of the First Meeting Medical Advisory Board of the National Pituitary Agency, April 27, 1963. *Federal Register*, January 8, 1963.

79 **"national resource"; "synonomous with hGH"** "Citation for the Ayerst Award of the Endocrine Society for 1975," *Endocrinology*, 97 (1) (July 1975).

80 **The same year that the National Pituitary Agency** Clarence J. Gibbs, Jr., "Spongiform Encephalopathies—Slow, Latent, and Temperate Virus Infections—in Retrospect," in Prusiner, Collinge, Powell, and Anderton, *Prion Diseases of Humans and Animals* (New York: Ellis Horwood, 1992), pp. 55, 58. The workshop was held in 1964.

80 **The Fore blamed *kuru*** For a fine account, see Jennifer Cooke, *Cannibals, Cows, and the CJD Catastrophe* (Sydney: Random House Australia, 1998).

80 **The list included** Gibbs, "Spongiform Encephalopathies." Some of the diseases that Gajdusek apparently suspected at the time were later ruled out as slow viruses, including infectious hepatitis, Parkinson's disease, and multiple sclerosis.

81 **Gajdusek reported in the journal** C. J. Gibbs, Jr., and D. C. Gajdusek, "Infection as the Etiology of Spongiform Encephalopathy (Creutzfeldt-Jakob Disease)," *Science*, 165 (September 5, 1969), pp. 1023–1025.

81 **The second coincidental event** P. Roos, H. R. Fevold, and C. A. Gemzell. "Preparation of Human Growth Hormone by Gel Filtration," *Biochimica et Biophysica Acta*, 74 (525) (1963).

81 **"simplified the collection"..."made the final product"** M. S. Raben, "Preparation of Growth Hormone from Pituitaries of Man and Monkey," *Science*, 125 (3253) (1957), pp. 883–884.

82 **He used an alkali** A. E. Wilhelmi, *Canadian Journal of Biochemistry and Physiology*, 39 (1659) (1961).

82 **Wilhelmi asserted it** Anne Stockell Hartree, "Preparation and Properties of Human Growth Hormone," in *Human Growth Hormone* (London: William Heinemann Medical, 1972).

82 **At least a half a dozen clinics** See Escamilla, "Clinical Studies," and M. L. Parker, I. K. Mariz, and W. H. Daughaday, "Resistance to Human Growth Hormone in Pituitary Dwarfism: Clinical and Immunologic Studies," *Journal of Clinical Endocrinology and Metabolism*, 24 (1964), pp. 997–1004.

83 **But Wilhelmi and colleagues concluded** J. B. Mills, R. B. Ashworth, A. E. Wilhelmi, and A. S. Hartree, "Improved Method for the Extraction and Purification of Human Growth Hormone," *Journal of Clinical Endocrinology and Metabolism*, November 1969, pp. 1456–1459.

CHAPTER 5. "NO PATIENT SEEMS TO HAVE CAUGHT ANYTHING"

84 **John Anthony Grossenburg came** Patricia (Patsy) Grossenburg, telephone interview with Susan Cohen, January 31, 2003.

86 **"what the native Sioux used to call"** Tom Brokaw, "Small Wonder," *Sports Illustrated* 50th Anniversary, sportsillustrated.cnn.com.

88 **From what he understood** Father John Anthony Grossenburg, telephone interview with Susan Cohen, January 18, 2003. There was further communication by telephone and e-mail over several years.

88 **Congratulatory letters poured** Li Papers.

88 **The university's press release** UCSF Office of Public Information press release, January 7, 1971. Li Papers.

89 **By comparison, the pituitary hormone** *Current Biography.*

89 **The synthetic hormone created** "Erroneous, Dr. Li....I Know, Dr. Niall," *Medical World News*, April 23, 1971, pp. 21–25.

89 **One science magazine described** Li Ibid.

90 **He had made a groundbreaking contribution** In 1975, the Pituitary Bank at UCSF, which had existed mostly to supply Li with some 46,000 human glands for his laboratory research, closed its doors for lack of funding. Final Report of the Pituitary Bank, 1975. Li Papers.

90 **In the United Kingdom** R. D. G. Milner et al., "Experience with Human Growth Hormone in Great Britain: The Report of the MRC Working Party," *Clinical Endocrinology*, 11 (1979), pp. 15–38.

90 **doctors measured their success** Douglas Frasier, interview with Susan Cohen, April 2004, San Francisco.

NOTES

90 **While the world's growth experts** Salvatore Raiti, interview with Susan Cohen, June 2003, Baltimore.

91 **Blizzard had generously** Blizzard, interview.

91 **Meanwhile, Salvatore Raiti eagerly hoped** Raiti, interview.

91 **"The challenge was"** Ibid.

92 **"hardly ever cause the appearance"** Ruth Illig, "Antibodies to Human Growth Hormone," in *Human Growth Hormone*, ed. A. Stuart Mason (London: William Heinemann Medical, (1972), pp. 144–157.

92 **In every study, the Roos method** Escamilla, "Clinical Studies."

92 **In contrast, pediatric endocrinologists...** "a dramatic resumption" Ibid.

92 **Elsewhere, an investigator** Ibid.

92 **In 1973, when Raiti oversaw...** "more stringent quality control" Salvatore Raiti, ed., *Advances in Human Growth Hormone Research: A Symposium Held in Baltimore, Maryland, October 9–12, 1973.* DHEW Publication No. [NIH] 74–612.

93 **"a strong argument"** Milner et al., "Experience."

93 **In 1973, the British** Cooke, *Cannibals.*

93 **There is no documented evidence** This statement is based on an interview with Judith Fradkin, who has reviewed the records, and with David Davis, who obtained some of them through the Freedom of Information Act. In the British court cases and Australian parliamentary investigations involving their national hormone programs, no such evidence emerged, either. In spite of numerous oral and written requests, NIH never complied with the Freedom of Information Act requests filed in the course of preparing this book, and so the authors want to state for the record that they have not personally reviewed all documented evidence.

93 **"The question of virus"** Quoted in David Davis, "When Good Intentions Go Wrong," *Atlanta Magazine*, August 2001.

94 **"We are presently going to modify"** Quoted in Emily Green, "A Wonder Drug That Carried Seeds of Death," *Los Angeles Times*, May 21, 2000.

94 **"tedious"..."high yield"** J. B. Mills, R. B. Ashworth, A. E. Wilhelmi, and A. S. Hartree, "Improved Method for the Extraction and Purification of Human Growth Hormone," *Journal of Clinical Endocrinology*, November 1969, pp. 1456–1459.

94 **In 1973, a South African chemist** S. W. Stroud, J. M. C. Hoog, and E. U. Bieler, "A Simple Method for the Extraction and Purification of Human Growth Hormone and Its Assay by Paper Chromotagraphy," *Journal of Clinical Endocrinology and Metabolism*, December 1973, pp. 860–866.

94 **An account of the achievement** Patrick Weech, "SA Discovery Aids Dwarfs," *Johannesburg Sunday Times*, February 1973.

95 **"color of Coca-Cola,"** Wayne Moore, telephone interview with Susan Cohen, May 7, 2003.

95 **He also undertook a study** Wayne Moore, "The Role of Aggregated hGH in the Therapy of hGH-Deficient Children," *Journal of Clinical Endocrinology and Metabolism*, 46 (1), pp. 20–27.

95 **"I don't think they knew"** Moore, interview.

95 **When Moore's paper appeared** Moore, "The Role of Aggregated hGH."

95 **As he prepared to leave** Raiti, interview.

96 **Parlow won the contract** Raiti confirmed that Parlow was the only bidder.

96 **a crusty Princeton- and Harvard-trained** The description of his falling-out with Wilhelmi and the quotation from Albert Parlow come from multiple conversa-

tions with him, two in person and many more over the telephone, from 2003 to 2008. The most extensive interview took place in his laboratory at UCLA Harbor Hospital on March 23, 2003.

98   **they found they could** C. J. Gibbs, Jr., and D. C. Gajdusek, "Infection as the Etiology of Spongiform Encephalopathy," *Science*, September 5, 1969, pp. 1023–1025.

98   **Whatever the mysterious infectious agent** R. D. Traub, D. C. Gajdusek, and C. J. Gibbs, "Precautions in Conducting Biopsies and Autopsies on Patients with Presenile Dementia," *Journal of Neurosurgery*, 41 (September 1974), pp. 394–395.

98   **Gajdusek and colleagues warned** Ibid.

99   **In a four-paragraph letter** P. Duffy et al., "Possible Person-to-Person Transmission of CJD," *The New England Journal of Medicine*, 299 (1974), pp. 692–693.

99   **Gajdusek's laboratory published** R. Traub, D. Gajdusek, and C. Gibbs, "Precautions in Autopsies on Creutzfeldt-Jakob Disease," *American Journal of Clinical Pathology*, 64 (1975), p. 287.

99   **Thus, by the mid-1970s** D. Gadjusek, et al., "Precautions in Medical Care of, and in Handling Materials from, Patients with Transmissible Virus Dementia (Creutzfeldt-Jakob Disease)," *The New England Journal of Medicine*, 297 (23) (December 8, 1977), pp. 1253–1258.

100   **Accepting his Nobel Prize** Gajdusek's lecture, delivered December 13, 1976, can be found online at http://nobelprize.org/nobel_prizes/medicine/laureates/1976/ gajdusek-lecture.html.

100   **Around midnight on October 5** Cooke, *Cannibals*.

101   **Dickinson had infected mice** Ibid.

101   **The next morning, he phoned** This story is also told in Richard Rhodes, "Infecting the Children," *Deadly Feasts: Tracking the Secrets of a Terrifying New Plague* (New York: Simon & Schuster, 1997).

102   **The committee agreed** Cooke, *Cannibals*.

102   **The council decided** Ibid. Judith Fradkin in her interview also reiterated that the British pediatric endocrinologists were never told about the possibility of CJD infection until after the first cases appeared.

102   **A few days after Dickinson** C. Bernouli, J. Siegfried, and G. Baumgartner, "Danger of Accidental Person-to-Person Transmission of Creutzfeldt-Jakob Disease by Surgery," *The Lancet*, 1 (1977), pp. 478–479.

102   **One of the virologists** Cooke, *Cannibals*.

103   **"The treatment was immensely satisfying,"** Quoted in Rhodes, *Deadly Feasts*.

103   **"Presumably the people"** Green, "A Wonder Drug." Emily Green broke this story.

103   **He worried that the Americans** Cooke, *Cannibals*.

104   **"'Just in case it hasn't happened'"** Ibid.

104   **Among children…tests found** S. J. Bhatia et al., "A Method of Screening for Growth Hormone Deficiency Using Anthropometrics," *American Journal of Clinical Nutrition*, 34 (2) (February 1981), pp. 281–288.

104   **At a Baltimore symposium** Raiti, *Advances in Human Growth Hormone Research*.

107   **John Crawford reported** J. D. Crawford et al., "Human Growth Hormone and Nonhypopituitary Disorders," in *Advances in Human Growth Hormone Research*, pp. 757–764.

107   **Another experimenter reported** Roberto Escamilla, "Non-Hypopituitary Dwarfs and Human Growth Hormone Therapy," in *Advances in Human Growth Hormone Research*, pp. 765–785.

107   **Money cautioned** J. Money, "Sex Education for Normal and Hypopituitary Patients," in *Advances in Human Growth Hormone Research*, pp. 786–805.

108 **The few psychological studies** Diane Rotnem et al., "Personality Development in Children with Growth Hormone Deficiency," *Journal of the American Academy of Child Psychiatry*, 16 (1977), pp. 412–426.

109 **When the Human Growth Foundation** Brian Stabler and Louis E. Underwood, eds., *Slow Grows the Child: Psychosocial Aspects of Growth Delay* (University of North Carolina and Lawrence Erlbaum Associates, 1986).

109 **those who assumed such children** This was the conclusion of the Galveston 1979 Symposium, as summarized in Stabler and Underwood, *Slow Grows the Child.*

109 **One such investigation of two dozen** Rotnem et al., "Personality Development."

110 **Trying to compensate** John S. Gillis, *Too Tall, Too Small* (Champaign, IL: Institute for Personality and Ability Testing, 1982).

110 **"Give me a guy less than five feet eight"** Pat Conroy, *The Great Santini* (Boston: Houghton Mifflin, 1976).

110 **"heightism": Even the English language** Gillis, *Too Tall.*

110 **The classic U.S. study** Marjaana Lindeman, "Height and Our Perception of Others: An Evolutionary Perspective," in *Growth, Stature, and Psychosocial Well-Being*, ed. Urs Eiholzer, Fritz Haverkamp, and Linda Voss (Seattle: Hogrefe & Huber, 1999), pp. 121–130.

110 **plight of the short male** Leonard H. Gross, "Short, Dark, and Almost Handsome," *Ms.*, 3 (1975).

111 **"the cardinal principle of date selection"** Lindeman, "Height and Our Perception of Others."

111 **while male and female monkeys** Keyes, *The Height of Your Life.*

112 **When early humans roamed** Ibid.

112 **irrational evolutionary leftover** Lindeman, "Height and Our Perception of Others."

112 **a 1954 study by psychiatrist Hugo Beigel** Keyes, *The Height of Your Life.*

112 **In 1966, two sociologists** Ibid.

112 **"Short People"** Lyrics found at http://www.shortsupport.org.

113 **Some short people failed** "Randy Newman—In His Own Words," http://www.superseventies.com/interview.

113 **They complained** "Short Like Me," *Health*, http://magnamags.com/health/archives/march2000/short/index.htm.

113 **Their angry reactions** These are described in Gillis, *Too Tall, Too Small*, and in Keyes, *The Height of Your Life.*

113 **A 1968 survey of one hundred graduates** "Short People—Are They Being Discriminated Against?" *U.S. News & World Report*, March 28, 1977.

113 **As for getting hired** Ibid.

114 **"Some people think"** Ibid.

114 **Conducting a survey** Ibid.

114 **In fact, most American men wanted** Gillis, *Too Tall, Too Small.*

114 **in 1979...press release** "First Successful Bacterial Production of Human Growth Hormone Announced," Genentech press release, July 11, 1979.

CHAPTER 6. "SOON. VERY SOON . . ."

115 **By the end of that first trading day** Stephen S. Hall, *Invisible Frontiers: The Race to Synthesize a Human Gene* (New York: Atlantic Monthly Press, 1987).

115 **The NPA was supplying** Maureen McKelvey, *Evolutionary Innovation: The Business of Biotechnology* (New York: Oxford University Press, 1996). To lessen confusion, we use KABI to refer to related companies that grew from the Swedish pharmaceutical firm KabiVitrum. In 1978, KABI also helped launch a biotech firm, KabiGen.

115 **As supplies had increased** "Teams Vie in Synthetic Production of hGH," *JAMA*, 242 (8) (August 24/31, 1979), pp. 701–702.

116 **Only another four hundred or so** McKelvey, *Evolutionary Innovation*.

116 **Their products cost about $5,000** Ibid.

116 **Bob Blizzard—who thought** S. Douglas Frasier, "The Not-So-Good-Old Days: Working with Pituitary Growth Hormone in North America, 1956 to 1985," *Journal of Pediatrics*, 131 (1) (July 1997), supplement, part 2, pp. S1–4.

116 **Defenders of the federal program** Colin Norman, "Virus Scare Halts Hormone Research," *Science*, 228 (1985), pp. 1176–1177.

116 **He said later that he'd filed** Boyer told this story to interviewer Sally Smith Hughes for the *Program in the History of the Biological Sciences and Biotechnology, Part 3: Genentech, Inc., and the Commercialization of Recombinant DNA Technology*. Interview with Herbert W. Boyer. Regional Oral History Office, The Bancroft Library, University of California, Berkeley.

117 **He'd break the circle** Ibid. Interview with Robert S. Swanson.

117 **Eli Lilly already dominated** Hall, *Invisible Frontiers*.

117 **Wearing jeans and playing pranks** Cynthia Robbins-Roth, *From Alchemy to IPO: The Business of Biotechnology* (Cambridge, MA: Perseus, 2000).

117 **As the soaring stock value** Swanson interview. Regional Oral History Office, The Bancroft Library, University of California, Berkeley.

118 **Genentech quietly paid** The UCSF professors who led recombinant growth hormone work at UCSF were Howard Goodman and John Baxter. An exciting account of the race to clone and express the human growth hormone gene is found in Hall, *Invisible Frontiers*.

118 **To help finance its growth hormone project** McKelvey. *Evolutionary Innovations*. The book provides a detailed account of KABI's thinking in this era.

119 **A sales effort would need** Swanson interview. Regional Oral History Office, The Bancroft Library, University of California, Berkeley.

119 **Swanson confidently predicted** Sally Smith Hughes interview of Daniel G. Yansura, Genentech senior scientist. Regional Oral History Office, The Bancroft Library, University of California, Berkeley. The name Protropin derived from the generic name for growth hormone, which is somatatropin.

119 **Ray Hintz was an experienced researcher** Raymond Hintz, interview with Susan Cohen, April 28, 2003, Palo Alto, California.

120 **These guinea pigs included** The details of this story were told to Susan Cohen not only by Raymond Hintz but also by Genentech scientists in 1984 and by Ron G. Rosenfeld, a pediatric endocrinologist who participated. Rosenfeld was interviewed by Susan Cohen in September 2003, in Palo Alto, California.

120 **Though Protropin was purer** As part of the process to persuade *E. coli* to make the hormone, scientists tacked on an extra amino acid called methionone. They were surprised to find that their final steps in the procedure did not remove all the methionone from the recombinant hGH, so that it was not exactly the same as the hormone produced by the human pituitary.

120 **Having none of the production experience** Michael Cronin, "Pioneering rGH Manufacturing: Pounds Produced per Mile of Height," *The Journal of Pediatrics*, 131 (1) (July 1997), supplement, part 2, pp. S5–7.

121 **"even a very small mistake"** Ibid.

121 **In September 1984, an FDA** Susan Cohen, "Engineering Heredity," *San Jose Mercury News, West Magazine*, November 11, 1985.

121 **"Soon. Very soon..."** Genentech, Inc., *Pediatrics*, 73 (1) (1984).

121 **They expected Protropin** Just one example of this anticipation can be found in Martin Benjamin, James Muyskens, and Paul Saenger, "Short Children, Anxious Parents: Is GH the answer?" *The Hastings Center Report*, 14 (1984), pp. 5–9.

121 **forestall or reverse aging** The belief was fueled by a study of the use of hGH in twelve elderly men, published in *The New England Journal of Medicine* in 1990.

121–122 **diagnosed only about 10 percent** Benjamin et al., "Short Children."

122 **The word "dwarf"** J. M. Tanner et al., "Effect of Human Growth Hormone Treatment for 1 to 7 Years on Growth of 100 Children, with Growth Hormone Deficiency, Low Birthweight, Inherited Smallness, Turner's Syndrome, and Other Complaints," *Archives of Diseases of Childhood*, 46 (1971), pp. 745–782.

122 **Adding its 2,450 recipients** Frasier, "The Not-So-Good-Old Days."

122 **"The trick of marketing"** Robbins-Roth, *From Alchemy to IPO*.

122 **"A great clinical development strategy"** Ibid.

123 **"little Johnny who"** Cohen, "Engineering Heredity."

123 **"We're really committed to this"** Ibid.

123 **As a Genentech marketing man** Ibid.

123 **Various laboratories used different methods** Louis Underwood, "Report of the Conference on Uses and Possible Abuses of Biosynthetic Human Growth Hormone," *The New England Journal of Medicine*, August 30, 1984, pp. 606–608.

123 **The traditionally accepted cutoff** Ibid.

124 **And Genentech hoped ... "the supply of growth hormone"** Cohen, "Engineering Heredity."

124 **Beyond treating deficiency** Ibid.

124 **A multicenter study investigated** Louis Underwood, "Growth Hormone Treatment for Short Children," *Journal of Pediatrics*, 104 (1984), pp. 237–238.

124 **"We hope we'll find"** Cohen, "Engineering Heredity."

124 **Raymond Hintz's personal favorite** J. M. Tanner et al., "Effect of Human Growth Hormone Treatment."

125 **Another experiment in the 1970s** J. M. Gertner et al., "Prospective Clinical Trial of Human Growth Hormone in Short Children Without Growth Hormone Deficiency," *The Journal of Pediatrics*, 104 (1984), pp. 172–176.

125 **In 1981, a researcher reported** Daniel Rudman et al., "Children with Normal Variant Short Stature: Treatment with Human Growth Hormone for Six Months," *The New England Journal of Medicine*, 305 (3) (1981), pp. 123–131.

125 **It seemed likely that GH treatment** Underwood, "Growth Hormone Treatment."

125 **"If you have a new treatment"** Raymond Hintz, interview with Susan Cohen, April 28, 2003.

125 **Most children brought** Benjamin et al., "Short Children."

126 **Children with familial short stature** Ibid.

126 **"The identification of short, otherwise healthy children"** Guy Van Vliet et al., "Growth Hormone Treatment for Short Stature," *The New England Journal of Medicine*, October 27, 1983, pp. 1016–1022.

126 **This did not prove** See Underwood, "Growth Hormone Treatment."

127 **Excessive GH in acromegalics** Benjamin et al., "Short Children."

127 **The editors would have liked** Selna Kaplan, interview with Susan Cohen in 1984, University of California, San Francisco.

127 **"If it ain't broke"** Ad Hoc Committee on Growth Hormone Usage, Lawson Wilkins Pediatric Endocrine Society, and Committee on Drugs, American Academy

of Pediatrics, "Growth Hormone in the Treatment of Children with Short Stature," *Pediatrics*, 72 (December 1983), pp. 891–894.

128 **"There is a group that feels"** Kaplan, interview, 1984.

128 **"It's a first case study, in a way"** Hintz, interview, 1984.

128 **In November 1983** The conference is summarized in Underwood, "Report of the Conference on Uses and Possible Abuses of Biosynthetic Growth Hormone," *The New England Journal of Medicine*.

129 **"In a society that values tallness"** Ibid.

129 **As Underwood wrote** Ibid.

129 **Even among the biggest success stories** C. M. Mitchell et al., "Psychosocial Impact of Long-term Growth Hormone Therapy," in Stabler and Underwood, eds., *Slow Grows the Child*, pp. 97–109.

129 **Children fantasized** Diane Rotnem et al., "Psychological Sequelae of Relative Treatment Failure for Children Receiving Growth Hormone Replacement," *Journal of the American Academy of Child Psychiatry*, July 1, 1979, pp. 505–520.

130 **"The need to perform"** Ibid.

130 **"narcissistically frustrating"** Ibid.

131 **Even this depended** Underwood, "Growth Hormone Treatment."

131 **"mainly children of upper-"** Benjamin et al., "Short Children."

131 **"the dilemma for the pediatrician"** Ibid.

132 **This literature, which almost unanimously** R. Richman et al., "Academic and Emotional Difficulties Associated with Constitutional Short Stature," in Stabler and Underwood, eds., *Slow Grows the Child*, pp. 13–24.

132 **"The child's adaptation to his or her size"** D. L. Rotnem, "Size Versus Age: Ambiguities in Parenting Short-Statured children," in Stabler and Underwood, eds., *Slow Grows the Child*, pp. 178–190.

132 **Investigating late bloomers** Richman et al., "Academic and Emotional Difficulties."

133 **The keynote speaker listened** L. Sawisch, "Psychosocial Aspects of Short Stature: The Day to Day Context," in Stabler and Underwood, eds., *Slow Grows the Child*, pp. 46–56.

CHAPTER 7. "ONLY GENENTECH IS NOT IN MOURNING"

137 **On Sunday, June 17, 1984** R. Hintz, "A Prismatic Case: The Prismatic Case of Creutzfeldt-Jakob Disease Associated with Pituitary Growth Hormone Treatment," *Journal of Clinical Endocrinology and Metabolism*, 80 (1995), pp. 2298–2301.

137 **Hintz had treated** Ibid. In this article, Hintz referred to the patient as "JRo"; the full name was used in Cooke, *Cannibals*.

137 **not a complainer** P. Brown, "Human Growth Hormone Therapy and Creutzfeldt-Jakob Disease: A Drama in Three Acts," *Pediatrics*, 1988, pp. 81, 85–92.

138 **"She noticed that when he got off"** Raymond Hintz, interview with Susan Cohen, April 28, 2003, Palo Alto, California.

138 **Joey did indeed have** Brown, "Human Growth Hormone Therapy."

138 **At a meeting to discuss** Hintz, "A Prismatic Case." The alert UCSF neurologist was Bruce Bond, who later wrote up his own account.

138 **Joey now stooped** Brown, "Human Growth Hormone Therapy."

138 **A UCSF pathology resident asked** Ibid. Hintz said he advised the family to comply.

138 **He'd attended an FDA conference** Hintz, "A Prismatic Case." Hintz added during an interview that he had discussed pituitary hGH informally with a colleague from KABI.

NOTES

139 **"The horror was even greater"** Hintz, interview, 2003.
139 **Hintz wrote letters** Hintz, "A Prismatic Case."
139 **"Because at that point"**, Hintz interview, 2003.
140 **There, it was decided to halt** Colin Norman, "Virus Scare Halts Hormone Research," *Science*, June 7, 1985.
140 **Leading those who argued** Blizzard, interview.
140 **But after hearing about Joey Rodriguez** Cooke, *Cannibals*.
140 **In Buffalo...Margaret MacGillivray** Brown, "Human Growth Hormone Therapy."
141 **"What we have is panic"** Quoted in *Science*, June 7, 1985.
141 **Commercial manufacturers, too** Frasier, "The Not-So-Good-Old Days."
141 **The head of the French program** Hintz, interview, 2003.
141 **Canada, which used** Hintz, "A Prismatic Case."
142 **"much too hastily"** Quoted in *Science*, June 7, 1985.
142 **Australia cut back, as programs** Cooke, *Cannibals*.
142 **"They weren't at that meeting"** Hintz, interview, 2003.
142 **At UCSF, Selna Kaplan** Kaplan, interview with the authors, May 15, 2003, University of California, San Francisco.
143 **"The most amazing thing"** Hintz, interview, 2003.
143 **"officially executed"; "among the spectators"** Brown, "Human Growth Hormone Therapy."
143 **enormous pressure on the FDA** *Science*, June 7, 1985.
143 **"as effective as pituitary GH"; "at an early date"** "Degenerative Neurologic Disease in Patients Formerly Treated with Human Growth Hormone: Report of the Committee on Growth Hormone Use of the Lawson Wilkins Pediatric Endocrinology Society, May 1985," *Journal of Pediatrics*, 107 (1) (July 1985), pp. 10–12.
144 **The FDA had responded** McKelvey, *Evolutionary Innovations*.
144 **Congress had passed the act** The Orphan Drug Act, Implementation and Impact, Department of HHS, Office of Inspector General, May 2001, OEI-09-00-00380.
144 **"We cannot regulate"** Quoted in Cohen, "Engineering Heredity."
144 **expensive...burdensome** McKelvey, *Evolutionary Innovations*.
144 **Genentech, already famous** Interview with David Goeddel conducted by the Regional Oral History Office, The Bancroft Library, University of California, Berkeley.
145 **Genentech bragged** McKelvey, *Evolutionary Innovations*.
145 **Now Genentech made them the first sales force** Robbins-Roth, *From Alchemy to IPO*.
145 **Genentech had stockpiled** McKelvey, *Evolutionary Innovations*.
145 **Kaplan, Hintz, Blizzard, and...Underwood** Blizzard, interview.
145 **Blizzard had calculated** R. Blizzard, "Growth Hormone as a Therapeutic Agent," *Growth, Genetics & Hormones*, 21 (4) (December 2005).
146 **The company financed** This paragraph is based on conversations with a variety of pediatric endocrinologists, as well as seeing Genentech's sponsorship of *Growth, Genetics & Hormones*, and at the Lawson Wilkins Pediatric Endocrinology meeting. Also oral history interviews of former Genentech employees.
146 **"a pressure point in our society"** M. Grumbach, "GH Therapy and the Short End of the Stick," *The New England Journal of Medicine*, July 28, 1988, pp. 238–241.
146 **"That's absolutely unacceptable!"** Quoted in Gina Kolata, "New Growth Industry in Human Growth Hormone?" *Science*, October 3, 1986.
147 **"For the first time in my life"** Ibid.
147 **"It really is a Brave New World"** Ibid.

147 **Genentech set out to influence** McKelvey, *Evolutionary Innovations.*
147 **at a Genentech-sponsored symposium** Louis E. Underwood and Barry M. Sherman, "Controversies in the Treatment of Short Stature," in Louis E. Underwood, ed., *Human Growth Hormone, Progress and Challenges* (New York: Marcel Dekker, 1988), pp. 145–191.
147 **The chapter described** Ibid.
148 **Case No. 1** Ibid.
149 **one pediatric endocrinologist...** "a nuisance" The pediatric endocrinologist was John S. Parks.
150 **By the end of 1986** McKelvey, *Evolutionary Innovations.*
151 **But Lilly had trouble** Ibid.
151 **The price of treating a child** Grumbach, "GH Therapy."
151 **By 1988...worldwide market** Ibid.
151 **Yet the doctors still did not** Ibid. Grumbach wrote that they agreed there was "no convincing evidence supporting the presence of disease in healthy children in the population who are at either extreme of the bell-shaped distribution for height."
153 **"Before considering its release"** Ibid.
153 **A closer look convinced** Ibid.
153 **The Lawson Wilkins Pediatric Endocrine Society concluded** David B. Allen et al. "Risk of Leukemia in Children Treated with Human Growth Hormone: Review and Reanalysis," *The Journal of Pediatrics,* July 1997, pp. 532–36.
153 **The postmarketing survey** McKelvey, *Evolutionary Innovations.*
153–154 **It didn't even pop in 1989** Barry Werth, "How Short Is Too Short? Marketing Human Growth Hormone," *The New York Times Magazine,* June 16, 1991.
154 **In 1990, Protropin sales** Ibid.
154 **"We do not usually call"** E. Bischofberger and G. Dahlstrom, "Ethical Aspects on Growth Hormone Therapy," *Acta Pædiatrica Scandinavica,* suppl. 362 (1989), pp. 14–17.
154 **However, because societal prejudices** L. Underwood and P. Rieser, "Is It Ethical to Treat Healthy Short Children with Growth Hormone?" *Acta Pædiatrica Scandinavica,* suppl 362 (1989), pp. 18–23.
155 **psychologist Brian Stabler** Brain Stabler, interview with Susan Cohen by phone for "Engineering Heredity," 1984.
155 **"family frustration"; "there is as yet little empirical"** Comments by Brian Stabler, "Controversies in the Treatment of Short Stature," in Underwood, ed., *Human Growth Hormone, Progress and Challenges.*
156 **Extreme differences** Leslie Martel and Henry Biller, *Stature and Stigma: The Biopsychosocial Development of Short Males* (Lexington, MA: Lexington Books, 1987).
156 **"A major goal of the present book"** Ibid.
159 **Gajdusek's laboratory warned** Paul Brown et al., "Potential Epidemic of Creutzfeldt-Jakob Disease from Human Growth Hormone Therapy," *The New England Journal of Medicine,* September 19, 1985, pp. 728–731.
159 **Cases slowly accumulated** Cooke, *Cannibals.*
159 **The average incubation** Judith Fradkin et al., "CJD in Pituitary GH Recipients in the U.S.," *JAMA,* February 20, 1991, pp. 880–884.
159 **Meanwhile, the federal government** Ibid.
160 **About 10,000 in all** Phillip Gorden, HHS letter to hGH families, January 22, 1988 (258 b. NIDDK fact sheet, December 1987). NIDDK CJD letters.
160 **Alfred Wilhelmi brought** Judith Fradkin, interview with Susan Cohen, June 2004, National Institutes of Health.

160 The mood among the officials Jane Demolay, public information officer, NIH.
160 Now they braced themselves Fradkin et al., *JAMA*, February 20, 1991.
160 "Dear Growth Hormone Recipient" Phillip Gorden letter to growth hormone recipients, Department of Health and Human Services, National Institute of Diabetes and Digestive and Kidney Diseases, January 22, 1988.
161 The enclosed fact sheet "Human Growth Hormone and Creutzfeldt-Jakob Disease," NIDDK Fact Sheet, December 1987, NIH Publication No. 88–2793.
162 Even if one vial of hGH Ibid.
163 The NIDDK wrote again Phillip Gorden, letter, December 6, 1989.
164 Patsy Grossenburg felt sick Patsy Grossenburg, interview.
164 Tony Grossenburg...had his Catholic faith Father Tony Grossenburg, telephone interview with Susan Cohen, July 14, 2007.
164 Fred Mahler had taken shots Fred and Gwen Mahler interview.
164 A young man named David Davis This account was drawn from articles written by David Davis; his interview with Susan Cohen in Burbank, California, in 2003; and multiple phone conversations.

CHAPTER 8. DEAR PARENT . . .
166 "make a stone grow" Ron Rosenfeld is credited with having first said this.
166 "I can only uglify you" Raymond Hintz, interview 2003.
167 Gordon B. Cutler, a pediatric endocrinologist Ernest D. Prentice et al., "Can Children Be Enrolled in a Placebo-Controlled Randomized Clinical Trial of Synthetic Growth Hormone," *IRB Human Subject Review*, January/February 1989, pp. 6–10.
167 With Lilly underwriting Andrew Kimbrell, "A Discriminating Drug," in *The Human Body Shop* (San Francisco: Harper, 1993).
167 He argued that only this type "NIH Hormone Test with Children Draws Criticism of Group," *The Wall Street Journal*, June 25, 1992.
167 Whether or not they personally Carol A. Tauer, "The NIH Trials of Growth Hormone for Short Stature," *IRB*, May/June 1994, pp. 1–9.
168 about half the American youngsters Ibid.
168 Besides the shots Ibid.
168 A Harris Poll in 1992 Jeremy Rifkin, "A Eugenic Civilization," *The Biotech Century: Harnessing the Gene and Remaking the World* (New York: Tarcher/Putnam, 1998).
169 In 1992, two groups petitioned "NIH Hormone Test."
169 "What about fat people?" David Brown, "Growth Hormone for Healthy Teens," *The Washington Post*, July 6, 1992.
169 "exploitative and abusive" "NIH Hormone Test."
169 "But in our society" Arthur S. Levine, quoted in *The Washington Post*, July 6, 1992.
170 "These kids are not normal" Michaela Richardson, quoted in *The Wall Street Journal*, June 25, 1992.
170 The Physicians Committee for Responsible Medicine...condemned Neal D. Barnard et al., "Concerns About Growth Hormone Experiments in Short Children," *Research Controversies & Issues: Ethics in Human Research*, Physicians Committee for Responsible Medicine website.
170 "Inappropriately muscular" Ibid.
170 The Physicians Committee for Responsible Medicine thought Ibid.
171 The panel did not question Sally Lehrman, "Challenge to Growth Hormone Trial," *Nature*, July 15, 1993, p. 179.

171 **He praised the "incredible" parents** Melvin Grumbach, interview with the authors, August 19, 2003, UCSF.

171 **At the time that the study was suspended** Barnard et al., Physicians Committee for Responsible Medicine.

171 **According to the NIH website** "Active Accrual, Protocols Recruiting New Patients," NIH Clinical Studies Research Studies Protocol Number 91-CH-0046.

172 **Especially since, as one newspaper reported** Brown, "Growth Hormone."

172 **"growth hormone doesn't work"; "could be dangerous"** "The NIA Trials."

172 **In Charlotte, North Carolina, in the early 1990s** This account draws from congressional testimony and newspaper reports.

173 **"Stature is relative"** John Trowle testimony (transcript) to House of Representatives, Committee on Small Business, Subcommittee on Regulation, Business Opportunities and Technology. Washington, D.C., October 12, 1994.

173 **The $217 million annual sales** Kolata, "Selling Growth Drug for Children," *The New York Times*, August 15, 1994.

174 **In 1993, the Human Growth Foundation** Ralph King, "Charity Tactic by Genentech Stirs Questions," *The Wall Street Journal*, August 10, 1994.

174 **That year, Eli Lilly** Ibid.

174 **But by 1991 it reportedly received** Barry Werth, "How Short Is Too Short?" *The New York Times Magazine*, June 16, 1991.

175 **"Is your child the right size for his age?"** A. L. Rosenbloom, "Height Screening in the Community: The Commercialization of Growth," *Clinical Pediatrics*, May 1990, pp. 288–292.

175 **As in Georgia, the letter** Kolata, *The New York Times*, August 15, 1994.

175 **A spokesman said that school officials** Ibid.

176 **"marketing effort"; "with a direct interest"** R. Wyden statement (transcript), Subcommittee on Regulation, Business Opportunities and Technology, October 12, 1994.

176 **Even before the hearing doors opened** Written statement of Genentech, Inc., U.S. House of Representatives, October 12, 1994.

176 **At the hearing, Mark Parker testified** Mark W. Parker testimony (transcript).

177 **"an unregulated form of drug advertising"** Steven Miles testimony (transcript).

177 **Yet Wyden heard testimony** Inspector General of the Department of Health and Human Services June Gibbs Brown testimony (transcript).

178 **The two who spoke at the hearing** The two pediatric endocrinologists were Margaret MacGillivray, representing the LWPES, and Alan Rogol, representing the Endocrine Society.

178 **"cosmetic endocrinology"; "unethical"** Alan D. Rogol testimony (transcript).

178 **"Scottie dogs have Scottie dog puppies"** We have been told the first pediatric endocrinologist to use this analogy was Robert Blizzard.

178 **In her view, drug manufacturers** FDA Deputy Commissioner Mary Pendergast testimony (transcript).

179 **Benjamin Dobrin, now a young man** Benjamin Dobrin testimony (transcript).

180 **"Carol and I basically felt"** Stanley Dobrin testimony (transcript).

180 **The Dobrins' pediatric endocrinologist** Kolata, *The New York Times*, August 15, 1994.

181 **Caremark, an Illinois-based home health care company** Kolata, *The New York Times*, August 15, 1994.

181 **Since Caremark then billed Medicaid** *U.S.A. v. David R. Brown*, U.S. District Court of Minnesota, Fourth Division, Case No. 4-94-95.

181 **the government argued that from January 1, 1989** Gibbs testimony (transcript), U.S. House of Representatives, October 12, 1994.

181 **About a month before going to trial** *U.S.A. v. David R. Brown*, U.S. District Court of Minnesota, Fourth Division, Case No. 4-94-95.

181 **But its officials** Associated Press, "Officials of Two Health Firms Acquitted," *Minneapolis Star Tribune*, October 4, 1995.

181–182 **Entering data into the postmarketing survey** Sheila M. Rothman and David J. Rothman, *The Pursuit of Perfection* (New York: Pantheon, 2003).

182 **During the Minneapolis trial** Ibid.

182 **Prosecutors had trouble finding** Ibid.

182 **"how psychologically affected the child is"** Ibid.

183 **Asked about his case** David R. Brown, interview with Susan Cohen, July 2003, Chicago.

183 **The FDA and the FBI interviewed** This account of the FDA's investigation comes from Tamar Nordenberg, "Investigators' Reports, Maker of Growth Hormone Feels Long Arm of Law," *FDA Consumer*, September/October 1999.

183 **Swiss-based Roche Holdings** Ariana Eunjung Cha, "Federal Jury Deadlocks over Accusations That Genentech Used Pilfered DNA," *San Jose Mercury News*, June 2, 1999.

183 **Raab adopted the strategy** G. Kirk Raab described this strategy in detail as part of the oral history project at the University of California, Berkeley.

184 **"an increased number of patients"** Genentech report of second-quarter results, July 14, 1993.

184 **The new CEO, Arthur D. Levinson** Described in the Raab oral history interview.

184 **Pharmacia's former vice president of marketing** Peter Rost eventually lost his job after Pfizer took over Pharmacia in 2003. His whistle-blower lawsuit was dismissed when a judge ruled that he had not shown that Pfizer had committed any fraud against the government. Pfizer did not dispute Pharmacia's off-label promotion of Genotropin between January 2000 and March 2003, which Pfizer reported to the Department of Justice, the FDA, and the Office of the Inspector General soon after acquiring Pharmacia.

184 **"paid for many hundreds of physicians"** Peter Rost, *The Whistleblower: Confessions of a Healthcare Hitman* (Brooklyn, NY: Soft Skull, 2006).

185 **"Needless to say, few of them"** Ibid.

185 **"It was too easy to make money"** This pediatric endocrinologist did not want to sound too critical of colleagues, and so asked not to be identified.

185 **"All of a sudden...these 747s"** Grumbach interview.

186 **Another pediatric endocrinologist remembers** This doctor asked not be identified.

187 **Physicians were attempting to modulate** R. Lanes and P. Gunczler, "Final Height After Combined GH and GRH Analogue Therapy in Short Healthy Children Entering into Normally Timed Puberty," *Clinical Endocrinology*, 49 (1998), pp. 197–202.

187 **They were identifying other substances, too** S. P. Taback, G. Van Vliet, and H. Guyda, "Pharmacological Manipulation of Height: Qualitative Review of Study Populations and Designs," *Journal of Clinical and Investigative Medicine*, 22 (April 1999), pp. 53–59.

187 **Yet with all this experimentation** Ibid. The following quotations come from this paper.

188 **In the spring of that year** Lawrence M. Fisher, "Genentech: Survivor Strutting Its Stuff," *The New York Times*, October 1, 2000.

188 **Genentech and the flagship product** Nordenberg, *FDA Consumer*.

189 **They took some vials** Justin Gills, "20 Years Later, Stolen Gene Haunts a Biotech Pioneer," *The Washington Post*, May 17, 1999.

189 **He testified that they had repeatedly** Jeff Fox, "Two Patent Disputes settled," *Nature Biotechnology*, January 2000.

189 **Genentech's accumulated recombinant hGH sales** "Genentech Pays Off UCSF," *Wired News*, November 19, 1999.

189 **In November 1999, the two parties** Ibid.

190 **Genentech paid $200 million** Fox, "Two Patent Disputes."

190 **The UCLA student newspaper reported** Timothy Kudo, "Regents Drop Case Against Genentech, Agree to Settle," *Daily Bruin*, November 22, 1999.

CHAPTER 9. "NEVER BEFORE IN THE HISTORY OF MEDICINE"

191 **The availability of recombinant growth hormone** This summary comes from D. Wyatt, D. Mark, and A. Slyper, "Survey of Growth Hormone Treatment Practices by 251 Pediatric Endocrinologists," *Journal of Clinical Endocrinology and Metabolism*, 80 (1995), pp. 3292–3297.

192 **Answering a survey in 1995** Ibid.

192 **Pediatric endocrinologists acknowledged** Leona Cutler et al., "Short Stature and Growth Hormone Therapy: A National Study of Physician Recommendation Patterns," *JAMA*, August 21, 1996, pp. 531–537.

193 **Douglas Frasier at UCLA** Douglas Frasier, interview with Susan Cohen, May 2004, San Francisco.

193 **"My advice to any family"** Margaret MacGillivray testimony (transcript), U.S. House of Representatives, October 12, 1994.

194 **The 1995 survey of physician practices** Wyatt et al., "Survey of Growth."

194 **When a study of Down-syndrome children** L. Underwood, "Growth Hormone Therapy in Children with Down Syndrome," Letter to the Editor, *Journal of Pediatrics*, May 1992, p. 833.

195 **"Adolescence is hard enough"** Ron Rosenfeld, interview with Susan Cohen, September 9, 2003, Lucille Packard Children's Hospital, Stanford University.

196 **In the early days, when Genentech** Ibid.

198 **To accelerate their growth** S. P. Taback et al., "Does Growth-Hormone Supplementation Affect Adult Height in Turner's Syndrome?" *The Lancet*, July 6, 1996, pp. 25–27.

199 **"lessening the chief visual cue"** I. Tesch, "Physician Recommendations Versus Insurance Coverage for Growth Hormone," letter, *JAMA*, September 23/30, 1998, p. 1052.

199 **There also had been no evaluation** Taback et al., "Does Growth-Hormone."

199 **Nonetheless, by 1998, U.S. doctors** Beth S. Finkelstein et al., "Insurance Coverage, Physician Recommendations, and Access to Emerging Treatments," *JAMA*, March 4, 1998, pp. 663–668.

199 **More than half of the pediatric endocrinologists** Ibid.

200 **When doctors answered questions** Cutler, "Short Stature."

200 **Eli Lilly's pamphlet** Quoted in Gladys White, "Human Growth Hormone: The Dilemma of Expanded Use in Children," *Kennedy Institute of Ethics Journal*, December 1993, pp. 401–409.

201 **"slow growers" ... "even transitory increases in height"** "Growth Hormone Deficiency in Children," Novo Nordisk fact sheet 609-919-7776.

202 **"Very Short Children Prone to Bad Behavior"** BBC News, September 1, 1998. Based on "Behavior Change After Growth Hormone Treatment of Children with

Short Stature," Brian Stabler et al., *Journal of Pediatrics*, September 1998, pp. 366–373.

202 **"simply as a result of being very short,"** Meinolf Noeker and Fritz Haverkamp, "Can the Clinical and Empirical Evidence Regarding Adjustment to Small Stature Be Reconciled?" in Urs Eiholzer, Fritz Haverkamp, and Linda Voss, eds., *Growth, Stature, and Psychosocial Well-Being* (Seattle: Hogrefe & Huber, 1999).

202 **As Linda Voss, a lead investigator** Linda Voss, "Short Stature—Does It Matter? A Review of the Evidence," in *Growth, Stature, and Psychosocial Well-Being*.

202 **Similarly, in the Netherlands** Jan Busschbach et al., "Some Patients with Idiopathic Short Stature See Their Short Stature as a Problem, but Others Do Not: Why This Difference?" in *Growth, Stature and Psychosocial Well-Being*.

202 **But multiple pieces of research** D. Sandberg, A. Brook, and S. Campos, "Short Stature: A Psychosocial Burden Requiring Growth Hormone Therapy?" *Pediatrics*, December 1994, pp. 832–840.

202 **They were not handicapped** John Kranzler et al., "Is Short Stature a Handicap? A Comparison of the Psychosocial Functioning of Referred and Nonreferred Children with Normal Short Stature and Children with Normal Stature," *Journal of Pediatrics*, 136 (2000), pp. 96–102.

202 **They not only were accepted** Jane Gilmour and David Skuse, "Peer and Self-Perception of Children with Short Stature—The Role of Cognition," in *Growth, Stature and Psychosocial Well-Being*.

202–203 **Kids who were just short** David Sandberg, "Experiences of Being Short: Should We Expect Problems of Psychosocial Adjustment?" in *Growth, Stature and Psychosocial Well-Being*.

203 **Looking at those with idiopathic short stature** L. T. Rekers-Momberg et al. "Quality of Life of Young Adults with Idiopathic Short Stature: Effect of Growth Hormone Treatment, *Acta Paediatrica*, 87 (1998), pp. 865–870.

203 **there was little evidence that short stature** D. Drotar and J. Robinson, "Impact of Short Stature on Quality of Life: Where is the Evidence?" in Brian Stabler and Barry Bercu, eds., *Therapeutic Outcome of Endocrine Disorders; Efficacy, Innovation, and Quality of Life* (New York: Springer, 2000).

203 **And little or conflicting evidence** See Gregory Zimet et al., "The Psychosocial Functioning of Adults Who Were Short as Children," in *Growth, Stature, and Psychosocial Well-Being*. D. E. Sandberg et al., "Quality of Life Among Formerly Treated Childhood-Onset Growth Hormone-Deficient Adults: A Comparison with Unaffected Siblings," *Journal of Clinical Endocrinology and Metabolism*, 83, (4) (1998), pp. 1134–1142.

203 **A 1990 study of salaries** Irene Hanson Frieze, Josephine E. Olson, and Deborah Cain Good, "Perceived and Actual Discrimination in the Salaries of Male and Female Managers," *Journal of Applied Social Psychology*, 20, pp. 46–67.

204 **The shortest kids in growth clinics** Noeker and Haverkamp, "Can the Clinical."

204 **One study explored whethers parents** Zimet, "The Psychosocial Functioning."

204 **Though the Lawson Wilkins Pediatric Endocrine Society** "Guidelines for the Use of Growth Hormone in Children with Short Stature: A Report by the Drug and Therapeutics Committee of the Lawson Wilkins Pediatric Endocrine Society," *Journal of Pediatrics*, December 1995, pp. 857–867.

204–205 **In 1998, both the American Association of Clinical Endocrinologists** American Association of Clinical Endocrinologists and the American College of Endocrinology, "AACE Clinical Practice Guidelines for Growth Hormone Use in Adults and Children," 1998.

205 **The Endocrinology Society in Britain** "Endocrinology and Short Stature," 1998.
205 **The American Academy of Pediatrics stated** Committee on Drugs and Committee on Bioethics, American Academy of Pediatrics, "Considerations Related to the Use of Recombinant Human Growth Hormone in Children," *Pediatrics*, January 1997, pp. 122–129.
205 **Even when offering the advice** Ibid.
205 **French research published** Susan Gilbert, "Growth Hormone Use in Children Found Ineffective in Large Study," *The New York Times*, September 23, 1997.
205 **The *British Medical Journal* editorialized** "Growth Hormone: Panacea or Punishment for Short Stature?" September 20, 1997, *British Medical Journal*, September 20, 1997, pp. 692–693.
205 **On the other hand, Raymond Hintz** R. I. Hintz et al., "Effect of Growth Hormone Treatment on Adult Height of Children with Idiopathic Short Stature," *New England Journal of Medicine*, February 18, 1999, pp. 502–507.
206 **"Hormone Boosts Height for Some Kids"** UPI, February 17, 1999.
206 **"Study Questions Growth Hormone Use in Children"** onhealth.webmd.com, February 19, 1999.
206 **Reviewing four decades of GH therapy** Harvey J. Guyda, "Four Decades of Growth Hormone Therapy for Short Children: What Have We Achieved?" *Journal of Clinical Endocrinology and Metabolism*, 84 (12) (1999), pp. 4307–4316.
206 **Given what was known** E. S. McCaughey et al., "Randomized Trial of Growth Hormone in Short Normal Girls," *The Lancet*, March 28, 1998, pp. 940–944.
206 **"The case for intervention"** Peter Hindmarsh, "Is There a Role for GH Therapy in Short Normal Children?" in John Monson, ed., *Challenges in Growth Hormone Therapy* (Oxford: Blackwell Science, 1999).
206 **The databases seemed to indicate** Arnold Slyper, "How Safe and Effective Is Human Growth Hormone at Pharmacological Dosing?" *Growth, Genetics & Hormones*, April 1998.
207 **To judge from Genentech's postmarketing surveillance** This summary relies heavily on David B. Allen, "Safety of Human Growth Hormone Therapy: Current Topics," *Journal of Pediatrics*, May 1996, pp. S8–13.
207 **Of course, these conclusions depended on** Hindmarsh, "Is There a Role."
207 **For example, only two or three** Ibid.
207 **Among those, one European study** Meir Lampit et al., "GH Dependence and GH Withdrawal Syndrome in GH Treatment of Short Normal Children: Evidence from Growth and Cardiac Output," *European Journal of Endocrinology*, 138 (1998), pp. 401–407.
207 **Because of that, in 1997** Bernard Silverman and Jason Friedlander, "Is Growth Hormone Good for the Heart?" *Journal of Pediatrics*, July 1997, pp. S70–74.
208 **There were theoretical causes of concern** Neal D. Barnard et al., "Concerns About Growth Hormone Experiments in Short Children," *Research Controversies & Issues: Ethics in Human Research*, Physicians Committee for Responsible Medicine website.
208 **pituitaries overproduce** Slyper, "How Safe."
208 **In 1997, scientists who implanted** Kathryn Jaehnig, "Tiny Mice, Long Life," Southern Illinois University, Carbondale, Public Affairs Office, Spring 1997.
208 **At the end of the decade, safety** See Monson, *Challenges in Growth Hormone Therapy*.
208 **The standard definition of growth hormone deficiency** Aetna Clinical Policy Bulletin No. 0170, Growth Hormone and Growth Hormone Releasing Hormone, September 23, 2003.

208 **Even so, as children who had** L.L.E. Bolt and D. Mul, "Growth Hormone in Short Children: Beyond Medicine?" *Acta Paediatrica Scandinavica*, 90 (2001), pp. 69–73.

208 **"very early and prolonged treatment"** Philippe Bareille, Fiona Frazer, and Richard Stanhope, "GH Replacement in Children: What Is the Optimum Dosing Schedule?" in *Challenges in Growth Hormone Therapy*.

209 **Patients tended to be very satisfied** A. Juul et al., "Diagnosis of Growth Hormone (GH) Deficiency and the Use of GH in Children with Growth Disorders," *Hormone Research*, 51 (1999), pp. 284–299.

209 **The insurance industry in the United States** J. E. Sabin and N. Daniels, "Making Insurance Coverage for New Technologies Reasonable and Accountable" (editorial), *JAMA*, March 4, 1998, 703–704.

209 **"Never before in the history of medicine"** Slyper, "How Safe and Effective."

CHAPTER 10. ABSENCE OF EVIDENCE IS NOT EVIDENCE OF ABSENCE

213 **Janet Cregan-Wood** Information about Cregan-Wood's experiences was gathered over a long period of time and entailed interviews with Christine Cosgrove in September 2003 in Melbourne, and ongoing e-mail correspondence. Much information in this chapter was taken from an unpublished manuscript written by Janet and her partner, Ed Wolf, about her experiences founding Tall Girls, which they graciously supplied for this book.

213 **headline in a Melbourne newspaper** Gary Hughes and Gerard Ryle, "Hormone Tests on Teenage Girls Referred to Inquiry," *The Age*, June 27, 1997. While researching a story about Wettenhall's involvement in testing vaccines on orphans for the Commonwealth Serum Laboratories, a company for which he worked, the two reporters came across the trial. Their article was a follow-up to the orphan stories, which "caused quite a storm over here [Australia]," according to Ryle in an e-mail to Christine Cosgrove, June 3, 2004.

214 **Over the weekend** Michelle Coffey and Andrew Cummins, "Tall Girls' Doctor Stands by Tests," *The Herald Sun*, June 28, 1997.

215 **"It was not known"** Wettenhall and Roche, "Tall Girls Assessment and Management," *Australian Paediatric Journal*, 1965, p. 214.

215 **On July 9** Graeme Barnes, scientific director, Royal Children's Hospital Research Foundation, "Medical Trials Worthy of Pride," *The Age*, July 9, 1997.

216 **On July 15** Janet Cregan-Wood, letter to the editor *The Age*, July 15, 1997.

219 **And in fact, two months later** Dr. Michael Wooldridge, "Review of Hormone Treatment for Tall Girls and Short Children Reveals No Evidence for Concern," Federal Department of Health and Family Services press release, October 9, 1997.

220 **The author of one paper** N. Kuhn et al., "Estrogen Treatment in Tall Girls," *Acta Paediatrica Scandinavica*, 66 (2) (1977), pp. 161–167.

220 **Doctors in the Netherlands** Stenvert L. S. Drop et al., "Sex Steroid Treatment of Constitutionally Tall Stature," *Endocrine Reviews*, 19 (5) (1998), pp. 540–558. In a telephone interview with Christine Cosgrove, March 20, 2003, Dr. Drop said the actual number of girls treated for tall stature in the Netherlands is unknown, but a reasonable guess would be between 100 and 150 per year during the 1970s and 1980s. Asked why estrogen treatment remained more popular in the Netherlands than in the United States, he suggested one reason might be that Dutch women did not play basketball.

220 **where the average girl and boy** Burkhard Bilger, "The Height Gap," *The New Yorker*, April 5, 2004, p. 38: "The Netherlands, as any European can tell you, has become a land of giants. In a century's time, the Dutch have gone from being among the smallest people in Europe to the largest in the world."

220 **"some have become mothers"** O. Trygstad, "Oestrogen Treatment of Adolescent Tall Girls: Short-term Side Effects," *Acta Endocrinol. Suppl.*, 279 (1986), pp. 170–173. In this study, the author reports that between 1980 and 1985, 680 girls in Norway were treated with high-dose estrogen to reduce their mature height.

220 **Massachusetts General's John Crawford** John Crawford, telephone interview with Christine Cosgrove, December 15, 2000.

223 **"I do not know of reproductive"** John Crawford to Laura Cooper, October 26, 1998.

225 **"We had a major task"** Alison Venn, interview with Christine Cosgrove, Melbourne, Australia. Information about the study was taken from interviews with Venn on several occasions, and with her researchers Fiona Bruinsma, Priscilla Pyett, Penny Jones, and Jo Rayner over several days in September 2003.

227 **After eighteen months** Much of the information about the study is found in "Oestrogen Treatment to Reduce the Adult Height of Tall Girls: Long-term Effects on Fertility," *The Lancet*, October 23, pp. 1513–1518.

227 **Some women recalled** Priscilla Pyett, telephone interview with Christine Cosgrove, October 31, 2002, and interview September 2003, Melbourne.

230 **What they had chosen to study** Venn, speaking to researchers at the National Institute for Environmental Health Studies, North Carolina, June 5, 2003.

230 **Worse, she told a group of DES daughters** Newbold spoke at the Action international Colloquium on DES, April 2, 2001, Washington, D.C.

234 **"It was shocking"** Neal Barnard, telephone interview with Christine Cosgrove, 2002. Barnard's study is "The Current Use of Estrogens for Growth-Suppressant Therapy in Adolescent Girls," *Journal of Pediatric and Adolescent Gynecology*, 15 (1) (2002), pp. 23–26.

234 **"My gripe is that"** Barnard, telephone interview.

CHAPTER 11. FRIENDLY FIRE

236 **As of 1991** Paul Brown, Michael Preece, and Robert Will, "'Friendly Fire' in Medicine: Hormones, Hemografts, and Creutzfeldt-Jakob Disease," *The Lancet*, July 4, 1992, pp. 24–27.

236 **In fact, the Public Health Service's** NIDDK letter to hGH recipients, February, 13, 1991.

237 **Publishing the original results** Judith Fradkin et al., "CJD in Pituitary GH Recipients in the U.S., *JAMA*, February 20, 1991, pp. 880–884.

237 **Parlow was certain** Numerous phone conversations with Albert Parlow, and interview, March 23, 2003, at UCLA Harbor Hospital.

237 **Raiti remembers that Parlow** Raiti, interview.

238 **"I let a lot of people"** Parlow, interview. G. Donald Whedon, who is deceased, headed the agency from 1962 to 1981. The original name of the agency, which opened in 1950, was the National Institute of Arthritis and Metabolic Diseases. It became the National Institute of Arthritis and Diabetes, Digestive and Kidney Diseases in 1972; the National Institute of Arthritis, Diabetes and Digestive and Kidney Diseases in 1981. Since 1986 it's been called the National Institute of Diabetes and Digestive and Kidney Diseases, more commonly known as NIDDK.

239 **By 1992, twenty-three CJD cases** Brown, Preece, and Will, "'Friendly Fire.'"

240 **This in spite of a reported** and "Two French Doctors Face Charges for Hormone Use," Reuters, *The New York Times*, July 22, 1993.

240 **"therapeutic misadventure,"** Brown, Preece, and Will, "'Friendly Fire.'"

240 **"friendly fire,"** Ibid.

240 **People who had been treated** Ibid.

240 **Publishing again in a medical journal** Judith Fradkin, "Creutzfeldt-Jakob Disease in Pituitary Growth Hormone Recipients," *The Endocrinologist*, 3 (2) (1993), pp. 108–114.

241 **Fradkin remembers Wilhelmi** Quotations from Judith Fradkin are from an interview, June 2003, NIDDK, Bethesda, Maryland.

241 **On March 23, 1995, the U.S. government** Phillip Gorden to growth hormone recipients, March 23, 1995.

242 **To confuse the matter** Gorden to growth hormone recipients, April 30, 1996.

242 **That was because experts** Gorden to growth hormone recipients, March 23, 1995.

242 **Former patients were told** Gorden to growth hormone recipients, April 30, 1996.

242 **It was a cluster** Gorden to growth hormone recipients, March 23, 1995.

243 **This additional evidence confirmed** Ibid.

243 **"We would like to offer"** Ibid.

243 **Back when Roland played Santa Claus** David Davis, "Growing Pains," *LA Weekly*, March 21, 1997.

243 **They had moved from Long Island** This account is based on, and relevant quotations are from, a telephone interview with Lucille Sluder, June 25, 2004, and on the description of events she wrote after Linda Sluder's death and sent to the authors.

245 **"Since I last wrote to you in early 1994"** Gorden to growth hormone recipients, April 30, 1996.

245 **"As each year goes by"** Ibid.

246 **"Hormone preparations"** Ibid.

247 **"HIV would be destroyed"** Ibid.

247 **This letter put the CJD death toll** Gorden to growth hormone recipients, March 31, 1997.

248 **"This is a painful situation"** Gorden to growth hormone recipients, June 1999.

248 **Debra McKenzie was a New Zealand victim** Cooke, *Cannibals*.

248 **It had been sent from Wilhelmi** The account of the lawsuit is based on a personal interview in Washington, D.C., with attorney Lewis Saul, who represented the McKenzie family in the United States, and on his files, which he generously shared.

249 **A few were settled for small amounts** Parlow, interview.

249 **"very complex information"** Fradkin, interview.

250 **"being young and dumb"** This account is based on multiple telephone conversations between Susan Cohen and David Davis; an interview, February 18, 2003, Glendale, California; and the articles that he has written.

251 **Davis's first story** Davis, "Growing Pains."

251 **"The hGH crisis, like many"** Ibid.

252 **"The people who got us into this mess"** Ibid.

253 **"I think there's a paternalism aspect"** David Davis, telephone interview.

253 **In 1998, he wrote about** David Davis, "A Mother's Life Cut Short," *Long Island Voice*, June 25–July 1, 1998.

253 **In 2000, Davis wrote about** David Davis, "Cut Short," *Mother Jones*, March 23, 2000.

253 **"I've wrestled with the specter"** David Davis, "When Good Intentions Go Wrong," *Atlanta Magazine*, August 2001.

254 **They were kept in the dark** Robert Owen, "The Human Growth Hormone Creutzfeldt-Jakob Disease Litigation," *Medico-Legal Journal*, 65 (2) (1997), pp. 47–64.

255 **At first, attorneys for the victims** Ibid.

255 **"suitable experts in the United States"** Lewis Saul, files.

255–256 **"the literature trail would have led"; "That CJD was transmissible"** Owen, "The Human Growth Hormone."

256 **"Awareness of the risk"** Ibid.

257–258 **That occurred, not in response to Dickinson** Ibid.

258 **Those new instructions, however** M. Allars, *Report of the Inquiry into the Use of Pituitary Derived Hormones in Australia and Creutzfeldt-Jakob Disease*, Australian Government Publishing Service, June 1994. The report was out of print and unavailable from the Australian government printing office when preparation for this book began. Thanks to Jennifer Cooke for transmitting some relevant portions. Much of it was also summarized in "Report on the CJD Settlement Offer, Commonwealth Government Response," Senate Community Affairs References Committee, March 31, 1998.

258 **the pituitary program that operated** "Human Growth Hormone and Creutzfeldt-Jakob Disease," NIH Publication No. 88-2793, December 1987.

258 **"negligent failure," and relevant quotations following** Owen, "The Human Growth Hormone."

259 **They knew recombinant human growth hormone** Richard Rhodes, "Infecting the Children," in *Deadly Feasts: Tracking the Secrets of a Terrifying New Plague* (New York: Simon & Schuster, 1997).

259 **"The saga perhaps demonstrates"** Owen, "The Human Growth Hormone."

259 **"the dreadful burden of guilt"** Ibid.

260 **"raised the issue of the danger"; "We both agree"** Parliament of Australia Senate Community Affairs Committee, *Report on the CJD Settlement Offer*, chapter 2, "Background," October 1997.

260 **But then, in July 1999** Ibid.

261 **A subcommittee of Australia's** Ibid., chapter 7, "Protection of Public Safety."

261 **"not to be blamed for their lack"** Ibid.

261 **"pushed aside the issue of risk of slow viruses"** Ibid.

261 **Another government scientist** Ibid.

261 **Two other prominent** Ibid. These were P. McCullagh and Wesley Whitten.

262 **"but making the leap"** Ibid.

262 **"a dangerous situation"; "Dracula in charge"** Ibid.

262–263 **"no one will ever be made accountable"; "sought kudos"** Ibid.

263 **In 1998, the Australian government** The government did not acknowledge that the hormone treatments were experimental. However, it did admit "some deficiencies in the operation and oversight" and added: "It is deeply regrettable that this tragedy has occurred." Commonwealth Government Response, Senate Community Affairs References Committee, *Report on the CJD Settlement Offer*, March 31, 1998.

263 Raymond Hintz remembered Hintz, interview. Hintz also mentioned this conference in his written account, "A Prismatic Case: The Prismatic Case of CJD Associated with Pituitary Growth Hormone Treatment," *Journal of Clinical Endocrinology and Metabolism*, 80 (1995), pp. 2298–2301.

263 "theoretical possibility" John Crawford, interview with both authors, May 2004, San Francisco.

263 Robert Blizzard, in the grand Blizzard, interview.

263 "I know how we did" Al Parlow, telephone communication with Susan Cohen.

264 "They took the program" Raiti, interview.

265 Father Tony Grossenburg rarely thought Grossenburg telephone interview.

265 Judith Fradkin believed they'd found Fradkin, interview.

265 report of a forty-seven-year-old man E. A. Croes et al., "Creutzfeldt-Jakob Disease Thirty-eight Years After Diagnostic Use of Human Growth Hormone," *Journal of Neurology, Neurosurgery and Psychiatry*, 72 (2002), pp. 792–793.

265 "The peak risk of CJD"; "size exclusion chromatography" A. J. Swerdlow et al., "Creutzfeldt-Jakob Disease in United Kingdom Patients Treated with Human Pituitary Growth Hormone," *Neurology*, 61 (2003), pp. 783–791.

CHAPTER 12. A DISEASE IS BORN

269 Gwen Mahler came thinking Fred and Gwen Mahler interview, March 28, 2003, Hyatt Hotel, Kansas City, Missouri.

270 Required in most states to keep Eli Lilly owns a continuing medical education company. For an excellent discussion of how the industry reaches doctors in this way, see the book by former *New England Journal of Medicine* editor Marcia Angell, *The Truth About the Drug Companies: How They Deceive Us and What to Do About It.*

272 a rare resistance to estrogen The man had an abnormal receptor, so that his body could not process estrogen. In males, some testosterone naturally converts to estrogen.

273 They carry risks Mary Lee, "Is Treatment with a Luteinizing Hormone-Releasing Hormone Agonist Justified in Short Adolescents?" *The New England Journal of Medicine*, editorial, March 6, 2003, pp. 942–945.

275 Yet even decades and more than 100,000 A. J. Swerdlow et al., "Risk of Cancer in Patients Treated with Human Pituitary Growth Hormone in the UK, 1959–185: A Cohort Study," *The Lancet*, July 27, 2002, pp. 273–277.

275 In 2000, A. J. Swerdlow A. J. Swerdlow, "Design and Interpretation of Studies of the Risk of Cancer and Other Long-term Morbidity and Mortality After Growth Hormone Treatment," *Growth Hormone & IGF Research*, 10 (2000), pp. 318–323.

276 Looking at 1,848 young people Swerdlow et al., "Risk of Cancer in Patients."

276 A commentary in the same issue Edward Giovannucci and Michael Pollak, "Risk of Cancer After Growth-Hormone Treatment," commentary, *The Lancet*, July 27, 2002, pp. 268–269.

276–277 The Lawrence Wilkins Pediatric Endocrinology Society issued "Special Editorial: Growth Hormone Treatment and Neoplasia—Coincidence or Consequence?" *Journal of Clinical Endocrinology and Metabolism*, December 2002, pp. 5351–5352.

279 He was Harvey Guyda...who'd been reluctant Harvey Guyda, interviews with Susan Cohen, June 2003, Holiday Inn Select, Bethesda, Maryland, and September 2004, Montreal.

281 **"the potential number of candidates"** FDA Briefing Document, Endocrinologic and Metabolic Drugs Advisory Committee, NDA 19-640/S-033 Humatrope, June 10, 2003.

282 **FDA staff also summarized** Ibid.

283 **"So why should one treat short stature?"** Quotations in this section are from the transcript of the Food and Drug Administration Center for Drug Evaluation and Research Endocrinologic and Metabolic Drugs Advisory Committee Meeting, June 10, 2003. Like the drug companies that ran the databases, pediatric endocrinologists testifying for the new indication talked about almost 250,000 treatment years to emphasize the extent of experience with hGH. The calculation is based on multiplying the years of shots by the number of recorded patients, however, and does not mean that a drug has been used for a long time or that it has been used safely in hundreds of thousands of patients.

289 **a lamb led to slaughter** Harvey Guyda, interview.

290 **The first was Nicole Costa** Patricia Costa, interview with Susan Cohen, April 2004, San Francisco.

298 **The FDA made its decision** David Orloff to Eli Lilly and Company, July 25, 2003.

299 **"a *very* loose wording"** Ron Rosenfeld, interview.

300 **She started this group** Mary Andrews, interview with Susan Cohen, July 2003, Chicago.

301 **Delaying puberty for three years** Deno Andrews, interview with Susan Cohen, July 2003, Chicago.

303 **The procedure involves chiseling** Deborah Stanitski, "Limb Lengthening in the Skeletal Dysplasias and Short Stature Conditions: State of the Art in 1997," *Growth, Genetics & Hormones*, June 1997.

303 **Deno Andrews was glad** Deno Andrews interview.

303 **a form of "child abuse"** Richard Stanhope, interview with both authors, July 2003, Chicago.

303 **Saturday night, the Smith family** Chip and Linda Smith, interview with both authors, July 2003, Chicago.

CHAPTER 13. NOW WHAT?

306 **new guidelines for practitioners** Thomas A. Wilson et al., "Update of Guidelines for the Use of Growth Hormone in Children: The Lawson Wilkins Pediatric Endocrinology Society Drug and Therapeutics Committee," *The Journal of Pediatrics*, October 2003, pp. 415–419.

308 **In 1997, a letter from the Division** Anne Reb to Eli Lilly and Company, July 11, 1997.

308 **In 2000, regulators told Genentech** Margaret Kober to Genentech, Inc., July 28, 2000.

308 **At the Moscone Center** Both authors attended this event.

313 **"are starting to push back"** David Allen, conversation, Moscone Center.

314 **Back in Buffalo.** Both authors spent several days at the Women and Children's Hospital of Buffalo in September 2004.

318 **Ritalin...which some studies** "Study: Ritalin Stunts Growth," WebMD, July 20, 2007, reporting on an article in *Journal of the American Academy of Child & Adolescent Psychiatry*, August 2007.

321 **In a 1994 article** D. E. Sandberg, "Short Stature: A Psychosocial Burden Requiring Growth Hormone Therapy?" *Pediatrics*, December 1994, pp. 832–840.

NOTES

NOTES

321 **"Adult height and degree of growth"** D. E. Sandberg et al., "Quality of Life Among Formerly Treated Childhood-Onset Growth Hormone–Deficient Adults: A Comparison with Unaffected Siblings," *Journal of Clinical Edocrinology and Metabolism*, 1998, pp. 4533–4534.

321 **"'Short stature' as an isolated"** D. E. Sandberg and Linda Voss, "The Psychosocial Consequences of Short Stature: A Review of the Evidence," *Best Pract. Res. Clin. Endocrinol. Metab.*, 16 (3) (September 2002), pp. 449–463.

322 **Short boys are...bullied** Linda Voss and Jean Mulligan, "Bullying in School: Are Short Pupils at Risk?" *British Medical Journal*, March 4, 2000, pp. 612–613.

322 **...more than 20 percent...suffer from bullying** Gwen Glew, "Bullying, Psychosocial Adjustment, and Academic Performance in Elementary School," *Archives of Pediatric and Adolescent Medicine*, November 2005, pp. 1026–1031.

322 **It's hard to get** John Bouclis, interview with both authors, September 20, 2004, Buffalo, New York.

322 **"The ideal child to measure"** L. Voss et al., "The Reliability of Height Measurement (The Wessex Growth Study)," *Archives of Diseases in Childhood*, 65 (1990), pp. 1345–1348.

322 **this can differ** Frank Falkner, "Recommendations for Monitoring Growth in Childhood: A Human Growth Foundation Committee Report, *International Child Health*, 6 (2) (1995), pp. 79–84.

323 **For decades doctors used charts** Howard Markel, "New Growth Charts Dispel the Myth That One Size Fits All," *The New York Times*, April 16, 2002.

324 **A recent study followed sixty-nine** E. Krajewska-Siuda, E. Malecka-Tendera, and K. Karjewski-Siuda, "Are Short Boys with Constitutional Delay of Growth and Puberty Candidates for rGH Therapy According to FDA Recommendations?" *Hormone Research*, e-publication, March 20, 2006, pp. 192–196.

328 **In fact, a recent study disputed** Nicola Persico, Andrew Postlewaite, and Dan Silverman, "The Effect of Adolescent Experience on Labor Market Outcomes: The Case of Height," PIER Working Paper 01-050, Penn Institute for Economic Research, University of Pennsylvania.

330 **In March 2004, a judge** John Pope, "Growth Hormone Ordered for Boy," *The Times-Picayune* (New Orleans), online, March 26, 2004.

332 **In 2004, he published** D. E. Sandberg, "Height and Social Adjustment: Are Extremes a Cause for Concern and Action?" *Pediatrics*, September 2004, pp. 744–750.

CONCLUSION: A NEW NORMAL?

335 **"And Ray and I well remember"** This and other quotations are from Ron Rosenfeld, interview, September 9, 2003, Stanford University.

337 **"Normal," she said, "changes."** Charmian Quigley, FDA hearing.

337 **thoughtful but anguished statement** Quotations are taken from the Little People of America website.

338 **Children in the Netherlands** See Paul Krugman, "America Comes Up Short," *The New York Times*, June 15, 2007.

341 **"'I didn't ask to be born'"** Margaret Atwood, "Arguing Against Ice Cream," *The New York Review of Books*, June 12, 2003.

342 **John Crawford, who treated hundreds of girls** John Crawford, interview.

344 **Laura...recently had another breast cancer scare** Laura Cooper, interview.

NOTES

EPILOGUE

345 **In Australia, Alison Venn's group** F. J. Bruinsma et al., "Concern About Tall Stature During Adolescence and Depression Later in Life," *Journal of Affective Disorders*, April 9, 2006, pp. 145–152.

345 **On a more positive note** H. L. Jordan et al., "Adolescent Exposure to High-Dose Estrogen and Subsequent Effects on Lactation," *Reproductive Toxicology*, November/December 2007, pp. 397–402.

345 **Investigators in Sweden** from Martin Ritzen, Karolinska Institute, e-mail, July 2, 2008.

346 **"Our response was that we are not"** Alison Venn, telephone communication.

346 **"By being specifically targeted"** John Scarlett, quoted in Aaron Lorenzo, "Increlex First to FDA Finish Line in Gaining Short Stature Approval," *BioWorld Today*, 16 (168) (September 1, 2005).

347 **"who form the basis"** Ibid.

347 **"building a franchise in short stature"** John Scarlett, quoted in *BioWorld Today*, 16 (39) (March 1, 2005).

347 **Tercica explained its business strategy** Quotations are from Tercica, Inc., TRCA Securities Registration Statement, filed January 21, 2005.

347 **There is increasing evidence** See Ingfei Chen, "In Aging, Being Small May Have Its Advantages," *The New York Times*, August 1, 2004; and "From the World's Oldest Mouse," *Popular Science*, July 2004.

347 **scientists continue to investigate** See A. Grimberg, "Mechanisms by Which IGF-1 May Promote Cancer," *Cancer Biol. Ther.*, 2 (6) (November/December 2003), pp. 630–635.

348 **UCLA pediatric endocrinologist Pinchas Cohen** Quoted in Chen, "In Aging." "Cohen, chief of pediatric endocrinology at Mattel Children's Hospital at the University of California, Los Angeles, said the mouse models were so complex and hard to understand that their relevance to growth hormone therapy remained 'entirely speculative.'"

348 **But recently, Cohen coauthored a study** K. R. Minkel, "'Methuselah' Mutation Linked to Longer Life," *Scientific American*, March 4, 2008.

348 **In September 2006, David Sandberg** David Sandberg, telephone interview.

348 **Two Princeton economists confirmed** Anne Case and Christina Paxson, "Stature and Status: Height, Ability, and Labor Market Outcomes." National Bureau of Economic Research (NBER) Working Paper No. 12466, August 2006.

349 **A comprehensive report on the National Hormone** National Hormone and Pituitary Program, "Information for People Treated with Human Growth Hormone." This report can be downloaded in either full-length or summary form at http://endocrine.niddk.nih.gov/pubs/creutz/update.htm.

349 **Freedom of Information Act requests** Requests filed for this book were not filled over three years, though documents were repeatedly promised. Freedom of Information Officer Lynelle Nelson, in a telephone conversation in June 2006, acknowledged that lawyers for at least two families of former patients had settled out of court before their FOIA requests were fulfilled.

350 **Worldwide, around two hundred** P. Brown et al., "Iatrogenic Creutzfeldt-Jakob Disease: The Waning of an Era," *Neurology*, 67 (August 2007), pp. 389–393.

350 **"watch for colon cancer"** National Hormone and Pituitary Program, "Information for People Treated with Human Growth Hormone": "We are asking the FDA to tell us if other people treated with hGH report colon cancer. We also ask that

you report colon cancer if it occurs so we can learn if there really is increased risk."

351 **Sales of all brands of hGH increased** See Arlene Weintraub with Michael Amdt, "My, How You've Grown," *Business Week* online, September 28, 2005.

351 **Other manufacturers continued** "The Oral Human Growth Hormone Program in Collaboration with Novartis, www.emisphere.com.

352 **Also in 2007, the Justice Department** "Pfizer Subsidiary Agrees to Plead Guilty for Offering Kickback and Pay $19.68 Million Criminal Fine; Second Subsidiary Agrees to Pay Additional $15 Million Penalty to Resolve Allegations of Illegal Promotion of Human Growth Hormone," United States Attorney's Office, District of Massachusetts, press release, April 2, 2007.

352 **"By defining the genes"** Joel Hirschhorn, pediatric endocrinologist at Children's Hospital Boston, and associate professor of genetics at Harvard Medical School, quoted in "Height Research Hits Growth Spurt," Broad Institute news release, September 2, 2007.

ABOUT THE AUTHORS

Susan Cohen is a freelance writer in Berkeley, California. She's been a reporter for the *San Jose Mercury News*, a contributing writer to the *Washington Post Magazine*, and a full-time faculty member of the University of California Graduate School of Journalism. Among her many journalism honors, she's won the Science in Society Award from the National Association of Science Writers and a John S. Knight Fellowship at Stanford University. Also an award-winning poet, she has two grown children and lives with her husband, Robert R. Youngs, an earthquake engineer.

Christine Cosgrove is a medical writer who has contributed numerous stories to WebMD, ReutersHealth, and a variety of other newspapers and magazines. She has worked as a reporter and editor for more than twenty-five years, beginning with United Press International in New York City, and later as a senior editor at *Parenting* magazine. She has a grown daughter and lives with her husband in Berkeley, where she also writes and edits for the University of California. As a tall teenager she was treated with DES in an effort to stunt her growth.